AF860934

ALLEN / HARPER

Laboratory Manual for Anatomy and Physiology

Abridged

Experiments Selected for
Anatomy and Physiology I
Manatee Community College

WILEY
CUSTOM SERVICES

To order books or for customer service, please call 1(800)-CALL-WILEY (225-5945).

Printed in the United States of America.

ISBN 0-471-69911-X

10 9 8 7 6 5 4 3 2 1

CONTENTS

Laboratory Safety Guidelines

1. Familiarize yourself with emergency exits, fire extinguisher and blanket, first aid kit, eyewash station, chemical shower, biohazard container, and broken glass container.
2. Do not eat or drink in the laboratory.
3. Notify your instructor immediately if you are pregnant or have medical conditions that need special laboratory precautions.
4. Secure long hair and loose clothing or jewelry for your own safety and that of the equipment used.
5. Decontaminate laboratory tops with an appropriate disinfectant prior to and at the completion of your lab activities as directed by your instructor.
6. Use safety glasses and laboratory coats or coverings when appropriate, especially during dissections, heating solutions, or handling dangerous chemicals.
7. Wear disposable gloves when working with body fluids, dissections, or chemicals.
8. Keep all laboratory equipment away from the edge of your laboratory work area.
9. Immediately notify your instructor of *all* spills, accidents, or damaged equipment.
10. Properly dispose of waste material, chemicals, or body fluids as directed by your instructor.
11. Wash your hands with soap and water before leaving the laboratory.
12. Follow other specific safety measures given in the laboratory exercises in this manual.

LABORATORY MANUAL FOR ANATOMY AND PHYSIOLOGY

CONNIE ALLEN
VALERIE HARPER
Edison Community College

John Wiley & Sons, Inc.

Senior Editor	Bonnie Roesch
Associate Editor	Mary O'Sullivan
Production Editor	Sandra Russell
Senior Marketing Manager	Clay Stone
Senior Designer	Kevin Murphy
Book Designer	Nancy Field
Photo Manager	Hilary Newman
Illustration Editor	Anna Melhorn
Production Management Services	TechBooks

Cover Photos
Body scan: ©Simon Fraser/Science Photo Library/Photo Researchers
Cardiac muscle tissue: ©Ed Reschke

This book was typeset in 10/12 Times Roman by TechBooks and printed and bound by Von Hoffmann Press. The cover was printed by The Von Hoffmann Corporation.

The paper in this book was manufactured by a mill whose forest management programs include sustained yield harvesting of its timberlands. Sustained yield harvesting principles ensure that the number of trees cut each year does not exceed the amount of new growth.

The procedures in this text are intended for use only by students with appropriate faculty supervision. In preparing the text, care has been taken to identify potentially hazardous steps and to insert safety precautions where appropriate. The authors and publisher believe the procedures to be useful tools if performed with the materials and equipment specified, in careful accordance with the instructions and methods in the text. However, these procedures must be conducted at one's own risk. The author and publisher do not warrant or guarantee the safety of individuals using these procedures and specifically disclaim any and all liability resulting directly or indirectly from the use or application of any information contained in this book.

This book is printed on acid-free paper. ∞

To order books or for customer service please, call 1(800)-CALL-WILEY (225-5945).

Library of Congress Cataloging in Publication Data:
Allen, Connie, Valerie Harper

ISBN 0-471-39464-5 (paper: alk. paper)

Printed in the United States of America.

10 9 8 7 6 5 4

I dedicate this book to my husband Jim and my daughter Michaela for their unwavering love, patience, and encouragement.

—Connie Allen

I dedicate this book to my husband Chuck, and our children Scott and Kate, for their love, support, and patience.

—Valerie Harper

PREFACE

Anatomy and physiology is a challenging course, and this laboratory manual is written to help students meet that challenge. It is written for students interested in allied health fields, such as nursing; physical, respiratory, or occupational therapy; radiology; and dental hygiene. Although this manual incorporates many illustrations from *Principles in Anatomy and Physiology, 10th edition,* by Gerard J. Tortora and Sandra R. Grabowski, it may be used with any two-semester anatomy and physiology textbook.

The design of this laboratory manual is based on the authors' experience as anatomy and physiology instructors and uses three learning styles: visual, auditory, and kinesthetic. When students label diagrams, they focus on the structure rather than just the dot at the end of a line. Writing out the structure's name and pronouncing it reinforces learning. Also, having students become subjects of laboratory exercises makes learning personal. Animal dissections give students an opportunity to physically manipulate structures, comparing location and texture, and to observe how structures are supported, protected, and attached by connective tissue.

Special features incorporated in this laboratory manual include:

- Just enough text is provided to introduce concepts in each section and to set up and support the laboratory section. The exercises are written so that students do not need their textbooks to complete the laboratory activities.
- New material is divided into small segments, starting with simple diagrams, illustrating the basic concepts and building up to more complex diagrams. Subsequent activities add to the students' knowledge in a stepwise fashion.
- Unlabeled four-color drawings, photographs, and photomicrographs are included for students to label either at home or in the laboratory. Students first write out the name of the structure to help memorize it. Then the completed diagrams will be used to identify structures on models. An answer key is provided at the back of the laboratory manual for the students to self-correct their diagrams.
- Word derivatives for bolded terms are given in the text.
- Phonetic pronunciation is included as new words are introduced. Students are directed to pronounce the name of a structure as they point to it on a model. Most students have difficulty pronouncing the anatomical terms, and need practice saying and hearing the words.
- Physiology experiments use students as subjects and can be completed with either simple, inexpensive equipment or more complex setups.
- Discussion Questions are within the activities to make the students think about the material presented.
- An Answer Key is provided at the end of the laboratory manual for the activities in each exercise. Students receive immediate feedback, and they are not dependent on the instructor for the correct answers.
- "Reviewing Your Knowledge" and "Using Your Knowledge" sections follow the activities at the end of each exercise. "Reviewing Your Knowledge" provides a thorough review of the material in the exercise, whereas "Using Your Knowledge" requires students to apply information learned. Either or both of these sections may be handed in to the instructors for a grade, because neither section has answers in the back of the laboratory manual. Answers to these two sections are in the online Instructor's Manual.
- Each exercise contains a list of objectives, materials needed for the exercise, a detailed paged outline, and easily identifiable laboratory activity sections.

Supplemental Materials:

- Instructor's Manual. Available on the book companion Web site at www.wiley.com/college/allen. Contains an Answer Key for "Reviewing Your Knowledge" and "Using Your Knowledge."
- Cat Dissection Manual. Contains dissection activities for use in the lab accompanied by full color photos and figures.
- Fetal Pig Dissection Manual. Contains dissection activities for use in the lab accompanied by full color photos and figures.
- Additional Student Exercises are located at www.wiley.com/college/allen.

ACKNOWLEDGMENTS

We deeply appreciate the support, instruction, and encouragement from the members of our editorial, production, and marketing team at Wiley, Bonnie Roesch, Mary O'Sullivan, Hilary Newman, Anna Melhorn, Sandra Russell, Kevin Murphy, Clay Stone, and at TechBooks, Stephanie Lentz. A special thanks goes to Mary O'Sullivan for all the encouragement, direction, and suggestions she gave us. Her steady, calm hand guided us through this whole project and we could not have done it without her. We also wish to thank Gerard Tortora and Sandra Grabowski for producing a wonderful textbook that provided many illustrations and ideas for our laboratory manual. Thank you Sandra Grabowski for reviewing our manuscript and providing suggestions.

A special thank you to William Benyak for reviewing all the exercises, making suggestions, giving clinical guidance, and for photographing the fetal pig dissection. We also wish to thank Donalie Benyak for her technical assistance with the dissection photography. A special thanks to Charles Harper for answering many clinical questions.

Many thanks to Michael Ross and his assistant Todd Barnash from the University of Florida for answering our histology questions and providing photomicrographs for the laboratory manual. We also wish to thank Kierstan Hong at Imagineering Art for the artwork she provided for our laboratory manual.

Thank you to our colleagues at Edison Community College, Paul Monagan, Bob Clemence, Sue Pilbeam, Colleen Swanson, Jody Gootkin, Richard McCoy, Jeff Davis, Florence Levin, John Berte, Dick Felden, Lyman O'Neil, Kitty Gronlund, Ken Laser, Greg Stancel, and Tony Contino who encouraged us, answered our questions, and provided critiques of exercises. We also wish to thank Sheila Stancel and James Newton for their encouragement.

Thank you to Chaim Jay Margolin of Regional Radiology Associates and David Michie of Clinical Physiology Associates for providing images for this manual.

Reviewers

A special thank you to all the reviewers. Their suggestions were extremely helpful in developing this laboratory manual.

Reviewers included the following: Susan Baxley, Troy State University; Elizabeth Becker, Elgin Community College; Moges Bizuneh, Ivy Technical State College; Joanna Borucinska, University of Hartford; Frank Cotty, Queensborough Community College; Rosemary Davenport, Gulf Coast Community College; Judith Davis, Florida Community College at Jacksonville; Chaya Gopalan, St. Louis Community College; Kerri L. Hoar, University of Wisconsin, La Crosse; Paul Krieger, Grand Rapids Community College; Raymond Lo, College of New Caledonia; Karen McCort, El Paso Community College; Sarah L. Milton, Florida Atlantic University; Charlene Newby, Lake Shore Technical College; Linda Nichols, Santa Fe Community College; Margaret Ott, Tyler Junior College; David Parker, Northern Virginia Community College; Betsy Peitz, California State University–Los Angeles; Kathleen Richardson, Portland Community College; Donna Ritch, University of Wisconsin, Green Bay; David S. Smith, San Antonio College; Robert Stinson, South Texas Community College; Jane Wallace, Chattanooga State Technical Community College; Stephen Williams, Glendale Community College; Clarence Wolfe, Northern Virginia Community College; Patricia Yokell, New Hampshire Technical College; Glenn Yoshida, Los Angeles Community College.

THE MICROSCOPE

OBJECTIVES

After completing this exercise, you should be able to:

- Understand and describe how to carry, clean, and use a light microscope.
- Identify the parts of the microscope.
- Demonstrate how to place a prepared slide on the microscope, and the proper focusing technique to observe a desired area of the slide under all magnifications.

MATERIALS

- compound microscope
- lens paper
- high quality cotton swab
- prepared slides of the letter "e"

INTRODUCTION

A compound light microscope is typically used in an anatomy and physiology class to see small structures like cells and groups of cells that make up tissues. This type of microscope can magnify images up to approximately one thousand times. Our laboratory manual has you perform most of the activities using prepared slides. If you are to make your own slides, that activity will include instructions for you.

A. Transporting the Microscope

The compound microscope is an expensive, precision instrument that must be handled with care. The term *compound* refers to the set of lenses used for magnification of the image. Demonstrate care in transporting, cleaning, using, and storing the microscope.

1. Pick up the microscope with two hands, one holding its arm and the other supporting the base with the cord in a secure position.
2. Carry the microscope upright so that a lens or eyepiece doesn't fall out and place the microscope on your lab bench in front of you.

B. Parts of the Microscope

1. Identify the parts of your microscope in Figure P1.
2. Compare your microscope with the one in Figure P1 and identify any differences with your lab partner.

Microscope Framework

- **Base**—The widest bottom part that supports the microscope.
- **Arm**—The straight or curved vertical part that connects the base to the upper portion.
- **Head** (or body tube)—extends from the arm and contains the ocular lens and the rotating nosepiece with the objective lenses.

NOTE: *All other microscope parts attach to these three basic parts of the framework.*

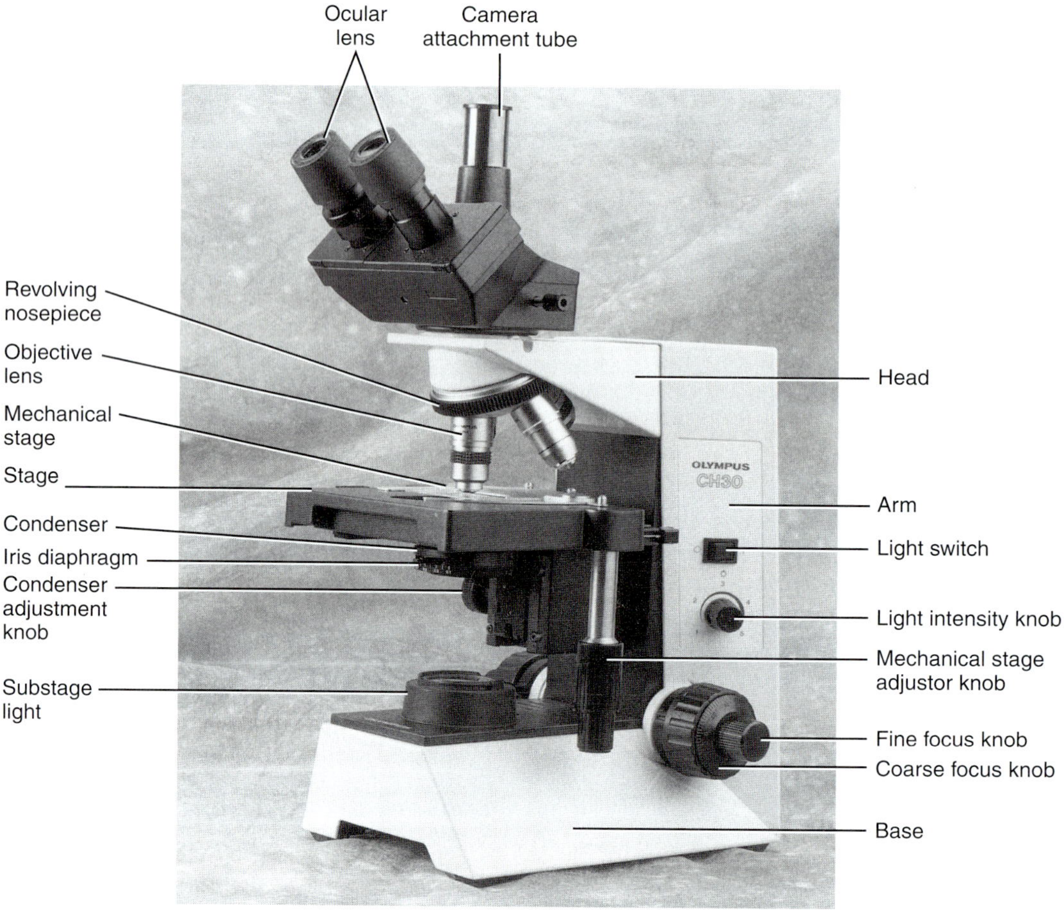

Parts of the microscope.

- **Ocular Lenses or Lens** (eyepieces)—One or two removable lenses that you look through to observe the microscope slide. Typically, these lenses have a magnification of 10x. Look at the eyepiece and record the magnification.

  ____

  One of the oculars may have a **pointer** used to identify a specific area on the slide when studying slides with others.
- **Objective lenses**—Usually a microscope will have three or four objective lenses mounted on a **revolving nosepiece.** Most microscopes for anatomy and physiology classes have objective lenses with magnifications of 4x (scanning), 10x (low), 45x (high dry), and 100x (oil immersion). List the magnifications of the objective lenses on your microscope.

  ____

  As the barrel of the objective lens increases in length, the magnifying power increases also.
- **Stage**—The flat platform located beneath the objective lenses on which the microscope slide is placed.
- **Mechanical stage** (or **spring clips**)—Holds the slide securely in place for viewing and can be moved with precision by using the **adjuster knobs.** If spring clips are on your microscope, adjust the slide beneath them by hand.
- **Coarse Focus Knobs**—On each side of the microscope toward the base is a large knob or dial with a smaller knob in the middle. You need to use only one of the large knobs, depending on if you are right or left handed. The large knob either moves the stage up and down with the objective lens in place, or moves the objective lenses up and down with the stage in place for coarse focusing. This knob is to be used with scanning or low power only.

- **Fine Focus Knob**—The smaller knob on each side of the microscope that is used for precision focusing.
- **Condenser**—Located just below the stage, this lens condenses light through the specimen on the slide above. If the condenser has an **adjustment knob** that raises and lowers the condenser, it usually needs to be in the highest position near the stage for the exercises that you will perform.
- **Iris diaphragm**—Located beneath the condenser, the iris diaphragm works similar to the iris of the eye. By adjusting its **lever,** the aperture changes diameter and regulates the amount of light that passes through the condenser.
- **Substage Light**—The light source is usually built into the base of the microscope and has a dial on one side to control the light intensity.

Determining Magnification

1. Total magnification is determined by multiplying your ocular lens power times the objective lens power.
2. Example:
   Ocular lens power = 10x; Objective lens power = 4x;
   Total magnification = 40x.
3. Multiply the powers of the lenses in your microscope to obtain the total magnification.

_____ scanning lens X ocular lens _____
= _____ total magnification

_____ low power lens X ocular lens _____
= _____ total magnification

_____ high dry lens X ocular lens _____
= _____ total magnification

_____ oil immersion lens X ocular lens _____
= _____ total magnification

C. Using the Microscope

1. Clean up your lab area and put non-essentials away to have plenty of room to use the microscope.
2. Unwind the cord and plug it in.
3. Clean the ocular, objective, and condenser lenses with only the *special lens paper* (optical safe) provided by your instructor. These lenses need the care of an expensive camera lens. Whenever the image on the slide cannot be focused clearly, the objective lens may need additional cleaning. If so, consult your instructor.
4. Turn on the light and adjust its intensity.
   Trouble shooting: If no light initially comes on, check two things before consulting your instructor.
   (a) Check the light dial to make sure it isn't on zero.
   (b) Check the safety switch on the electrical outlet by pushing in the reset button. If the light still doesn't work, plug your microscope into an outlet that you know works.

Scanning Objective Lens

5. Click the scanning or low power objective lens into place so it is over the light aperture on the stage. This objective lens has the shortest barrel. Make sure you feel the click, or your field of view will be black.
6. Obtain a prepared slide with the letter "e" from your instructor and place it on the stage, securing it in the mechanical stage clamps or stage clips.
7. Practice moving the slide back and forth in addition to up and down using the mechanical stage knobs.
8. Using the mechanical stage knobs, position the letter "e" over the light hole in the stage and turn the light on a middle setting.
9. Check to see that the condenser lens is raised completely up to the stage.
10. If your *stage is moveable,* the coarse focus knob will move the stage. Raise the stage up as far as it will go. If your *objective is moveable,* use the coarse focus knob to lower the objective lens until it stops. The slide and objective lens will not actually touch.
11. If you have a binocular microscope, adjust the two oculars as you would a pair of binoculars so the two oculars are a comfortable distance for your eyes.
12. Looking through the ocular lens(es), adjust the coarse focus knob to focus in the letter "e".

> **CAUTION:** *Do not use the coarse focus knob with high dry or oil immersion lenses.*

13. Using the mechanical stage knobs, bring the letter "e" directly into the center of the **field of view** (the lighted circular area you see as you look through the oculars).
14. Does the letter "e" look normal to you? What is different about it? ______________________________

____

15. While observing the "e", use your mechanical stage knob to move the "e" away from you. Now move it back toward you, to your right and to your left. What did you notice that seemed different about these movements? ______________________________

____

Low Power Objective Lens

16. Reposition the letter "e" directly in the middle of the field of view and switch to the low power objective lens.
17. Most microscopes are **parfocal** so when you move to a higher magnification, it is almost in focus. Use the fine focus to sharpen the image.
18. Use the iris diaphragm lever to adjust the amount of light and improve the contrast of your image.

High Dry Objective Lens

19. Center the area you want to view and repeat this procedure with the high dry objective lens. Be sure to focus with the FINE FOCUS KNOB ONLY.

Oil Immersion Lens

20. Most anatomy and physiology slides do not need the magnification of the oil immersion lens. Your instructor will inform you if and when you will use this objective lens.
21. Center the area you want to view and then obtain a container of oil made especially for the microscope.
22. With the slide focused at high dry, move the objective lens out of the way and apply a drop of oil directly on the part of the slide you wish to study.
23. Click the oil immersion lens into place, open the iris diaphragm as needed, and focus with the FINE FOCUS KNOB ONLY.

D. Cleaning Up

24. Turn off the substage light. The bulb light is extended if it cools before moving the microscope.
25. Remove the slide and clean oil from the objective lens (and also the high dry objective lens if you passed it through the oil) with lens paper or a high quality cotton swab. Your instructor may ask you to use an additional cleaner.
26. Clean the slide with lens paper and also the stage, if necessary.
27. Position the scanning objective lens back in place and carefully wrap the cord around the base of the microscope, making sure it isn't pulled too tightly.
28. Place the dust cover over the microscope.
29. Using both hands and the proper technique, return the microscope to the appropriate cabinet.

EXERCISE 1

ANATOMICAL LANGUAGE

OUTLINE

OBJECTIVES

After completing this activity, students will be able to:

- Describe the anatomical position
- Identify major body regions
- Use anatomical terms correctly
- Use directional terms correctly
- Identify planes and sections

MATERIALS

- human models or anatomical charts
- articulated skeleton
- 5 sheep brains for 1 class demonstration
- apples (1 per group)
- plastic tubing (1 foot piece per group)

Students often complain that they are not just learning anatomy and physiology, but are learning a new language. This is so true. In this exercise, you will learn anatomical language that will be used throughout the course and also to communicate effectively with other health care professionals.

A. ANATOMICAL POSITION

The anatomical position is the position that is assumed when referring to the location of body parts with relation to one another. In the anatomical position, the body is erect and facing forward; the arms are straight and at the sides of the body with the palms facing forward; the legs are straight with the feet facing forward and flat (see Figure 1.1 on the following page).

ACTIVITY 1 Anatomical Position

1 Assume the anatomical position.

2 Have your laboratory partner determine if you are in the correct position.

B. BODY REGIONS

The main body regions are described in Table 1.1. It is important that you learn the correct boundaries for each region. Two common misconceptions are that the arm is the area between the shoulder and wrist and that the leg includes the thigh. The arm is located between the shoulder and elbow, and the forearm is located from the elbow to wrist. The thigh is located between the groin and knee, and the leg is located between the knee and ankle.

ACTIVITY 2 Body Regions

1 Label Figure 1.1 with the appropriate body regions. Use terms from Table 1.1.

2 Identify body regions on models or anatomical charts. Use terms from Table 1.1.

3 Pronounce the terms as you point to them.

TABLE 1.1 Body Regions

BODY REGION	DESCRIPTION
Head	
Face	Portion of head not normally covered by scalp
Skull	Bony portion of head
Neck	Body area between head and trunk
Trunk	Central body area to which head and limbs are attached
Chest	Area of trunk between neck and abdomen; contains heart and lungs; diaphragm forms boundary between chest and abdomen
Abdomen	Area of trunk between chest and pelvis; contains digestive organs; hip bones form lower boundary of abdomen
Pelvis	Area of trunk below abdomen; contains internal reproductive organs and urinary bladder
Back	Posterior portion of trunk between neck and buttocks
Upper limb	
Shoulder	Curved area where arm attaches to upper border of trunk
Armpit	Under arm area where upper limb attaches to trunk
Arm	Area of upper limb between shoulder and elbow
Forearm	Area of upper limb between elbow and wrist
Wrist	Portion of hand that connects hand to forearm
Hand	Includes wrist and digits
Lower limb	
Buttocks	Rounded area on posterior surface where thigh attaches to trunk
Groin	Area where lower limb attaches to the pelvis
Thigh	Area of lower limb above the knee
Leg	Area of lower limb between knee and ankle
Ankle	Portion of foot that connects foot to leg
Foot	Includes ankle and digits

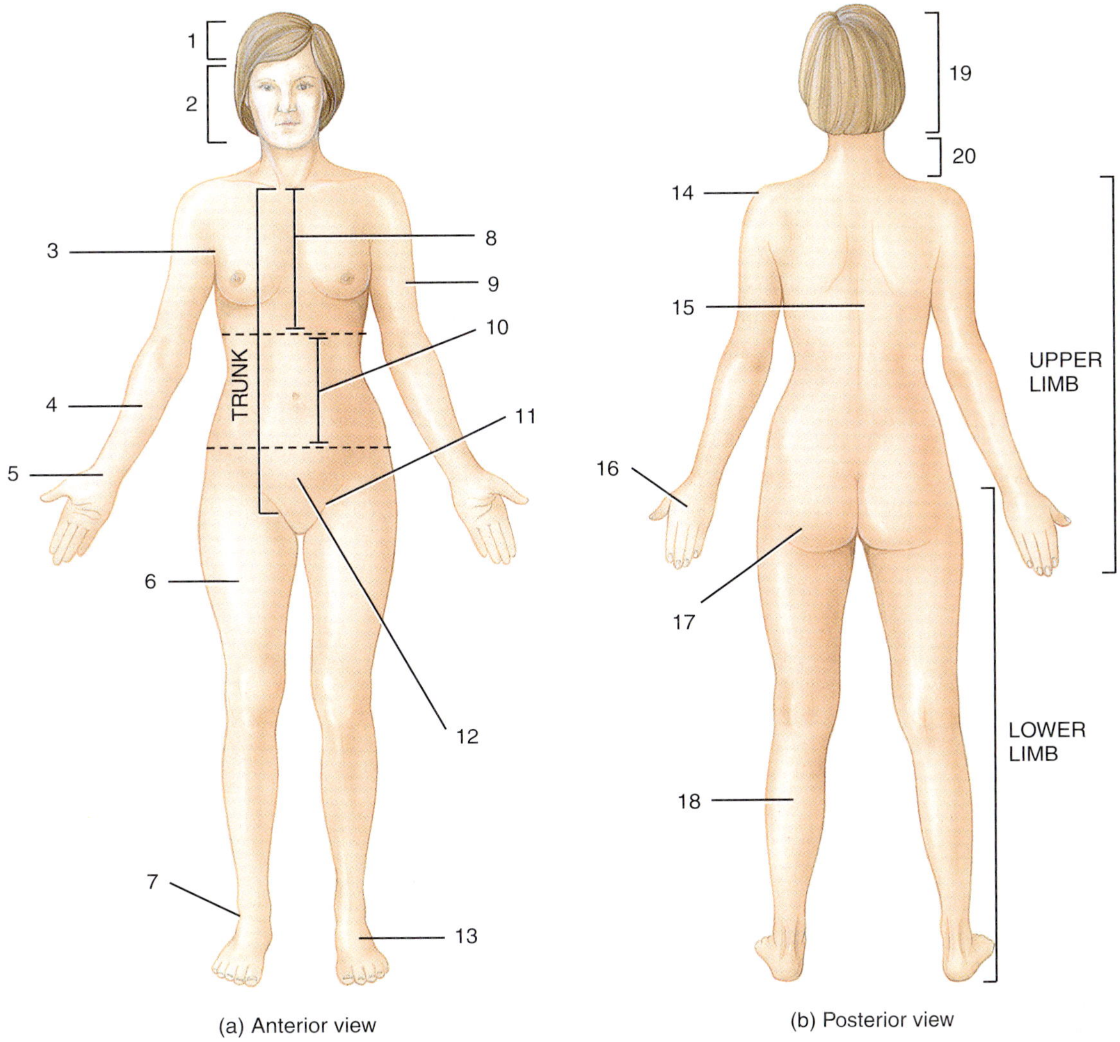

(a) Anterior view

1 ______________________

2 ______________________

3 ______________________

4 ______________________

5 ______________________

6 ______________________

7 ______________________

8 ______________________

9 ______________________

10 ______________________

11 ______________________

12 ______________________

(b) Posterior view

13 ______________________

14 ______________________

15 ______________________

16 ______________________

17 ______________________

18 ______________________

19 ______________________

20 ______________________

FIGURE 1.1 Body regions.

C. ANATOMICAL TERMS

Anatomical terms describe body regions, specific body areas, and landmarks. These terms are often part of the names of muscles, bones, nerves, and blood vessels. Most of these words are derived from Latin or Greek. Many words have one or more word roots with a prefix and/or a suffix added. For example, in the word *antebrachial, ante-* is a prefix meaning before or in front of; the word root *brach-* means arm; *-al* is a suffix meaning pertaining to. Table 1.2 contains anatomical terms with four different suffixes that all mean "pertaining to." These suffixes are: *-al*, *-ic*, *-ar*, and *-ary*. When suffixes like these are added to word roots, they form an adjective. Nouns have different endings, such as *-um*, *-us*, *-is*, or *-a*. For example, sternum is a bone (noun) and sternal is an adjective. Another example is umbilicus (noun) and umbilical (adjective). Learning these terms at this time will help you throughout the course. Anatomical terms and their definitions are found in Table 1.2.

ACTIVITY 3 Anatomical Terms

1 Label Figure 1.2 with the appropriate anatomical terms. Use terms from Table 1.2.

2 Identify the specific body regions, areas, and landmarks on models or anatomical charts.

3 Pronounce the anatomical terms as you point to them on models or anatomical charts.

TABLE 1.2 Anatomical Terms

TERM	DEFINITION	TERM	DEFINITION
AXIAL	Pertaining to the central part of the body, the head and trunk	• Axillary	Pertaining to the armpit
Cephalic (se-FAL-ik)	Pertaining to the head	• Brachial (BRAY-key-ul)	Pertaining to the arm
• Facial	Pertaining to the face	• Cubital	Pertaining to the elbow
• Frontal	Pertainig to the forehead	• Antecubital	Pertaining to the anterior (front) surface of the elbow
• Orbital	Pertaining to the eye	• Olecranal (oh-LEK-ra-nul)	Pertaining to the posterior (back) surface of the elbow
• Otic (OH-tik)	Pertaining to the ear	• Antebrachial	Pertaining to the forearm
• Nasal	Pertaining to the nose	• Carpal	Pertaining to the wrist
• Buccal (BUCK-al)	Pertaining to the cheek	• Manual	Pertaining to the hand
• Oral	Pertaining to the mouth	• Palmar	Pertaining to the palm of the hand
• Mental	Pertaining to the chin	• Digital	Pertaining to the digits (fingers or toes)
• Cranial	Pertaining to the skull	**Lower Appendage**	Lower limb
• Occipital (ox-SIP-i-tal)	Pertaining to the back of head	• Inguinal (ING-won-ul)	Pertaining to the groin where the thigh attaches to the pelvis
Cervical	Pertaining to the neck	• Gluteal	Pertaining to the buttocks
Thoracic	Pertaining to the chest	• Femoral	Pertaining to the thigh
• Pectoral (PEK-tore-al)	Pertaining to the breast	• Patellar	Pertaining to the anterior (front) surface of the knee
• Sternal	Pertaining to the breast bone	• Popliteal (pop-lih-TEE-ul)	Pertaining to the posterior (back) surface of the knee
Abdominal	Pertaining to the abdomen	• Crural	Pertaining to the anterior (front) surface of the leg
• Ventral	Pertaining to the belly	• Sural	Pertaining to the posterior (back) surface of the leg
• Umbilical	Pertaining to the navel	• Fibular or peroneal	Pertaining to the lateral side of the leg
• Coxal (COX-al)	Pertaining to the hip	• Tarsal	Pertaining to the ankle
Pelvic	Pertaining to the pelvis	• Pedal	Pertaining to the foot
• Pubic	Pertaining to the genital area	• Calcaneal (kal-KANE-ee-ul)	Pertaining to the heel
Dorsal	Pertaining to the back	• Plantar	Pertaining to sole of foot
• Scapular	Pertaining to the shoulder blade region		
• Vertebral	Pertaining to the spine		
• Lumbar	Pertaining to the lower back or loin region		
APPENDICULAR	Pertaining to the extremities or limbs		
Upper Appendage	Upper limb		
• Acromial (a-KROM-ee-al)	Pertaining to the highest point of the shoulder		

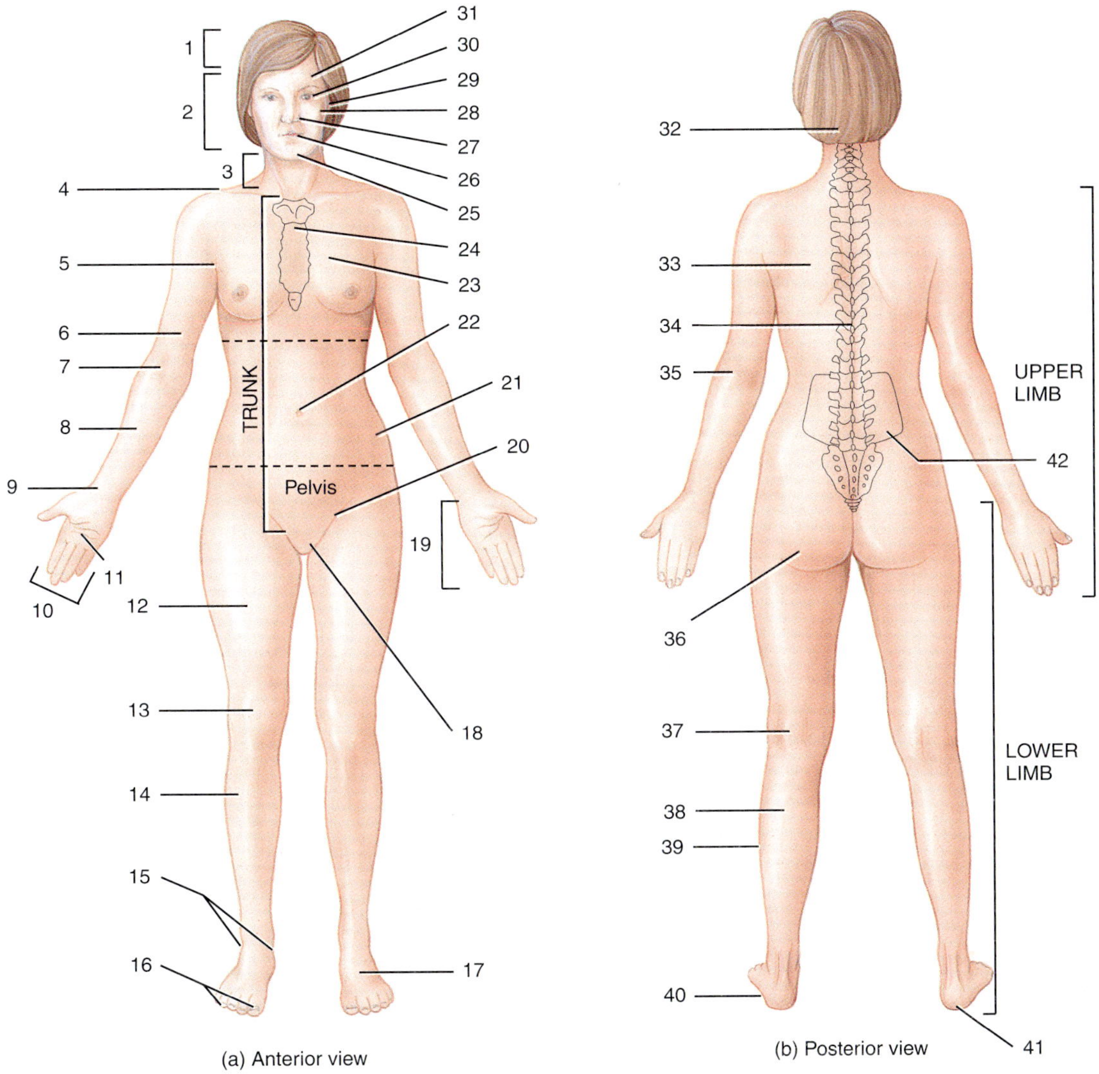

(a) Anterior view

1 ______________

2 ______________

3 ______________

4 ______________

5 ______________

6 ______________

7 ______________

8 ______________

9 ______________

10 ______________

11 ______________

12 ______________

13 ______________

14 ______________

15 ______________

16 ______________

17 ______________

18 ______________

19 ______________

20 ______________

21 ______________

22 ______________

23 ______________

24 ______________

25 ______________

26 ______________

27 ______________

28 ______________

29 ______________

30 ______________

31 ______________

(b) Posterior view

32 ______________

33 ______________

34 ______________

35 ______________

36 ______________

37 ______________

38 ______________

39 ______________

40 ______________

41 ______________

42 ______________

FIGURE 1.2 Anatomical terms.

TABLE 1.3 Directional Terms

DIRECTIONAL TERM	DEFINITION	EXAMPLE OF USE
Superior	Above	The head is superior to the neck.
Inferior	Below	The neck is inferior to the head.
Anterior	Closer to front of body	The lips are anterior to the teeth.
Posterior	Closer to back of body	The teeth are posterior to the lips.
Medial	Closer to midline of body	The nose is medial to the eyes.
Lateral	Farther from midline of body	The eyes are lateral to the nose.
Ipsilateral	On same side of body	The right arm and right leg are ipsilateral.
Contralateral	On opposite sides of body	The right arm and left arm are contralateral.
Proximal	Nearer to point of attachment of limb to trunk	The elbow is proximal to the wrist.
Distal	Farther from point of attachment of limb to trunk	The wrist is distal to the elbow.
Superficial	Closer to surface of body	The skin is superficial to muscles.
Deep	Farther from surface of body	The muscles are deep to the skin.

D. Directional Terms

The directional terms are listed in Table 1.3, along with an example of how they are used. Note that opposite terms are paired. Directional terms are used to describe the location of body structures relative to other structures. An example of a directional term is *inferior,* which means below. It would be correct to say that the neck is inferior to the head, but incorrect to say that the neck is inferior.

Note that the directional terms *proximal* and *distal* only apply to structures on the limbs. These terms refer to the location of structures relative to the point of attachment of the limb to the torso, whether they are closer to the point of attachment (proximal) or farther away (distal).

ACTIVITY 4 Directional Terms

1 Complete the sentences using directional terms.

a. The sternum (breastplate) is _______________ to the vertebrae (spine).

b. The mouth is _______________ to the chin.

c. The heart is _______________ to the lungs.

d. The fingers are _______________ to the wrist.

e. The right lung and the liver are _______________.

f. The skin is _______________ to the bones.

2 Label Figure 1.3 with directional terms.

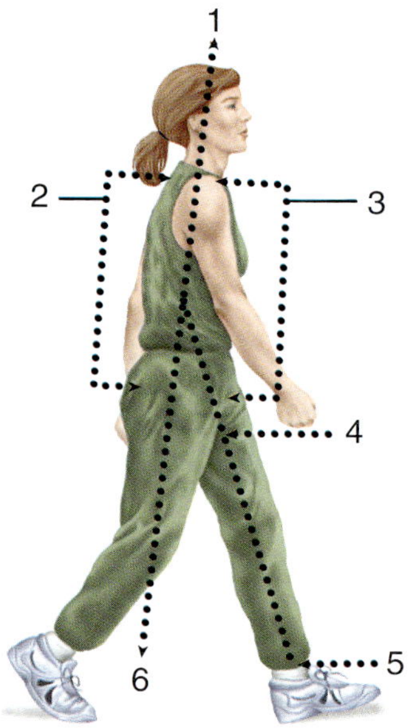

- Superior 1 ______________________
- Inferior 2 ______________________
- Anterior 3 ______________________
- Posterior 4 ______________________
- Proximal 5 ______________________
- Distal 6 ______________________

FIGURE 1.3 Directional terms.

E. BODY PLANES AND SECTIONS

Planes divide the body or organs into sections to observe internal structures (Figure 1.4). **Sagittal** (*sagitta* = arrow) **planes** pass vertically through the body or organs, and divide it into right and left sections (**sagittal sections**). A **midsagittal** plane passes vertically through the midline and divides the body into right and left halves. A **frontal** or **coronal plane** passes vertically through the body or organs and produces anterior and posterior sections (**frontal sections**). A **transverse plane** passes horizontally through the body and produces superior and inferior sections (**transverse sections**). Transverse sections are also called cross-sections. **Oblique planes** pass through the body at an angle. The type of plane will determine which type of sections are obtained and the structures that can be viewed in the sections.

Often, we look at sections of organs and tissues to observe structures. Sections that are produced by a plane running along the long axis of a long narrow structure, such as a blood vessel, are called **longitudinal sections**. Sections that are produced by a plane running perpendicular to the long axis are called **cross-sections**.

CLINICAL NOTE: *Transverse sections observed with CT scans or MRIs are called axial sections.*

ACTIVITY 5 Planes and Sections

1 Label the planes in Figure 1.4.

2 Cut sagittal, frontal, and transverse planes through an apple.
- Work in a group.
- Draw a face on the apple.
- Cut sagittal, frontal, and transverse planes through the apple to make sagittal, frontal, and transverse sections.
- Keep sections together to form a whole apple to show to your instructor.

3 Cut longitudinal and transverse planes through a tube.
- Tube-like structures are found throughout the body. Examples of these are blood vessels and kidney tubules that twist and bend as they travel through the body. A slice of tissue may contain a tube in longitudinal section, one in cross-section, and one in oblique section.
- Twist the tube so that one plane will divide the tube into a longitudinal section and a cross-section.
- Make the cut so that you can see the tube in longitudinal section and in cross-section.
- Show the sections to your instructor.

4 Demonstration of sagittal, frontal, transverse, and oblique sections on sheep brains.
- Your instructor will display five sheep brains; one whole brain and four brains that have been cut into different sections.
- Before you start, determine the anterior, posterior, superior, and inferior surfaces of the brain.
- Decide which brain has been cut into sagittal, frontal, transverse, or oblique sections.

Brain 1—Whole brain

Brain 2 ______________ section

Brain 3 ______________ section

Brain 4 ______________ section

Brain 5 ______________ section

- Compare the appearance of the different sections.

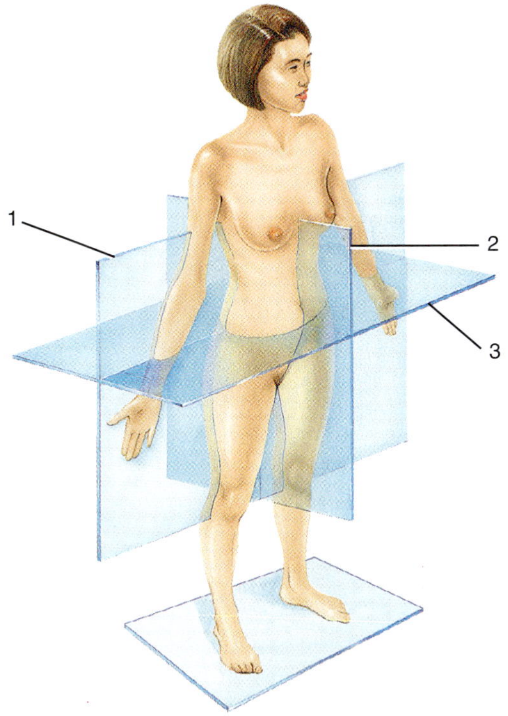

- Frontal
- Sagittal
- Transverse

1 ______________

2 ______________

3 ______________

FIGURE 1.4 **Body planes.**

Name ______________________ Date ______________ Section ______________

EXERCISE 1

REVIEWING YOUR KNOWLEDGE

A. Anatomical Position

The person in Figure 1.5 is not in anatomical position. List four differences from anatomical position.

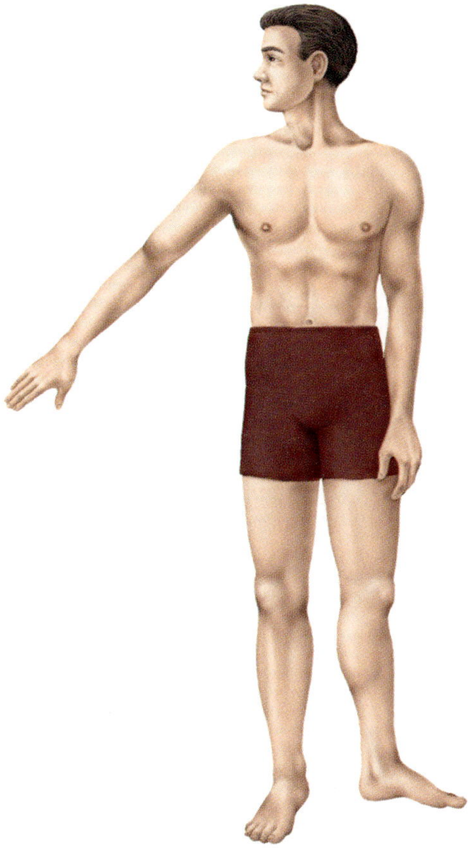

1 ______________________________

2 ______________________________

3 ______________________________

4 ______________________________

FIGURE 1.5 Person not in anatomical position.

B. Anatomical Terms

Write the anatomical terms that the phrase describes.

______________ **1.** Pertaining to the navel

______________ **2.** Pertaining to the area between neck and abdomen

______________ **3.** Pertaining to the ear

______________ **4.** Pertaining to the palm of hand

______________ **5.** Pertaining to the high point of shoulder

______________ **6.** Pertaining to the anterior surface of elbow region

______________ **7.** Pertaining to the face; anterior portion of head

______________ **8.** Pertaining to the nose

______________ **9.** Pertaining to the neck

______________ **10.** Pertaining to the posterior surface of knee

______________ **11.** Pertaining to the wrist

______________ **12.** Pertaining to the area between the elbow and the wrist

______________ **13.** Pertaining to the back

______________ **14.** Pertaining to the armpit area

______________ **15.** Pertaining to the mouth

______________ **16.** Pertaining to the anterior surface of knee

______________ **17.** Pertaining to the breastplate

_______________ **18.** Pertaining to the hip

_______________ **19.** Pertaining to the side of the leg

_______________ **20.** Pertaining to the calf

_______________ **21.** Pertaining to the area between shoulder and elbow

_______________ **22.** Pertaining to the fingers or toes

_______________ **23.** Pertaining to the hand

_______________ **24.** Pertaining to the breast area

_______________ **25.** Pertaining to the cheek

_______________ **26.** Pertaining to the heel

_______________ **27.** Pertaining to the sole of foot

_______________ **28.** Pertaining to the groin where thigh attaches to pelvic region

_______________ **29.** Pertaining to the head

_______________ **30.** Pertaining to the chin

_______________ **31.** Pertaining to the foot

_______________ **32.** Pertaining to the eye

_______________ **33.** Pertaining to the genital area

_______________ **34.** Pertaining to the area between hip and knee

_______________ **35.** Pertaining to the area that includes bones enclosing the brain, but excluding facial bones

_______________ **36.** Pertaining to the forehead

_______________ **37.** Pertaining to the spine

_______________ **38.** Pertaining to the inferior back of the head

_______________ **39.** Pertaining to the anterior surface of leg

_______________ **40.** Pertaining to the area of back between ribs and buttocks

_______________ **41.** Pertaining to the belly; anterior area between diaphragm and pelvis

_______________ **42.** Pertaining to the anterior trunk below the abdomen

_______________ **43.** Pertaining to the area of back that contains shoulder blades

_______________ **44.** Pertaining to the posterior surface of elbow region

C. Planes

Complete the sentences using the planes listed.

- Frontal
- Sagittal
- Transverse

1. The _______________ plane divides body or organ into right and left sections.

2. The _______________ plane divides body or organ into anterior and posterior sections.

3. The _______________ plane divides body or organ into superior or inferior sections.

4. Which planes when passed through the body would result in two sections, with each section containing a piece of the heart and a piece of each lung?

_______________ and _______________

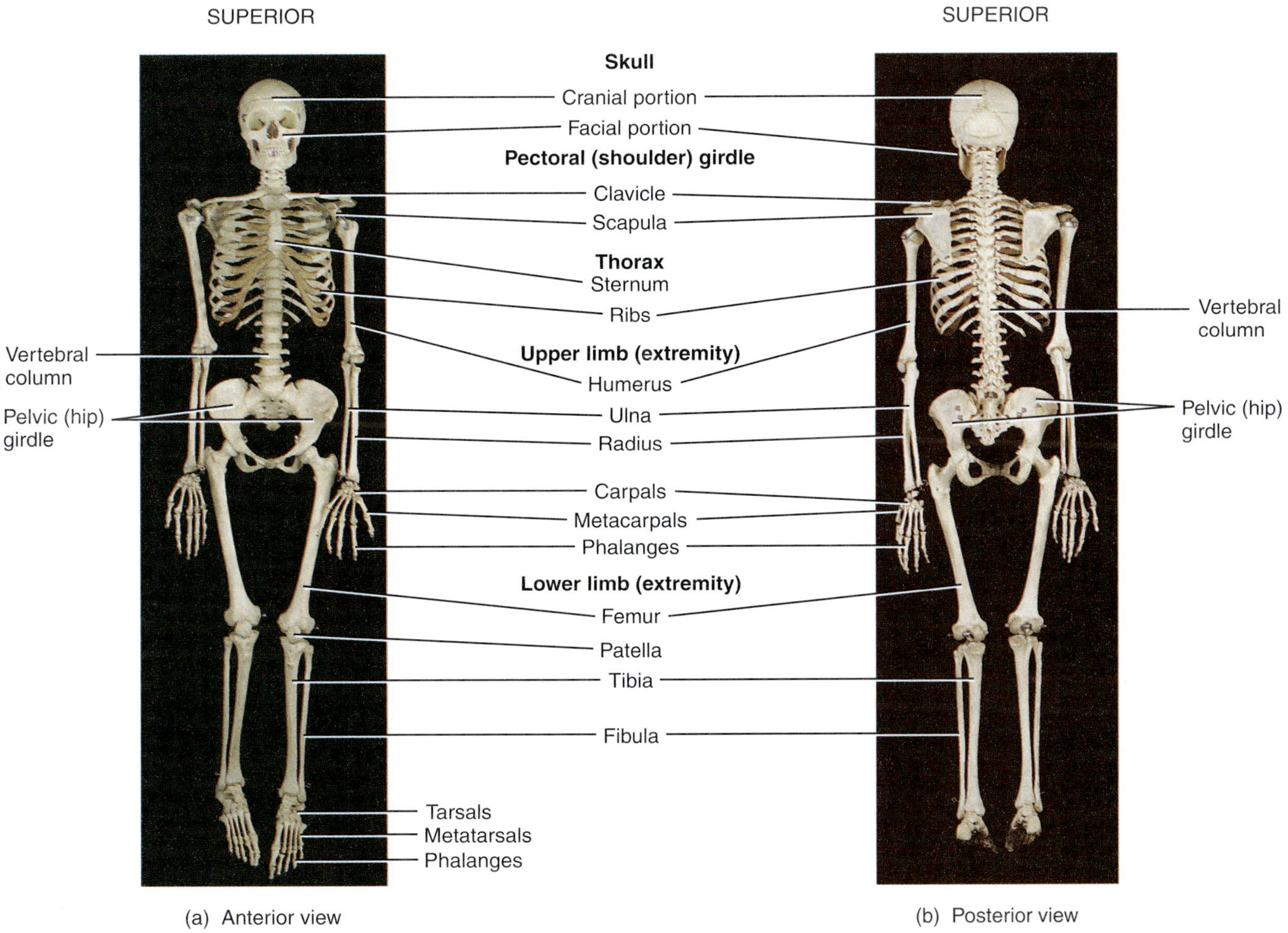

FIGURE 1.6 **Human skeleton.**

D. Directional Terms

Complete the sentences using directional terms. Use Figure 1.6 for reference.

1. The clavicle is ______________ to the ribs.
2. The ribs are ______________ to the sternum.
3. The humerus is ______________ to the radius.
4. The ulna is ______________ to the radius.
5. The tibia is ______________ to the femur.
6. The right humerus and the right radius are ______________.
7. The pelvic girdle is ______________ to the ribs.
8. The sternum is ______________ to the vertebral column.
9. The scapula is ______________ to the clavicle.
10. The right fibula and the left fibula are ______________.

Name ____________________ Date ______________ Section ______________

EXERCISE 1

USING YOUR KNOWLEDGE

A. Body Regions, Anatomical Terminology, and Directional Terms

1. A 26-year-old female presented with an irregularly shaped and colored mole in the right lumbar region, just lateral to the vertebrae. Indicate on Figure 1.7 where this mole is likely to be found.

2. A 10-year-old male presented to the emergency room with a laceration on the left forearm just distal to the antecubital region. Indicate on Figure 1.7 where the laceration is likely to be found.

3. A 22-year-old female was identified by a tattoo on the fibular surface of the left leg just proximal to the tarsal region. Indicate on Figure 1.7 where the tattoo is likely to be found.

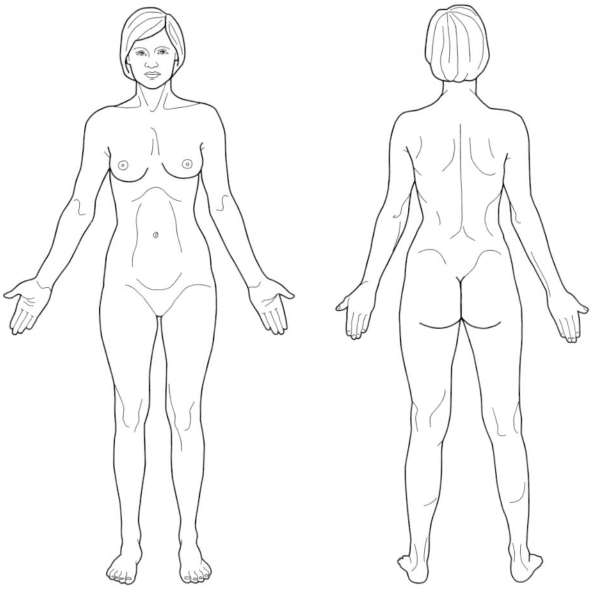

(a) Anterior view (b) Posterior view

FIGURE 1.7 **Body regions, anatomical language, and directional terms.**

Using the names of the structures in italics, answer questions 4–8.

4. Is the *pectoralis* major muscle anterior or posterior to the *subscapularis* muscle?

5. Is the *buccinator* muscle superior or inferior to the *frontalis* muscle?

6. Are the *thoracic* vertebrae medial or lateral to the *scapulae*?

7. Is the biceps *brachii* muscle proximal or distal to the extensor *digitorum* muscle?

8. The humerus bone is located in the arm. Is the *olecranon* process of the humerus on the distal or proximal end of the humerus?

B. Body Planes and Sections

Figure 1.8 contains three different sections through the thorax. Indicate which section (view a, b, or c) is a

9. Sagittal section ______

10. Transverse (axial) section ______

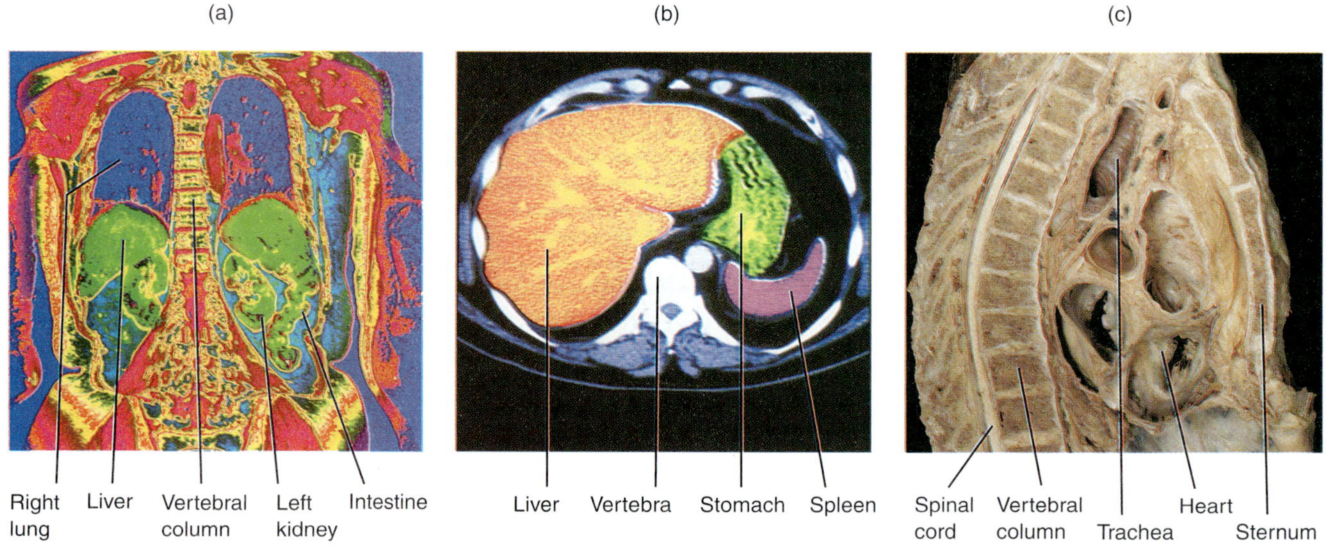

FIGURE 1.8 Sections through the thorax.

EXERCISE 2

ORGAN SYSTEMS

OUTLINE

OBJECTIVES

After completing these activities, you will be able to:

- Name the organ systems and describe their function
- Identify selected organs from each organ system
- Identify the body cavities and the organs they contain
- Identify the serous membranes
- Identify the abdominopelvic quadrants and the organs found in each quadrant

MATERIALS

- torso models or charts
- male and female reproductive models
- masking tape

A. Overview of Organ Systems

Organ systems work together to provide the cells of the body with an optimal environment for their needs. Maintenance of this optimal environment, within limits, is called **homeostasis** (*homeo-* = sameness; *-stasis* = standing). All organ systems cooperate to maintain homeostasis, and failure to maintain homeostasis results in disorders and disease. Organ system functions and major organs are summarized in Table 2.1.

ACTIVITY 1 Identifying Organ Systems

Identify the organ systems in Figure 2.1 using the organ system list provided.

B. Identification of Selected Organs on a Torso Model

You will be identifying organs from anterior to posterior and answering questions concerning their position relative to the organs around them. Refer to the directional terms in Exercise 1.

TABLE 2.1 Functions and Major Organs of the Organ Systems

ORGAN SYSTEM	FUNCTION
Cardiovascular	Transports nutrients, chemical messengers, gases, and wastes in blood Major organs: heart and blood vessels
Respiratory	Adds oxygen to blood and removes carbon dioxide from blood; maintenance of carbon dioxide levels helps regulate pH Major organs: nose, pharynx (throat), trachea, bronchi, lungs
Digestive	Breaks down food into units that can be absorbed into the body; eliminates solid wastes Major organs: mouth, pharynx, esophagus, stomach, intestines, pancreas, liver
Urinary	Removes nitrogenous wastes; maintains body fluid volume, pH, and electrolyte levels through urine production Major organs: kidneys, ureters, urinary bladder, urethra
Integumentary	Provides a protective barrier for the body, aids in production of vitamin D, and contains sensory receptors for pain, touch, and temperature Major organs: skin and skin structures (hair, nails, sweat and oil glands)
Lymphatic and Immune	Returns fluid to cardiovascular system; detects, filters, and eliminates disease-causing organisms, including cancer cells Major organs: lymphatic vessels, lymph nodes, spleen
Skeletal	Protects major organs; provides levers and support for body movement Major organs: bones
Muscular	Moves bones and maintains posture Major organs: skeletal muscles
Nervous	Controls cell function with electrical signals Major organs: brain, spinal cord, nerves
Endocrine	Controls cell function with hormones Major organs: hypothalamus, pituitary, thyroid, pancreas, adrenal glands, ovaries, testes
Reproductive	Produces gametes; female uterus provides environment for development of fetus Major organs in the male: testes, epididymis, ductus deferens, penis Major organs in the female: ovaries, uterine tubes, uterus, vagina

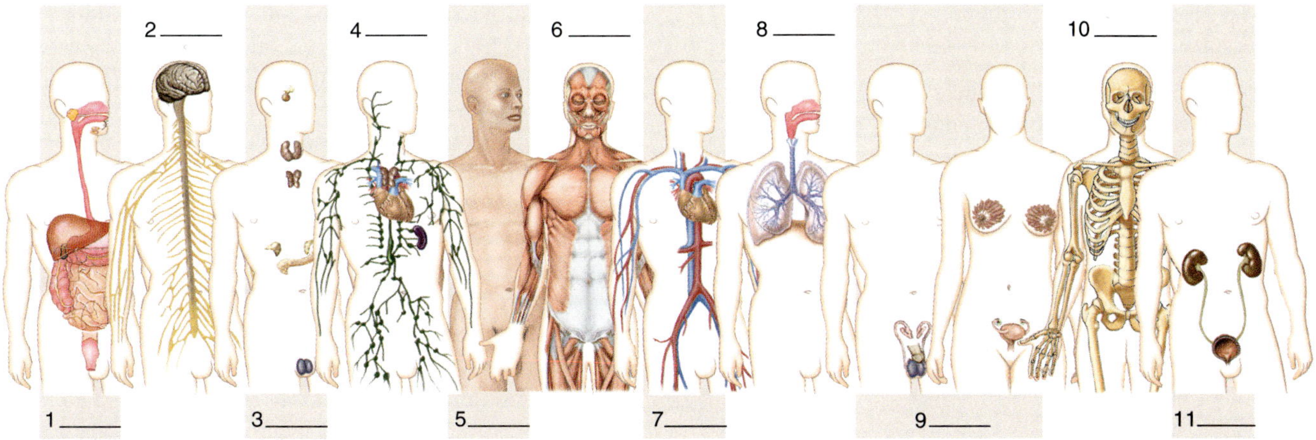

- cardiovascular
- digestive
- endocrine
- integumentary
- lymphatic and immune
- muscular
- nervous
- reproductive
- respiratory
- skeletal
- urinary

1 ______________________
2 ______________________
3 ______________________
4 ______________________
5 ______________________
6 ______________________
7 ______________________
8 ______________________
9 ______________________
10 ______________________
11 ______________________

FIGURE 2.1 Organ systems and selected organs.

ACTIVITY 2 Organ Systems and Organs

1 Identify the following organs on the anterior surface of a torso model. Identify all the organs without removing any organs from the model.
- brain
- heart
- large intestine
- liver
- lungs
- small intestine
- stomach
- trachea

2 Remove the lungs, heart, liver, and stomach.
Identify the following organs.
- bronchi (right and left)
- esophagus
- gallbladder (inferior surface of liver)
- pancreas
- spleen
- superior vena cava

3 Remove the large intestine and small intestine.
Identify the following organs.
- abdominal aorta
- adrenal glands
- appendix (lower right side of large intestine)
- inferior vena cava
- kidneys
- ureters
- urinary bladder

4 Identify the female reproductive organs on a female reproductive model or chart. Observe the position of the urinary bladder relative to the uterus.
- ovaries
- uterine tubes
- uterus

5 Identify the male reproductive organs on a male reproductive model or chart.
- penis
- scrotum
- testes

6 Answer the questions about the position of each organ.

1. The stomach is ______ to the small intestines.
   a. superior b. inferior c. medial d. lateral
2. The liver is ______ to the lungs.
   a. superior b. inferior c. medial d. lateral

3. The heart is ______ to the lungs.
   a. superior b. inferior c. medial d. lateral
4. The trachea is ______ to the esophagus.
   a. superior b. inferior c. anterior d. posterior
5. The pancreas is ______ to the stomach.
   a. medial b. anterior c. superior d. posterior.
6. The gallbladder is on the ______ surface of the liver.
   a. superior b. inferior c. posterior d. lateral
7. The stomach is ______ to the spleen.
   a. lateral b. medial c. superior d. inferior
8. The abdominal aorta and inferior vena cava are ______ to the kidneys.
   a. medial b. lateral c. superior d. inferior
9. The adrenal glands are ______ to the kidneys.
   a. anterior b. posterior c. superior
   d. inferior
10. The urinary bladder is ______ to the uterus.
    a. posterior and superior
    b. anterior and inferior
    c. medial and superior
    d. lateral and posterior

C. Body Cavities

The two main cavities of the body are the dorsal and ventral body cavities. The **dorsal body cavity** is located near the posterior surface of the body. It has two main subdivisions: the **cranial cavity** that contains the brain and the **vertebral** (*vertebra* = back) **canal** that contains the spinal cord. The cranial and the vertebral cavities are continuous.

The **ventral body cavity** is located near the anterior surface of the body and has two subdivisions, the thoracic cavity and the abdominopelvic cavity, that are separated by the **diaphragm.** The **thoracic cavity** is a space enclosed by the ribs, sternum, and vertebral column. This cavity is subdivided into three smaller cavities: the **pericardial cavity** (*peri-* = around; *-cardia* = heart), and two **pleural cavities** (*pleura* = rib). The pericardial cavity surrounds the heart, and each pleural cavity contains a lung. The **mediastinum** (*media* = middle; *-stinum* = partition), a central area within the thoracic cavity, extends from the neck to the diaphragm and from the sternum to the vertebral column. The organs located in the mediastinum are the heart, thymus gland, large blood vessels, esophagus, and trachea. The pleural cavities are located on either side of the mediastinum.

The **abdominopelvic cavity** consists of two continuous cavities: the abdominal cavity and the pelvic cavity. The **abdominal cavity** is the superior portion located between the diaphragm superiorly and the brim of the pelvis inferiorly. This cavity contains the stomach, liver, gallbladder, pancreas, small intestine, kidneys, and part of the large intestine. The **pelvic cavity** is the inferior portion of the abdominopelvic cavity that contains the reproductive organs, the urinary bladder, part of the large intestine, and the rectum. It is important to note that the testes are not located in the ventral body cavity but are outside the body wall. Blood vessels, lymphatic vessels, and nerves are found in all body cavities.

ACTIVITY 3 Body Cavities

1 Label the dorsal and ventral body cavities, their subdivisions, and the diaphragm on Figure 2.2a and Figure 2.2b.

2 Locate the dorsal body cavity and its subdivisions on a skeleton.

3 Locate the ventral body cavity, its subdivisions, and the diaphragm on a torso model.

4 Complete Table 2.2 by listing the organ(s) found in each body cavity.

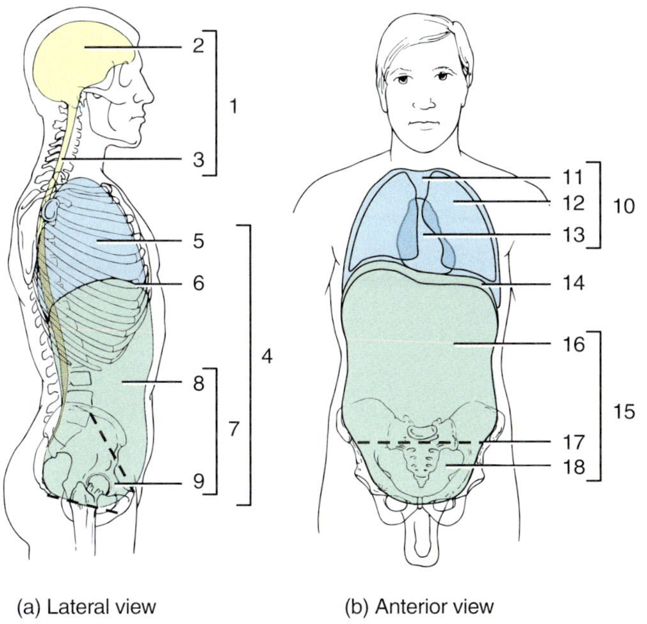

(a) Lateral view

- abdominal cavity
- abdominopelvic cavity
- cranial cavity
- diaphragm
- dorsal cavity
- pelvic cavity
- thoracic cavity
- ventral cavity
- vertebral canal

1 ____________________
2 ____________________
3 ____________________
4 ____________________
5 ____________________
6 ____________________
7 ____________________
8 ____________________
9 ____________________

(b) Anterior view

- abdominal cavity
- abdominopelvic cavity
- brim of pelvis
- diaphragm
- mediastinum
- pelvic cavity
- pericardial cavity
- pleural cavity
- thoracic cavity

10 ____________________
11 ____________________
12 ____________________
13 ____________________
14 ____________________
15 ____________________
16 ____________________
17 ____________________
18 ____________________

FIGURE 2.2 Body cavities.

TABLE 2.2 Body Cavities

BODY CAVITY	ORGANS
Dorsal body cavity	
Cranial cavity	
Vertebral canal	
Ventral body cavity	
Thoracic cavity	
Pleural cavities (2)	
Pericardial cavity	
Abdominopelvic cavity	
Abdominal cavity	
Pelvic cavity	

D. Serous Membranes

Most of the organs in the ventral body cavity are covered with **serous** (*serum* = any clear, watery fluid) **membranes.** Serous (SEAR-us) membranes are composed of two layers: the visceral layer and the parietal layer. The **visceral** (*viscera* = internal organs) **layer** covers the organ, whereas the **parietal** (*paries* = wall) **layer** attaches to and covers the ventral body wall. Between these two layers is serous fluid. The clear, watery **serous fluid** prevents friction as the organs move within the ventral body cavity.

The serous membranes are named for the cavities they surround. The serous membrane covering the lungs is the **pleura,** the membrane covering the heart is the **pericardium,** and the membrane covering the abdominal organs is the **peritoneum** (*peri-* = around; *teinein* = to stretch).

ACTIVITY 4 Serous Membranes

1. Label the serous membranes and cavities in the thoracic cavity on Figure 2.3.
2. Label the serous membranes and cavities in the abdominal cavity on Figure 2.4.

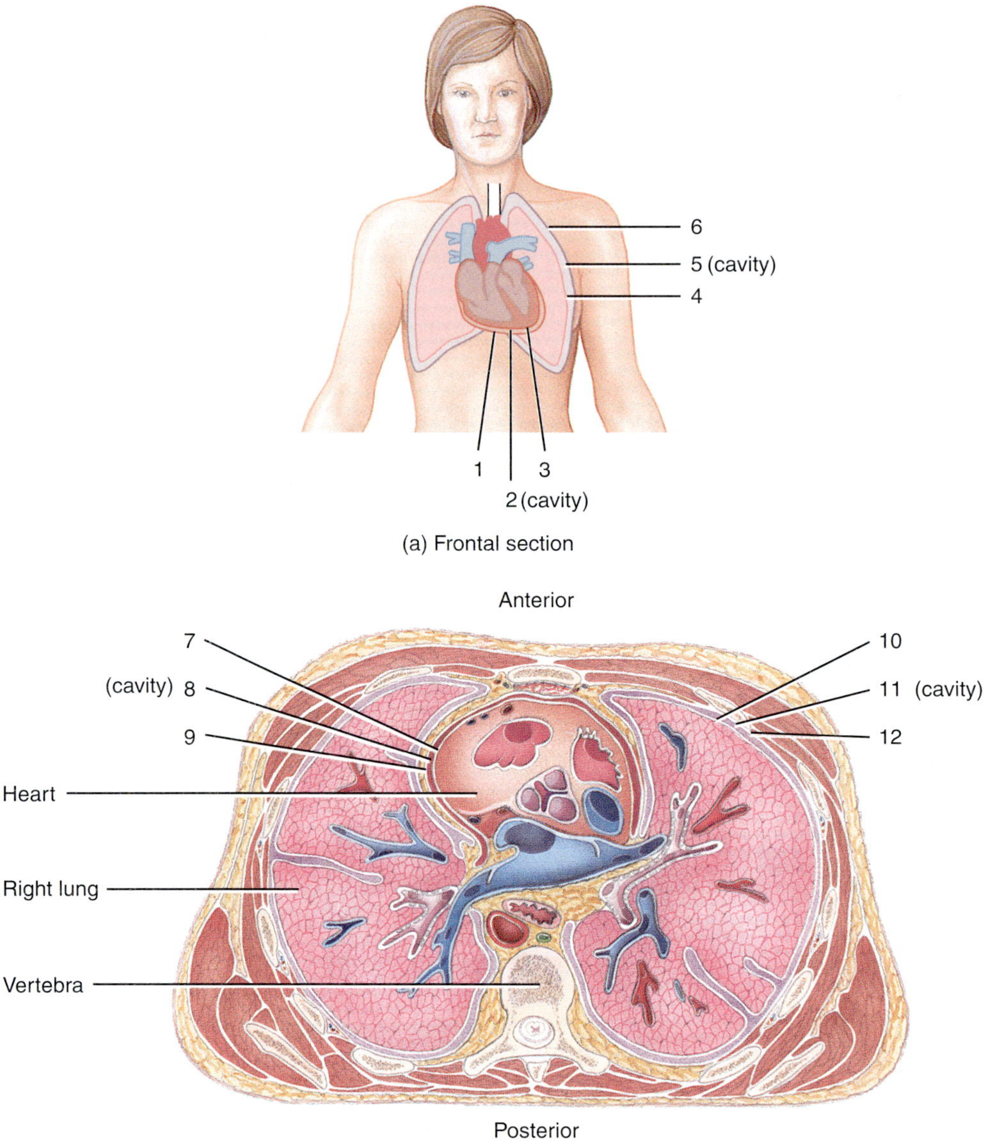

(a) Frontal section

(b) Transverse section

(a) Frontal section

- parietal pericardium (pa-RYE-e-tul per-i-CAR-dee-um)
- parietal pleura (PLEUR-uh)
- pericardial cavity (peri-CAR-dee-ul)
- pleural cavity
- visceral pericardium (VIH-sir-ul)
- visceral pleura

1 ____________________

2 ____________________

3 ____________________

4 ____________________

5 ____________________

6 ____________________

(b) Transverse section

- parietal pericardium
- parietal pleura
- pericardial cavity
- pleural cavity
- visceral pericardium
- visceral pleura

7 ____________________

8 ____________________

9 ____________________

10 ____________________

11 ____________________

12 ____________________

FIGURE 2.3 Serous membranes of the thoracic cavity.

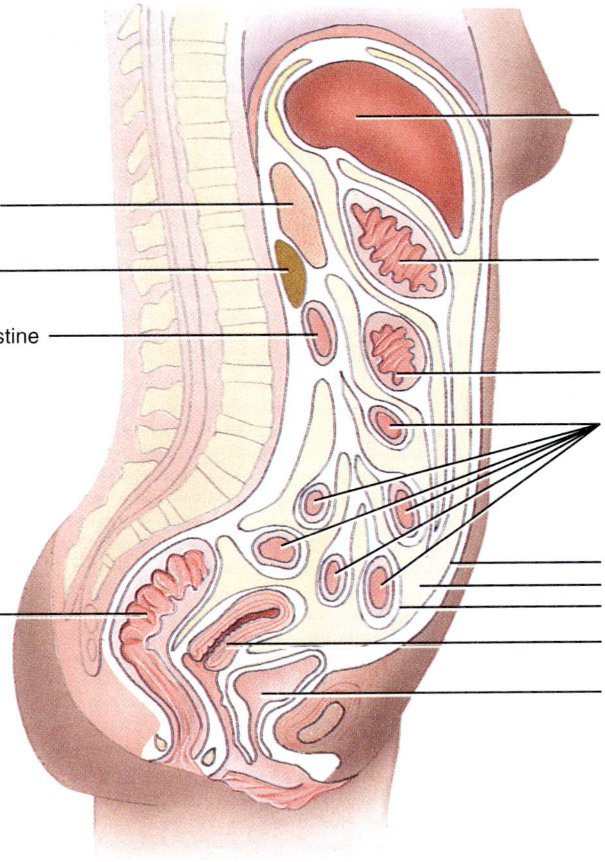

(a) Sagittal section through lower body

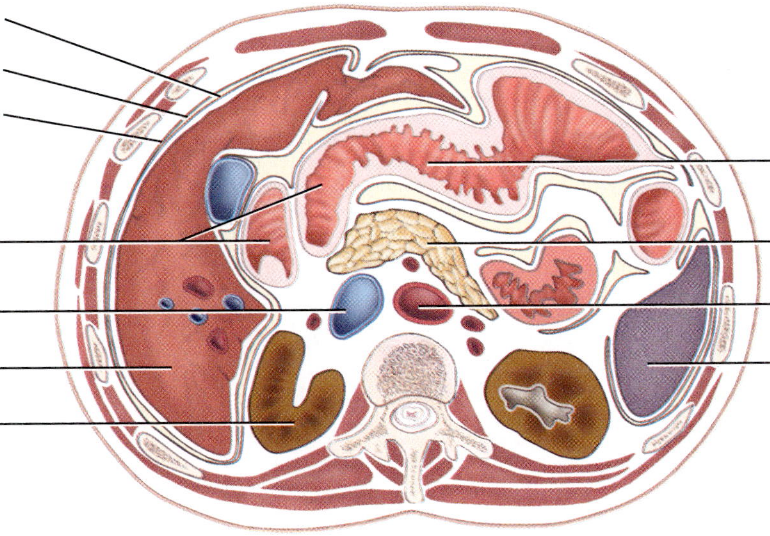

(b) Transverse section through abdomen

(a) Sagittal section

- parietal peritoneum (per-i-toe-NEE-um)
- peritoneal cavity (per-i-toe-NEE-ul)
- visceral peritoneum

1 ______________________

2 ______________________

3 ______________________

(b) Transverse section

- parietal peritoneum
- peritoneal cavity
- visceral peritoneum

4 ______________________

5 ______________________

6 ______________________

FIGURE 2.4 Serous membranes of the abdominal cavity.

E. Abdominopelvic Regions and Quadrants

Anatomists divide the abdominopelvic cavity into nine **regions** to describe the location of various organs. Two vertical and two horizontal lines are drawn to form a tic-tac-toe grid. The two vertical lines are drawn midclavicular and medial to the nipples beginning at the diaphram and extending inferiorly through the pelvic area. The upper horizontal line is drawn across the abdomen inferior to the ribs across the inferior portions of the liver and stomach. The lower horizontal line is drawn a little inferior to the top of the hipbones. These nine regions from the top right to the lower left are: **right hypochondriac, epigastric, left hypochondriac, right lumbar, umbilical, left lumbar, right inguinal** (iliac), **hypogastric** (pubic), and **left inguinal** (iliac).

Clinicians are more apt to divide this cavity into four **quadrants** that are formed by transverse and sagittal planes running through the umbilicus (navel). These quadrants are useful clinically when trying to describe abnormalities or determining which organ may be the cause of pain. Because the abdominopelvic quadrants are used more often clinically, this exercise will concentrate on abdominopelvic quadrants and their organs. The four quadrants are: **right upper quadrant (RUQ), left upper quadrant (LUQ), right lower quadrant (RLQ),** and **left lower quadrant (LLQ).**

ACTIVITY 5 Abdominopelvic Quadrants

1 Draw lines on Figure 2.5 separating the abdominopelvic area into regions or quadrants as advised by your instructor. Label the areas.

2 Using two pieces of masking tape, divide the abdominopelvic cavity of a torso into quadrants.

3 Using a torso model (or diagram), identify in which abdominopelvic quadrant(s) each organ is located. Use the abbreviations RUQ, LUQ, RLQ, LLQ.

- appendix ______________
- large intestine ______________
- liver ______________
- ovaries ______________
- pancreas ______________
- small intestine ______________
- spleen ______________
- stomach ______________

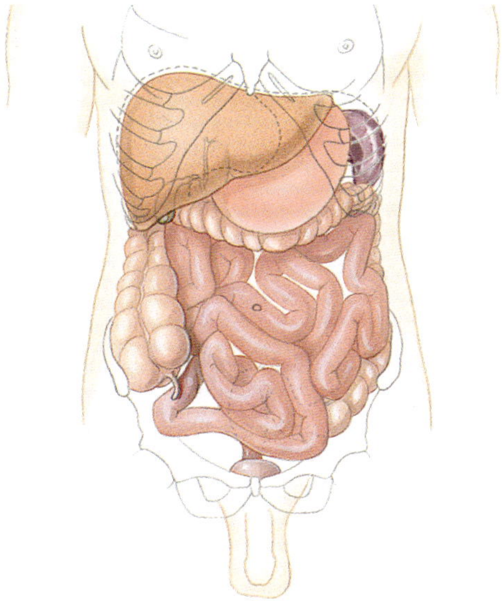

FIGURE 2.5 Abdominopelvic area.

Name ______________________ Date ______________ Section ______________

EXERCISE 2

REVIEWING YOUR KNOWLEDGE

A. Function of Organ Systems

Identify the organ system whose function is described below.

______________ 1. Maintains blood oxygen and carbon dioxide levels

______________ 2. Controls muscles and glands by electrical impulses

______________ 3. Controls cell function by hormone action

______________ 4. Movement of bones, blood, and food

______________ 5. A waterproof barrier that blocks the entrance of pathogens into the body and the loss of water from the body

______________ 6. Transports nutrients, oxygen, and carbon dioxide throughout the body

______________ 7. Breaks down food into absorbable nutrients

______________ 8. Regulates composition of blood by eliminating nitrogenous wastes, excess water, and minerals

______________ 9. Protection of body organs and framework for body

______________ 10. Produces gametes (sperm and egg)

______________ 11. Returns fluid that has leaked out of blood vessels into tissue, and provides protection against pathogens that have entered the body

B. Organ Identification

Identify the correct organ system for the following organs.

Organ System **Organ**

______________ 1. spleen

______________ 2. liver

______________ 3. trachea

______________ 4. blood vessels

______________________ 5. hair

______________________ 6. kidney

______________________ 7. uterine tube

______________________ 8. pituitary gland

______________________ 9. spinal cord

______________________ 10. testes

C. Body Cavities

Identify all the cavities for each organ as follows: dorsal (D), ventral (VN), cranial (C), vertebral (VR), thoracic (T), pleural (PL), pericardial (PC), abdominal (A), or pelvic (P). All structures are present in more than one cavity, and some are in three cavities.

________ 1. brain

________ 2. spinal cord

________ 3. heart

________ 4. lungs

________ 5. bronchi

________ 6. stomach

________ 7. intestine

________ 8. liver

________ 9. kidneys

________ 10. uterus

________ 11. urinary bladder

________ 12. ovaries

D. Serous Membranes

Complete the information below regarding serous membranes.

1. ______________________ Attaches heart to body cavity

2. ______________________ Covers the surface of the lungs

3. ______________________ Covers the surface of the abdominal organs

4. ______________________ The lubricating liquid in ventral body cavities

E. Abdominopelvic Quadrants

Name the quadrant(s) that the following organs predominantly occupy: RUQ, LUQ, RLQ, and LLQ.

________ 1. liver

________ 2. stomach

________ 3. spleen

________ 4. ascending colon

________ 5. gallbladder

________ 6. appendix

________ 7. left kidney

________ 8. right ovary

Name ______________________ Date ______________ Section ______________

EXERCISE 2

USING YOUR KNOWLEDGE

A. Homeostatic Imbalances of Organ Systems

Using your textbook, identify the organ system that is homeostatically imbalanced in the following diseases or disorders.

Organ System	Disease
______________________	**1.** muscular dystrophy
______________________	**2.** multiple sclerosis
______________________	**3.** myocardial ischemia
______________________	**4.** infectious mononucleosis

B. Body Cavities

Identify *all* the cavities entered for each procedure, beginning with the largest cavity and ending with the most specific body cavity. (A) abdominal; (C) cranial; (D) dorsal; (P) pelvic; (PC) pericardial, (PL) pleural; (T) thoracic; (VN) ventral; and (VR) vertebral.

_______ **5.** coronary bypass surgery

_______ **6.** cholecystectomy (gallbladder removal)

_______ **7.** spinal tap

C. Serous Membranes and Abdominopelvic Quadrants

8. John Doe, a 44-year-old male, went to the emergency room complaining of severe pain in his RLQ. The doctor palpated the area and determined that the pain was originating from an organ in that quadrant. Which organ might be involved?

a. liver; b. appendix; c. gallbladder; d. spleen; e. stomach

9. Ana Tomy, a 23-year-old female, went to the doctor with the chief complaint of RLQ pain. Circle the organ that is most likely the cause.

a. descending colon; b. ovary; c. gallbladder; d. pancreas; e. kidney

D. Organ Identification

Identify the organs in the color enhanced medical images in Figure 2.6.

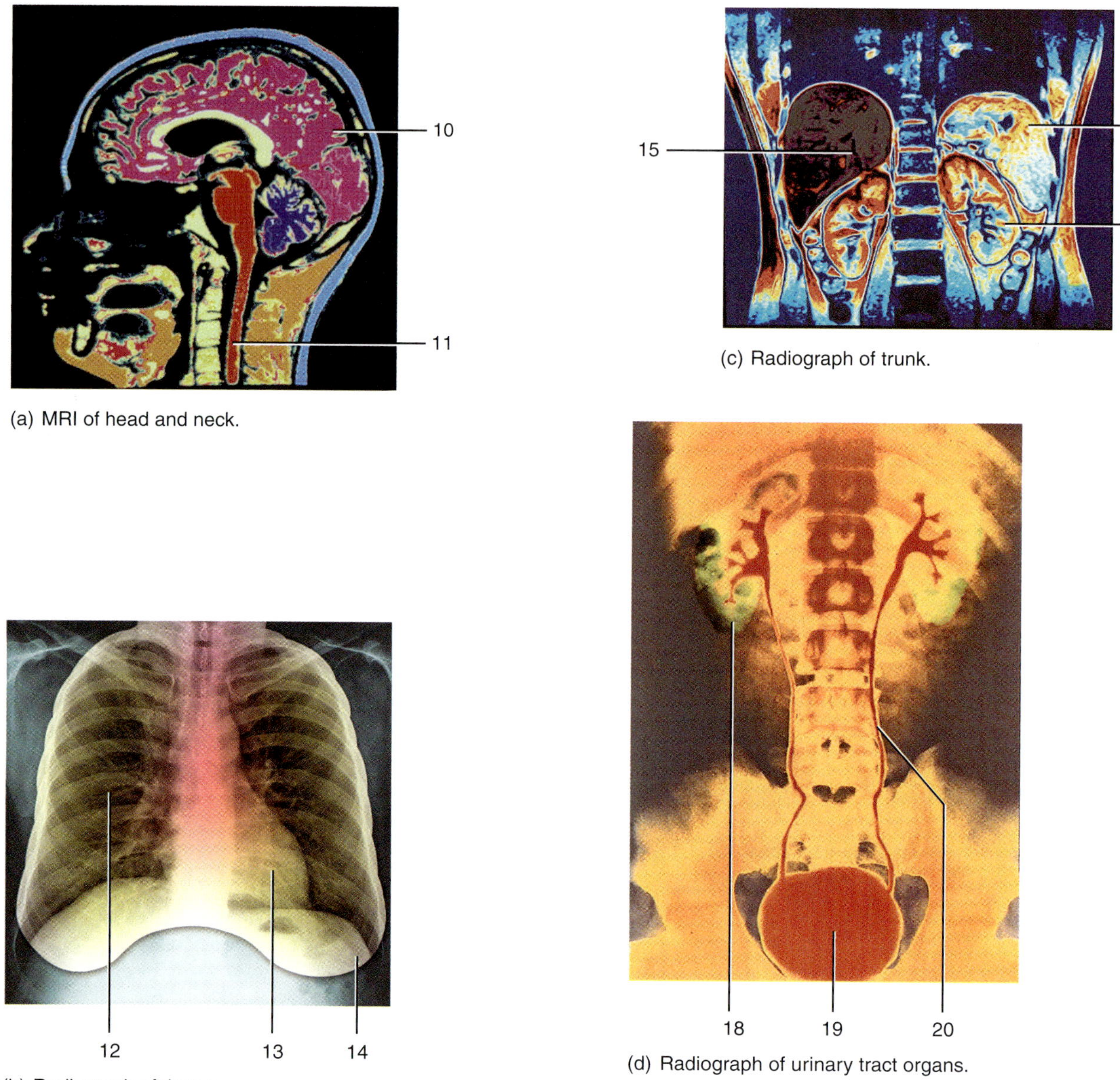

(a) MRI of head and neck.

(b) Radiograph of thorax.

(c) Radiograph of trunk.

(d) Radiograph of urinary tract organs.

FIGURE 2.6 Identification of organs on medical images.

10. ______________________

11. ______________________

12. ______________________

13. ______________________

14. ______________________

15. ______________________

16. ______________________

17. ______________________

18. ______________________

19. ______________________

20. ______________________

EXERCISE 3

CELL STRUCTURE AND FUNCTION

OUTLINE

OBJECTIVES

After completing this exercise, you should be able to:

- Identify cellular organelles on a diagram, model, or chart
- Describe the function of the plasma membrane and cellular cell organelles
- Identify cells and their main structures on prepared microscope slides
- Describe diffusion, osmosis, filtration, and phagocytosis
- Distinguish between and define hypotonic, hypertonic, and isotonic solutions
- Identify the stages of mitosis

MATERIALS

Activities 1–2 Cell Structure and Function

- diagram, chart, or model of a cell
- compound microscopes and lens paper
- prepared slides of human smooth muscle cells, motor neurons, sperm, and blood
- microscope slides, coverslips, flat toothpicks and dropper bottle of dilute methylene blue

Activities 3–8 See materials listed under each activity

A. Cellular Structures and Organelles

Cells are the smallest structural and functional units of living organisms. Cells are enclosed by a plasma membrane which controls the movement of substances into and out of the cell. Cytoplasm fills the interior of the cell and contains cytosol (a viscous fluid) and organelles. Like an automobile, a cell has different parts or organelles (little organs) that perform different functions. A "generalized" animal cell is shown in Figure 3.1, and functions of cellular organelles are described in Table 3.1.

The human body contains many different types of cells with different functions. These differences in function are reflected in cell structure. These cells differ from the generalized animal cell in shape, size, or in number and type of organelles present. In this activity you will observe smooth muscle cells, motor neurons, sperm cells, and red and white blood cells. **Smooth muscle cells** are located in the walls of hollow muscular organs and move substances through these organs when they contract (shorten in length). **Motor neurons** receive information from other neurons and send signals to muscle cells causing them to contract. **Sperm cells** carry genetic information through the female reproductive tract and try to insert this genetic information into an egg (fertilization). **Red blood cells** contain large amounts of hemoglobin, a red pigment that binds oxygen, and **white blood cells** defend the body from pathogens and cancerous cells. The differences in function of these cells are reflected in differences in their size, shape, and cellular organelles.

ACTIVITY 1 Cell Structures and Organelles

1 Point to each cellular organelle shown in Figure 3.1 on a cell model or chart.
2 Pronounce the name of each organelle and describe its function as you point to it.
3 Using a compound microscope, observe each prepared slide of human tissue or cells (smooth muscle, motor neuron, sperm, and blood smear). Use Figure 3.2 to help you locate the cells.
4 Answer discussion questions with your lab partners.

TABLE 3.1 Function of Cellular Structures

STRUCTURE	FUNCTION
PLASMA MEMBRANE	Mediates entrance and exit of substances into and out of the cell.
• Microvilli	Folds of the plasma membrane that increase its surface area.
CYTOPLASM	Area of the cell that includes the cytosol and organelles.
Cytosol	Fluid portion of cytoplasm that surrounds organelles
Organelles	
• Nucleus (NOO-klee-us)	Contains the cell's hereditary information in genes; directs cellular activities
Nucleolus (noo-KLEE-o-lus)	Assembly site for ribosomes
Chromatin (KROH-mah-tin)	Long thin strands within nucleus. Each strand composed of one DNA molecule and associated proteins.
• Centrioles	Needed to form cilia and flagella; active in mitosis and meiosis
• Mitochondria (my-toh-KON-dree-a)	Makes ATP via aerobic cellular respiration
• Smooth endoplasmic reticulum	Phospholipid and carbohydrate synthesis; detoxifies toxic substances
• Ribosomes (RYE-bow-some)	Protein synthesis site.
• Rough endoplasmic reticulum (endo-PLAZ-mik re-TIC-u-lum)	Processes secretory proteins that are made on the ribsomes
• Golgi complex (GOAL-jee)	Membranous sacs; stores, alters, and packages cellular exports
• Lysosomes (LY-so-some)	Digests worn-out organelles and substances that enter the cell
• Cytoskeleton	Three kinds of protein filaments; maintain cell shape and movement
• Cilia	Move fluids particles along a cell surface or move a one-celled organism
• Flagella	Longer than cilia; move cell. In humans, only found on sperm cells.

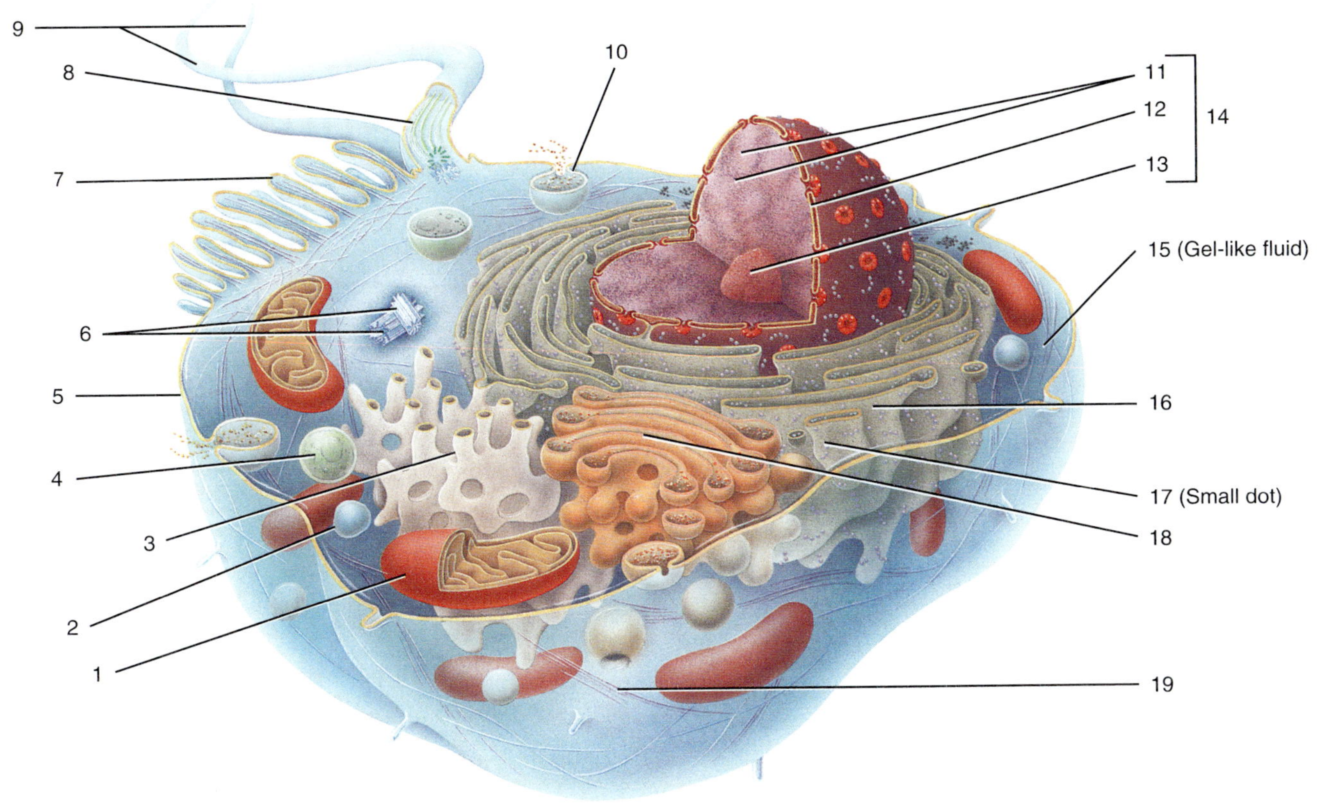

1 mitochondrion
2 peroxisome
3 smooth endoplasmic reticulum
4 lysosome
5 plasma membrane
6 centrioles
7 microvillus
8 cytoskeleton
9 flagella
10 secretory vesicle
11 chromatin
12 nuclear membrane
13 nucleolus
14 nucleus
15 cytoplasm
16 rough endoplasmic reticulum
17 ribosome
18 Golgi complex
19 cytoskeleton

FIGURE 3.1 **Sectional drawing of a cell.**

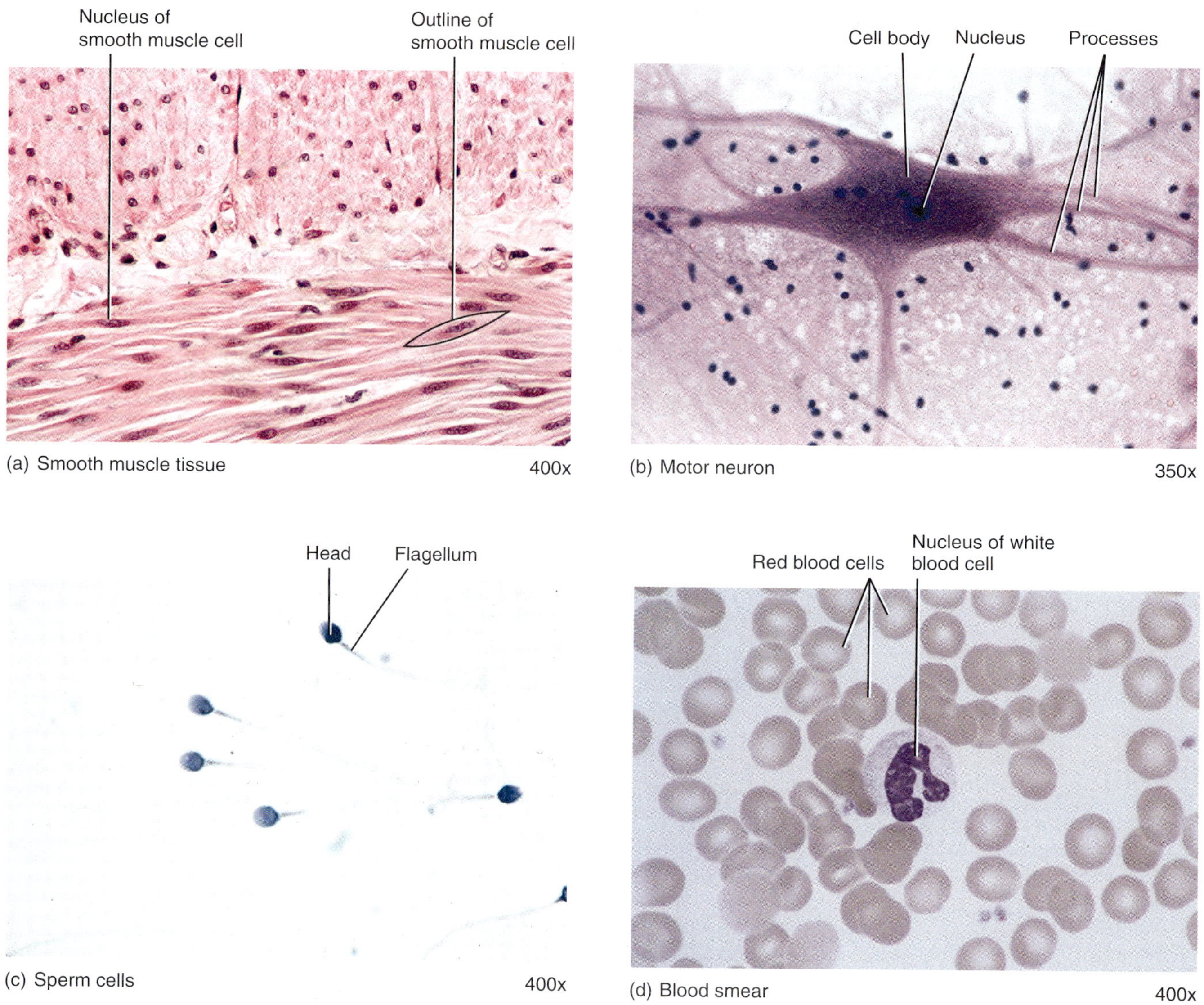

FIGURE 3.2 Cell Specialization.

DISCUSSION QUESTIONS: CELL SPECIALIZATION

1 Using the figure letters a–d, rank the size of each cell type in your slides from *largest* to *smallest* using the high-power objective lens.

(Largest) 1st ______ 2nd ______ 3rd ______ 4th ______ (Smallest)

2 Describe each cell's shape and list the organelles that can be seen with the light microscope in each type of cell.

a. Smooth muscle cell ____________________

b. Motor neuron (nerve cell) ____________________

c. Sperm cell ____________________

d. Red blood cell ____________________

e. White blood cell ____________________

3 How does the shape of a cell affect its function?

4 What were the main differences you observed in the cells?

Cells that line the interior of the mouth fit closely together like floor tile and form a thick cell layer that protects the underlying tissue from abrasion and microbes (bacteria and viruses). The superficial cells continually slough off and are replaced by underlying cells. Gently scraping the lining of the cheek removes the superficial cells that are about to slough off.

ACTIVITY 2 Cheek Smear

1 Prepare a cheek smear slide and observe it under the compound microscope.
- Obtain a toothpick, a clean microscope slide, and a coverslip.
- Place a drop of 0.9% saline on the microscope slide.
- Gently scrape the flat end of the toothpick (no blood, please!) on the inner lining of your cheek.
- Mix the sample in the drop of saline on the slide.
- Dispose of the toothpick as your instructor directs.
- Add *one drop* of dilute methylene blue to the cells on your slide.
- Cover the sample with a coverslip as directed by your instructor.
- Using low power, locate the blue-stained cells. Switch to high power to observe the organelles.

2 Compare the cells on your slide with Figure 3.3.

3 Place microscope slides in a 10% bleach solution as your instructor directs. Clean your lab top with a 10% bleach solution.

4 Answer discussion questions with your lab partners.

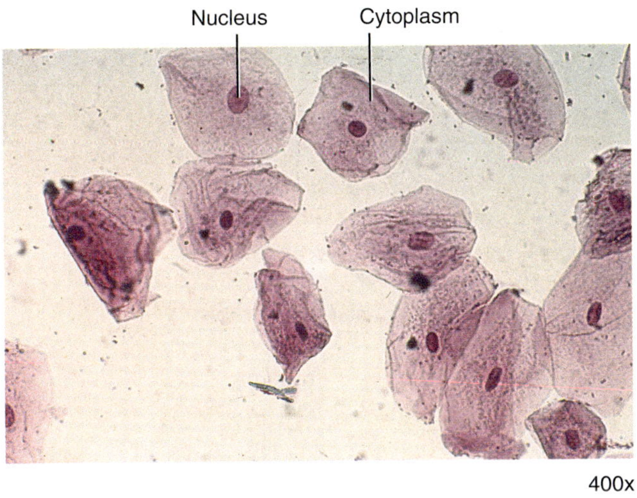

FIGURE 3.3 Cheek cells.

DISCUSSION QUESTIONS: CHEEK SMEAR

1 Why was stain added to the cheek cells?

2 What organelle did you identify?

3 Did you observe small bacteria on your cells?

4 Is your mouth sterile?

5 Is it unusual to see bacteria on cheek cells?

B. Passive Transport Across the Plasma Membrane—Diffusion, Osmosis, and Filtration

The plasma membrane with its unique design is responsible for selectively allowing substances into and out of the cell (selectively permeable membrane). Table 3.2 describes the variety of methods the cell uses to move substances across the cell membrane, either actively or passively. **Active processes** require ATP (energy) to get the work done. **Passive processes** do not require the cell to expend energy because the kinetic energy of the particles causes them to move from an area of their higher concentration to an area of their lower concentration.

A **solvent** is a dissolving medium, typically a liquid and always water in living organisms. **Solutes** are the substances dissolved in a solvent. When two different solute concentrations are on either side of a selectively permeable membrane, there is a **concentration gradient** of the solute.

1. Diffusion

In **diffusion**, there is a net movement of substances from a region of their greater concentration to a region of their lesser concentration. Diffusion can occur in solids, liquids, or gas, and across the plasma membrane of cells. In the following activity, diffusion of two crystals through a solid (agar) will be studied. Methylene blue has a molecular weight of 320, and potassium permanganate has a molecular weight of 158. The two crystals move at different rates through the agar, which is made up mostly of water.

ACTIVITY 3 Diffusion

Materials: 2 agar petri dishes per group, small millimeter rulers, forceps, methylene blue crystals, potassium permanganate crystals

1 Using the molecular weight of the two crystals, predict which crystal will move faster. Circle your answer: *methylene blue or potassium permanganate*

TABLE 3.2 Movement of Substances across Cell Membranes

TRANSPORT PROCESS	DESCRIPTION
Passive Processes	Do not use ATP
• Diffusion	Movement of molecules or ions by kinetic energy from their greater concentration to their lesser concentration (down a concentration gradient) until equilibrium is reached
• Osmosis	Movement of *water molecules* by diffusion across a selectively permeable membrane; movement is from a hypotonic solution into a hypertonic solution; water moves until equilibrium is reached
• Facilitated diffusion	Movement of a substance down its concentration gradient using a transmembrane protein for transport
• Filtration	Flow of liquid (and solutes smaller than the pores) through the pores of a filter or plasma membrane; movement due to hydrostatic pressure
Active Processes	Cells use ATP to move substances across the plasma membrane
• Active transport	Movement of a substance against its concentration gradient using a transmembrane protein and ATP for transport
• Vesicular transport	Movement of substances into or out of a cell using vesicles that form at or fuse with the plasma membrane
Endocytosis	Movement of substances into a cell via vesicles forming at the plasma membrane
Phagocytosis	A type of endocytosis; specialized movement of solid particles into a cell by pseudopodia forming a vesicle around the particles; "cell eating"
Pinocytosis	A type of endocytosis; drops of fluid brought into a cell by an invagination of the plasma membrane forming a small vesicle; "cell drinking"
Exocytosis	Movement of substances out of a cell via fusion of secretory vesicles with the plasma membrane

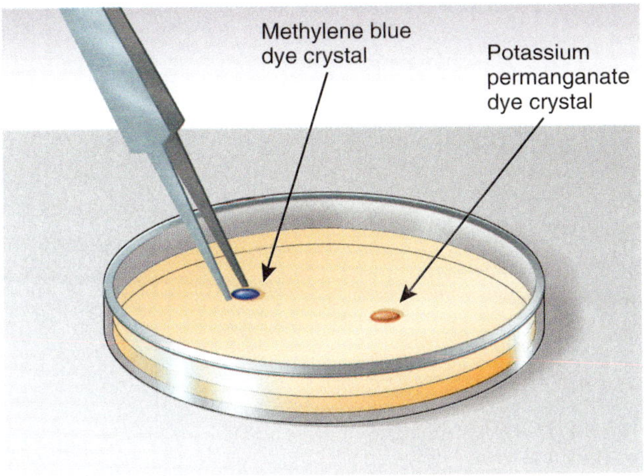

FIGURE 3.4 Diffusion in agar plate set-up.

2 Obtain materials for this activity (see material list).

3 Measure the diffusion rates of methylene blue and potassium permanganate.
- Carefully using forceps, place a large crystal of methylene blue on the surface of an agar petri dish (see Figure 3.4). Be careful not to drop any extra crystals on the agar surface.
- Using the same technique, place a similar sized crystal of potassium permanganate on the other side of the petri dish.
- Using a millimeter (mm) ruler, measure the crystals' diameter of diffusion at 15-minute intervals for at least 1 hour (or longer if desired).
- After each observation, record the diffusion diameter of each crystal in millimeters (mm) in Table 3.3.

4 Answer the discussion questions with your lab partners.

DISCUSSION QUESTIONS: DIFFUSION

1 Which substance moved faster?

2 Why did that substance move faster?

2. Osmosis

Osmosis is the net movement of water molecules through a selectively permeable membrane from a solution with a lower solute concentration (**hypotonic**) into a solution with a higher solute concentration (**hypertonic**). The terms hypotonic (*hypo-* = deficient; *-tonos* = stretching) solutions or hypertonic (*hyper-* = excessive) solutions are used only when two solutions are compared. Water will move into the hypertonic solution until the solute concentrations of the two solutions equalize to become **isotonic** solutions (*iso-* = same) or if enough pressure is applied to stop the flow of water. In this activity, a sucrose solution is added to a dialysis membrane bag. Dialysis membranes contain small pores which allow water and small solutes to cross. If water enters the bag, the weight of the bag will increase and if water leaves the bag, its weight decreases.

TABLE 3.3 Diffusion Results

TIME (MIN)	DIFFUSION OF METHYLENE BLUE (DIFFUSION DIAMETER IN MM)	DIFFUSION OF POTASSIUM PERMANGANATE (DIFFUSION DIAMETER IN MM)
15		
30		
45		
60		
75		

ACTIVITY 4 Osmosis Through a Nonliving Dialysis Membrane

NOTE: *Set this experiment up first at the beginning of class, so the students can observe and record changes throughout the lab time. The results become more dramatic the longer this experiment runs.*

Materials: dialysis tubing 12 cm long, 2 dialysis clips, scissors, Congo red or red food coloring, 40% sucrose solution, 500 ml beakers, distilled water, gram scale

1 Label Figure 3.5.

2 Predict the direction of water movement in Fig. 3.5 by circling the correct italicized choice.
- The net movement of water will be *into* or *out of* the dialysis bag (see Figure 3.5).

3 Obtain materials for this activity (see materials list).

4 Observe osmosis through a dialysis membrane and record your results in Table 3.4.

Set-up
- Cut a 12-cm piece of dialysis tubing and soak the bag in water for 3 minutes to make it easier to open.
- Fold over one end of the dialysis tubing and secure it with a dialysis clip.
- Rub the open end of the dialysis tubing between your thumb and finger to separate the sides, and fill the dialysis tubing more than three-quarters full with the red 40% sucrose solution.
- Pushing the air out of the bag, fold over the end of the bag and clip it with a dialysis clip. The dialysis bag now looks like a large "cell."
- Check to see that no liquid is leaking out of either end of the dialysis bag.

Experimental Procedure
- Rinse the bag to remove excess sucrose solution, dry and weigh it. Record the beginning weight in Table 3.4.
- Submerge the dialysis bag in a beaker of distilled water.
- Record the time in Table 3.4.
- Dry and weigh the dialysis bag after 15-minute, 30-minute, and 45-minute intervals. If your lab lasts longer, you may do a 60-minute measurement also.
- Record each measurement in Table 3.4.

5 Answer discussion questions with your lab partners.

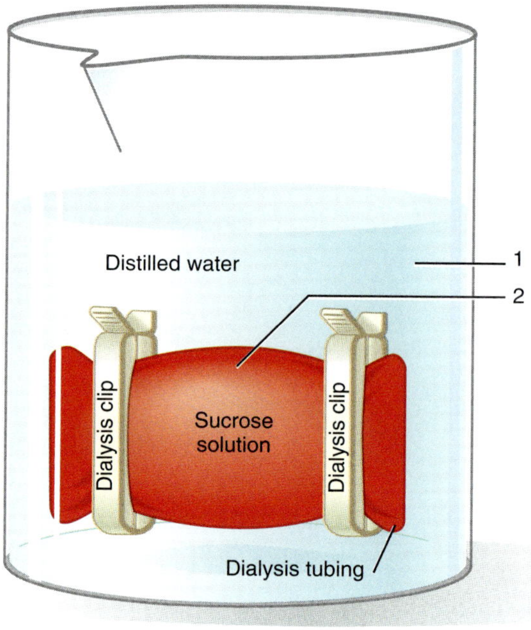

- hypertonic solution (hy-per-TOHN-ik)
- hypotonic solution (hy-poh-TOHN-ik)

1 ____________________

2 ____________________

FIGURE 3.5 Dialysis bag set-up.

TABLE 3.4 Dialysis Bag Results

TIME (min)	CHANGE IN WEIGHT OF SUCROSE SOLUTION (grams)
0 min	Start weight:
15 min	
30 min	
45 min	
60 min	

DISCUSSION QUESTIONS: DIALYSIS BAG

1 What was the direction of osmosis?

2 Why was distilled water used instead of tap water?

3 Why was the red dye added to the sucrose solution?

4 Did net water movement stop? Did the two solutions become isotonic? Explain.

5 Did any red sucrose solution leave the bag and enter the beaker water?

6 Explain why the bag gained weight since sucrose, Congo red and water crossed the dialysis membrane. (Hint: MW of sucrose is 342, Congo red is 697, and water is 18).

Osmosis in Living Red Blood Cells

Red blood cells (RBCs) are good examples to use for this osmosis experiment because their shape changes dramatically when they are exposed to hypotonic or hypertonic solutions. Their normal shape is a round biconcave disk with a smooth plasma membrane. Under the microscope, they look two-toned, with the center being lighter because of the concavity and thinness of the center. If the cell loses most of its water by osmosis when put in a hypertonic solution, it becomes **crenated** or shriveled with spiked edges. If the cell gains a significant amount of water by being placed in a hypotonic solution, it swells and may eventually burst—a process called **hemolysis** (*hemo-* = blood; *-lysis* = break down). As a basis for comparing various solutions to blood, the salt content (NaCl) of blood is 0.9% and is the same salt content as a physiologic saline solution.

NOTE: *Remember . . . salt shrivels and water swells (a cell).*

Safety Precautions

- Clean laboratory tabletops before and after conducting your experiments.
- Wear safety glasses and disposable gloves when handling body fluids or animal blood.

ACTIVITY 5 Osmosis in Living Cells

Materials: animal blood (uncoagulated), disposable gloves, clean microscope slides, coverslips, 4 medicine droppers/group, compound microscope, filter paper, distilled water, 0.9% saline solution, 5% saline solution, and 10% bleach solution (clean up)

1 With your lab group, discuss and identify which solutions for this experiment are hypotonic, hypertonic, or isotonic to the RBCs. The isotonic solution is also called physiologic saline.
- 0.9% saline solution ____________
- 5% saline solution ____________
- distilled water ____________

2 With your lab partners, predict the net movement of water in all three types of solutions.
Circle your choices for all three situations:
- In the isotonic solution, the RBCs will *swell*, *crenate*, or *not change shape*.
- In the hypotonic solution, the RBCs will *swell*, *crenate*, or *not change shape*.
- In the hypertonic solution, the RBCs will *swell*, *crenate*, or *not change shape*.

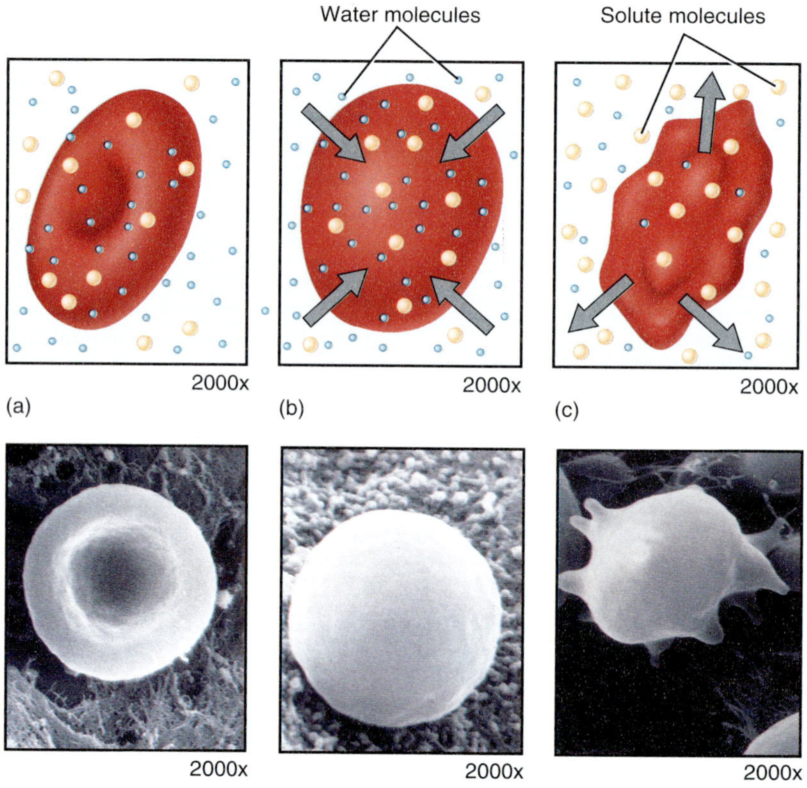

(a) shape ______ type of solution ______

(b) shape ______ type of solution ______

(c) shape ______ type of solution ______

FIGURE 3.6 **Osmosis in RBCs.**

3 In Figure 3.6, identify the shape of the RBC (normal, swollen, or crenated) and the type of solution the RBC is in (isotonic, hypertonic, and hypotonic).

4 Observe osmosis in RBCs.

Set-up

- Obtain materials
- Take out a compound microscope
- Put on gloves

Experimental Procedure:

Slide #1: 0.9% saline solution

- Place a drop of animal blood on a slide with a medicine dropper and cover with a coverslip. With a different medicine dropper, add a drop of 0.9% saline solution to the blood. Tilt the slide to intermix the two solutions, and cover with a coverslip.
- Using high power, observe the slide for changes in cell shape. Blood cells are very tiny and difficult to see under low power.
- Record shape of red blood cells and the type of solution in which it was placed.
  shape ______ type of solution ______

Slide #2: 5% saline solution

- Place a drop of animal blood on a 2nd slide and cover with a coverslip. Observe the RBCs using high power. On one side of the coverslip, add one drop of 5% saline with a clean medicine dropper. Place filter paper or a small piece of paper towel on the opposite side of the coverslip to absorb the liquid and pull the 5% saline solution into the RBCs.
- Immediately observe the 2nd slide under high power and watch for changes in cell shape. You may have to wait a few minutes for cell changes to occur.
- Record shape of RBCs and type of the solution.
  shape ______ type of solution ______

Slide #2 Again: distilled water

- Using slide #2 again, add one drop of distilled water to the same edge of the coverslip that was used for the saline solution.
- Hold a piece of filter paper at the opposite edge of the coverslip, observe the paper absorb the saline solution, and watch as the distilled water is drawn under the coverslip and into the RBCs.
- Immediately observe the slide under high power and watch if the RBCs change shape.

- Record shape of RBCs and type of solution.
  shape ______ type of solution ______

Clean Up

- Place blood-stained items (slides, coverslips, and droppers) in a 10% bleach solution or as directed by your instructor.
- Place gloves in an autoclavable bag or location indicated by your instructor.
- Wash down the lab counters with 10% bleach solution in a squirt bottle and wipe with paper towels wet with 10% bleach solution. Allow to air dry.
- Wash your hands with soap and water before leaving the lab area.

5 Answer discussion questions and conclusions with your lab partners.

DISCUSSION QUESTIONS: OSMOSIS IN RBCs

1 Does distilled water contain any solutes?

2 Does tap water contain any solutes?

3 Compare what would happen if the RBCs were placed in tap water instead of distilled water.

4 Osmosis was observed using which solution(s)?

3. Filtration

Filtration is the separation of substances passed through a filter or membrane from a region of higher pressure to a region of lower pressure. In the human body, filtration occurs in the kidneys and capillaries. Liquid and dissolved solutes flow through the pores of a filter or membrane, keeping solutes larger than the pores on the original side. In this activity, you will observe **selectivity** of the filtration membrane and a **change in filtration rate.** Keep in mind that the plasma membrane is part of a living cell and can have active processes going on simultaneously with passive processes, such as filtration.

ACTIVITY 6 FILTRATION

Materials: filter paper, funnel, ring stand with ring, 250 ml beaker, distilled water, 5% powdered charcoal solution, and 1% copper sulfate solution

1 With your lab partners, predict which substances will pass through the filter: water, copper sulfate (blue) or charcoal.

_________________ will pass through the filter.

_________________ will not pass through the filter.

2 Obtain materials for this activity (see materials list).

3 Set up and conduct the experiment (see Figure 3.7).

- Decide who will be the timer, the counter, and the recorder in your group.
- Fold the circular filter paper in half twice, and open it to form a cone. Place the cone in the funnel and place the funnel in a ring on the ring stand. Put the beaker under the funnel.

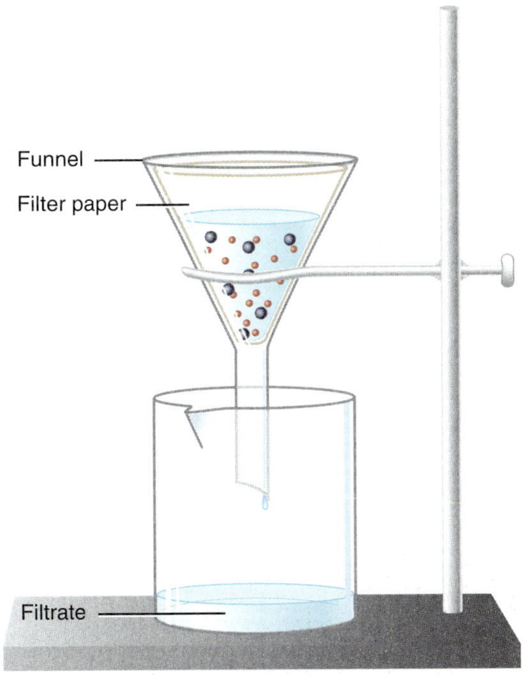

FIGURE 3.7 Filtration set-up.

TABLE 3.5 Filtration Results

TIME (SEC)	#DROPS
15	
30	
45	
60	
90	

- Stir or mix the filtrate solution comprised of water, copper sulfate (blue), and powdered charcoal, and pour it into the funnel to just below the top of the filter paper. Watch so the edges of the filter paper do not capsize or that the solution doesn't go over the top.
- As soon as the liquid slows down enough to count individual drops, count number of drops in 15, 30, 45, 60, and 90 seconds.
- Record your information on Table 3.5.
- Observe the filtrate (liquid) in the beaker. If it is blue, the copper sulfate was filtered, and if it is black, the charcoal was filtered.
- Compare your results with your predictions.

4 Answer the discussion questions with your lab partners.

DISCUSSION QUESTIONS: FILTRATION

1 What cell structure does the filter paper represent?

2 What is the force that drives the filtration?

3 Did you see a difference in the filtration rate during the activity? Explain.

C. Active Transport Across the Plasma Membrane—Phagocytosis

Phagocytosis (*phage-* = to eat) or "cell eating" is an active process that involves bringing solid material into the cell via vesicles that form from cellular extensions of the plasma membrane called **pseudopodia** (*pseudo* = false; *-podia* = feet). Although one-celled organisms like amoebas are involved in this activity, the human body also has cells that move in an amoeboid fashion and are involved in phagocytosis.

ACTIVITY 7 Phagocytosis in Amoebas

Materials: *Amoeba proteus* culture, amoeba food (*Tetrahymena pyriformis*), clean glass slides and coverslips, medicine droppers, and compound microscope

1 Observe phagocytosis in amoebas.
- Obtain a compound microscope, a microscope slide, coverslip, amoeba culture, and amoeba food.
- Using a medicine dropper, place one drop of amoeba (starved) culture on a clean microscope slide.
- Place one drop of amoeba food in the drop of amoeba culture on the slide. Cover with a coverslip.
- Observe the amoebas first under low power and then under a higher power.
- Watch the amoebas change shape as they move. Observe them as they extend out their "false feet" to engulf the food.

2 Answer the discussion question with your lab partners.

DISCUSSION QUESTION: PHAGOCYTOSIS

How would you describe the shape of an amoeba?

D. Somatic Cell Division: The Cell Cycle and Mitosis

Somatic (*soma-* = body) **cell division** occurs when one cell divides to produce two identical cells. Cell division is needed for growth of the individual and cell replacement.

The cell cycle begins when a cell is produced by cell division and ends when the cell divides. The length of the cell cycle differs according to the type of cell, with some cells dividing more frequently than others. The **cell cycle** can be divided into two basic periods: **interphase,** a longer period during which the cell conducts its normal activity, grows and prepares for cell division, and the **mitotic phase,** when the cell is dividing. The mitotic phase consists of **mitosis,** or nuclear division, and **cytokinesis,** or cytoplasmic division. The four stages of mitosis are: prophase, metaphase, telophase and anaphase (Table 3.6).

To observe interphase and the stages of mitosis, you will examine a prepared microscope slide containing several whitefish blastula. The **blastula** is an active growth stage of embryonic development that has many dividing cells.

ACTIVITY 8 Mitotic Phases

Materials: 3-dimensional models of mitosis, whitefish blastula slides, compound microscope, lens paper

1. Observe the three-dimensional models of the mitotic phases, noting the changes in each phase.
2. Identify interphase, each phase of mitosis, and cytokinesis in Figure 3.8a–e.
3. Obtain a prepared whitefish blastula slide and hold it up to the light. Notice that there are many blastulae circles placed on each slide. It will be necessary to view several of the blastulae circles to find all of the phases.
4. Using a compound microscope, begin looking at your slide with the low power objective lens. Use the high power objective lens to identify interphase, the stages of mitosis, and cytokinesis.

TABLE 3.6 Phases of Somatic Cell Cycle

PHASE	DESCRIPTION OF ACTIVITY
INTERPHASE (*inter-* = between)	Normal cell work; cell metabolically active and growing, DNA replicates; chromosomes not visible
MITOTIC PHASE	Parent cell divides into two daughter cells
Mitosis (*mitos-* = thread)	Nuclear division
• Prophase (*pro-* = first)	Nucleolus and nuclear membrane disappear; chromatin condenses into chromosomes; centrioles move to opposite poles; spindle fibers form
• Metaphase (*meta-* = next)	Chromosomes line up at metaphasal plate; spindle fibers attach to centromeres of chromatids
• Anaphase (*ana-* = apart)	Chromatids of chromosomes separate; move to opposite poles
• Telophase (*telo-* = end)	Cell reverses prophase activities
Cytokinesis (*cyto-* = cell; *kinesio-* = movement)	Cytoplasmic division into two daughter cells

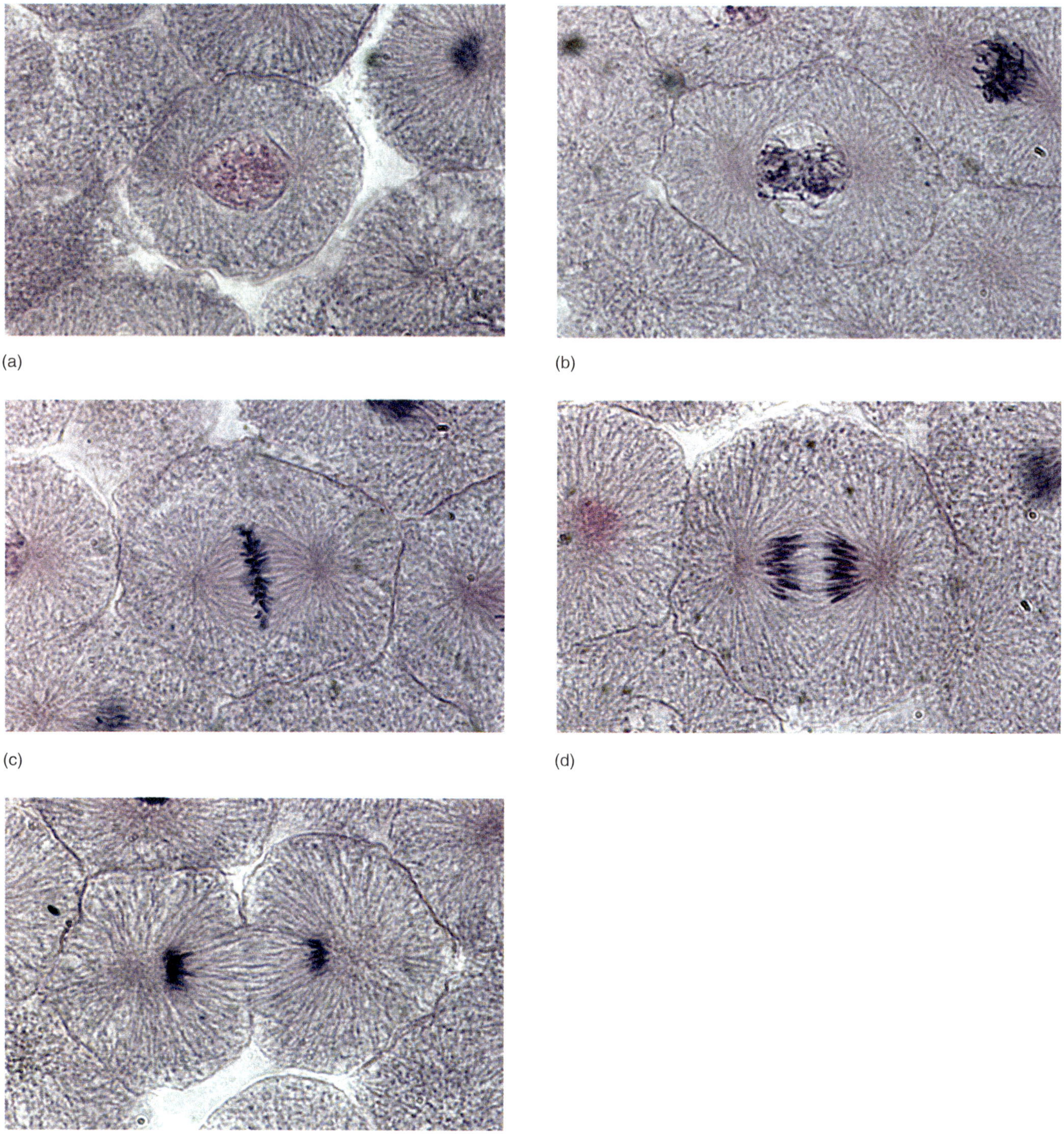

(a) (b) (c) (d) (e)

- anaphase (AN-a-faze)
- interphase (IN-ter-faze)
- metaphase (MEH-ta-faze)
- prophase (PRO-faze)
- telophase and cytokinesis (TELL-o-faze and cyto-kih-NEE-sis)

a ______________________

b ______________________

c ______________________

d ______________________

e ______________________

FIGURE 3.8 **Mitotic phases.**

Name ______________________ Date ______________ Section ________________

EXERCISE 3

REVIEWING YOUR KNOWLEDGE

A. Cellular Structures and Organelles

Fill in the blank with the name of the cell structure or organelle that fits the description.

_________________ 1. hair-like projections for cellular movement

_________________ 2. intracellular fluid

_________________ 3. energy production by cellular respiration

_________________ 4. protein synthesis site

_________________ 5. carbohydrate and lipid synthesis site

_________________ 6. small vesicle with digestive enzymes

_________________ 7. organelles needed to form cilia and flagella

_________________ 8. threadlike strand of DNA with associated proteins

_________________ 9. synthesis of secretory proteins

_________________ 10. stores, packages, and exports protein product

_________________ 11. contains genes that control cellular activities

_________________ 12. site for synthesis of ribosomes

_________________ 13. maintains cell shape and cell movements

_________________ 14. mediates transport of substances into or out of the cell

B. Phases of the Cell Cycle

Match the description with the phase of the cell cycle.

____ **1.** anaphase	A. cytoplasmic division
____ **2.** cytokinesis	B. cell performing normal functions; longest phase
____ **3.** interphase	C. nuclear division
____ **4.** metaphase	D. chromatid pairs line up at equatorial plate
____ **5.** mitosis	E. chromatin condenses into chromosomes; nucleus disappears
____ **6.** prophase	F. spindle fibers break up; nucleus reappears; chromosomes unravel to form chromatin
____ **7.** telophase	G. centromeres divide; chromosomes move to opposite poles

C. Transport across the Plasma Membrane

Match the definition with the term.

____ **1.** concentration gradient	A. to shrink or shrivel
____ **2.** crenate	B. water moving through selectively permeable membrane
____ **3.** diffusion	C. false feet of an amoeba or phagocytic white blood cell
____ **4.** hemolysis	D. substance dissolved in a solution
____ **5.** hypertonic solution	E. to burst a red blood cell
____ **6.** hypotonic solution	F. difference between solute concentrations across a membrane
____ **7.** isotonic solution	G. same solute concentration on both sides of membrane
____ **8.** osmosis	H. cell eating of large solid particles
____ **9.** pseudopodia	I. lower concentration of solutes than in cytosol of cell
____ **10.** phagocytosis	J. a fluid that can contain dissolved substances
____ **11.** solute	K. higher concentration of solutes than in cytosol of cell
____ **12.** solvent	L. random mixing of particles from their greater concentration to their lesser concentration

Name ______________________ Date ______________ Section ______________

EXERCISE 3

USING YOUR KNOWLEDGE

A. Cellular Organelles and Their Function

1. A cell makes and secretes a protein-based hormone. This particular cell would have a great amount of Golgi complex and:

A. SER B. RER C. mitochondria D. lysosomes

2. Cells that make steroids (lipids) would have more:

A. SER B. RER C. mitochondria D. ribosomes

3. Cells that need large amounts of ATP would have many:

A. Golgi complexes B. ribosomes C. SER D. mitochondria

4. Amoebas use what organelles for amoeboid movement and phagocytosis?

A. mitochondria B. cytoskeleton C. lysozome D. Golgi complex

B. Movement of Substances

5. In the filtration experiment, hydrostatic pressure was the force driving filtration. What is the force driving filtration in the kidney? ______________________

C. Osmosis

6. A. A test tube with blood in it has a particular solution added to it. After several minutes, the solution is not clear anymore, but becomes red. What happened to the blood cells? ______________________

B. Which solution was added to the blood to obtain these results?

A. 0.9% saline B. 5% saline C. distilled water

7. A 0.8% saline solution would be ______ to the cytosol of a cell.

A. hypotonic B. hypertonic C. isotonic

8. If a 50% sugar solution had been used in the dialysis bag in Activity 4, there would be a faster rate of osmosis.

A. true B. false

9. If you placed a peeled apple or potato in a 5% salt solution, it would:

A. gain weight B. lose weight C. stay the same weight

10. A person's hands become wrinkled after spending a long, relaxing time in the tub. Tub water does not have as many solutes in it compared with the human body. Explain why the hands look wrinkled.

A. The tub water is *hypotonic* to body cells and water *enters* the cells.

B. The tub water is *hypotonic* to body cells and water *leaves* the cells.

C. The tub water is *hypertonic* to body cells and water *enters* the cells.

D. The tub water is *hypertonic* to body cells and water *leaves* the cells.

EXERCISE 4

TISSUES

OUTLINE

OBJECTIVES

After completing this exercise, you should be able to:

- Identify the four primary tissue types
- Compare and contrast primary tissue structure and function
- Identify examples of epithelial and connective tissue types and state where they are located
- Compare and contrast the structure and function of epithelial and connective tissue types
- Identify the three types of epithelial membranes

MATERIALS

- compound microscope and lens paper
- prepared epithelial tissue slides: whole mount of mesothelium, simple squamous (tissue sections of mesothelium), simple cuboidal (kidney), simple columnar nonciliated (small intestine), stratified squamous nonkeratinized (esophagus), transitional (relaxed urinary bladder), ciliated pseudostratified columnar (trachea)
- prepared connective tissue slides: areolar, reticular, adipose, dense regular (tendon), dense irregular (skin), elastic, hyaline cartilage (trachea), bone, blood
- colored pencils

There are four primary tissues: epithelial, connective, muscle, and nervous. **Epithelial tissue** covers surfaces, lines cavities, and forms glands. **Connective tissue** supports and protects other tissues. **Muscle tissue** causes movement and **nervous tissue** receives and generates nerve impulses. In this exercise we compare the structure and function of the four primary tissues and examine specific epithelial and connective tissue types.

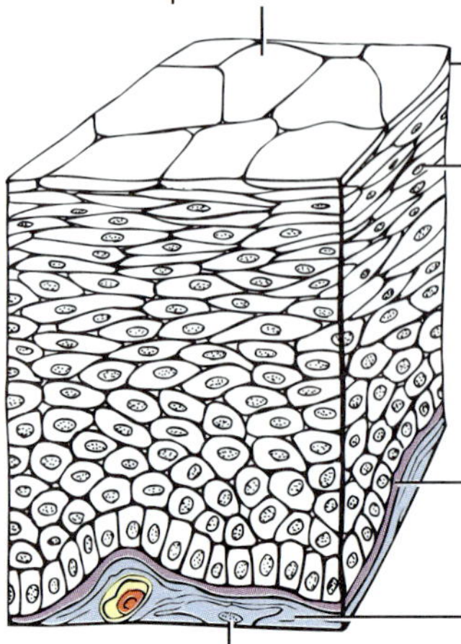

FIGURE 4.1 Epithelial tissue lining the mouth.

OVERVIEW OF PRIMARY TISSUES

A. Epithelial Tissue Overview

There are two categories of epithelial tissues—covering and lining epithelium and glandular epithelium. **Covering and lining epithelium** covers the surface of the body and some organs, and lines all hollow body structures. This epithelium forms barriers that protect and control what substances can cross into adjacent tissues. **Glandular epithelium** forms glands that produce and secrete products needed by the body. **Exocrine** (*exo-* = outside; *-crine* = secrete) glands secrete their product through a duct onto a body surface such as the skin or lumen of a hollow organ. **Endocrine** (*endo-* = within) glands are ductless glands that produce and secrete hormones into the extracellular space surrounding the gland. The hormones then diffuse into blood vessels to be distributed.

Epithelial tissues exhibit **cellularity** (most of the tissue consists of cells and not extracellular material) and are supported by underlying connective tissue. Epithelial and connective tissues are separated by a **basement membrane,** which is produced by both tissues. Epithelial cells are packed together in an orderly fashion, and tight junctions may occur between cells. **Tight junctions** prevent material from passing between cells and allow the epithelium to control what crosses into underlying tissues. Covering and lining epithelium faces a space such as the **lumen** (*lumen* = light) of a blood vessel or intestine. The epithelial cell surface adjacent to the space is called the **apical** (*apex* = tip) **surface,** whereas the epithelial cell surface adjacent to the basement membrane is the **basal surface.** Apical and basal surfaces differ in structure and function.

Epithelial tissue is avascular (does not contain blood vessels) and receives its nutrients by diffusion from the underlying connective tissue. Only those epithelial cells that are close to the basement membrane receive enough nutrients to enable them to divide and regenerate the epithelial layer(s).

Epithelial tissue types differ in the number of epithelial cell layers and in the shape of the cell in the apical cell layer.

ACTIVITY 1 Epithelial Tissue

1 Examine and color Figure 4.1, which depicts the surface and side view of epithelial tissue lining the mouth. Color the apical and basal layers of the epithelium using contrasting colors.
2 Label the photomicrograph of the epithelial tissue lining the mouth in Figure 4.2. Notice that the epithelial and connective tissue layers stain differently.
3 Answer discussion questions with your lab partners.

DISCUSSION QUESTIONS: EPITHELIAL TISSUE

1 Do the cells in the apical and basal layers in Figure 4.2 have the same shape?

2 Compare the amount of space between cells in the epithelial tissue layer and the underlying connective tissue layer in Figure 4.2.

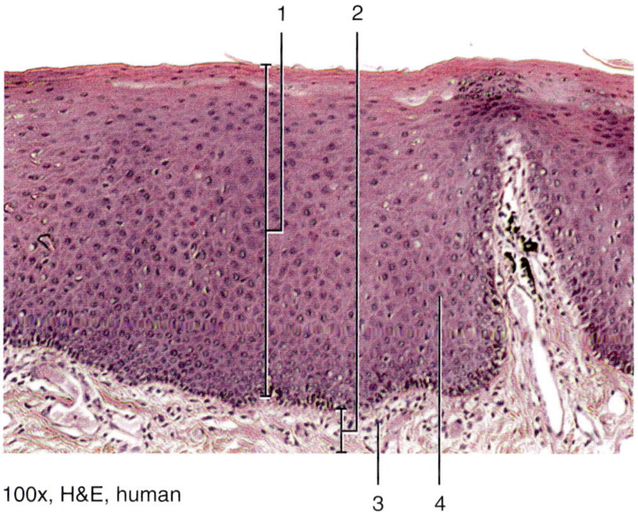

- connective tissue
- epithelial tissue
- nucleus of epithelial cell
- nucleus of connective tissue cell

1 ____________

2 ____________

3 ____________

4 ____________

FIGURE 4.2 Sectional view of epithelial tissue lining the mouth.

B. Connective Tissue Overview

Connective tissue is the most abundant tissue in the body and has a variety of functions. It supports epithelial tissue and connects it to other tissues. Connective tissue forms tendons (connect muscle to bone) and ligaments (connect bone to bone). Connective tissue also provides coverings that support and protect muscle and nervous tissue. Bone, the hardest connective tissue, protects body organs and provides a framework for movement of muscles. Adipose tissue (fat) insulates body tissues and stores lipids, and blood provides a liquid medium for transportation of substances throughout the body.

Most connective tissues are not very cellular, usually containing more extracellular material (matrix) than cells. **Extracellular matrix** consists of **ground substance** and **fibers** that are synthesized and secreted by connective tissue cells. Connective tissues are classified according to the nature of the ground substance and the amount and type of fibers present in the extracellular matrix. Characteristics of the extracellular matrix determine the function of individual connective tissues. Connective tissue of tendons and ligaments has an extracellular matrix filled with fibers that give them strength and resiliency. Extracellular matrix of connective tissue that supports epithelial tissues contains a loose arrangement of fibers and a ground substance that permits diffusion of nutrients to the epithelium. Bone has a hard extracellular matrix that offers protection and support. Blood has a fluid extracellular matrix that is used to transport substances throughout the body.

Most connective tissues are vascular and regenerate easily. However, the connective tissue in tendons is poorly vascularized, and cartilage (a type of connective tissue) is avascular. These poorly vascularized or nonvascularized connective tissues do not heal easily when damaged.

ACTIVITY 2 Connective Tissue

1. Examine and color Figure 4.3, which depicts the most common type of connective tissue (areolar). Color the ground substance and fibers using contrasting colors.
2. Label the photomicrograph of connective tissue in Figure 4.4. Notice that there are different fiber and cell types in this connective tissue.
3. Answer discussion questions with your lab partners.

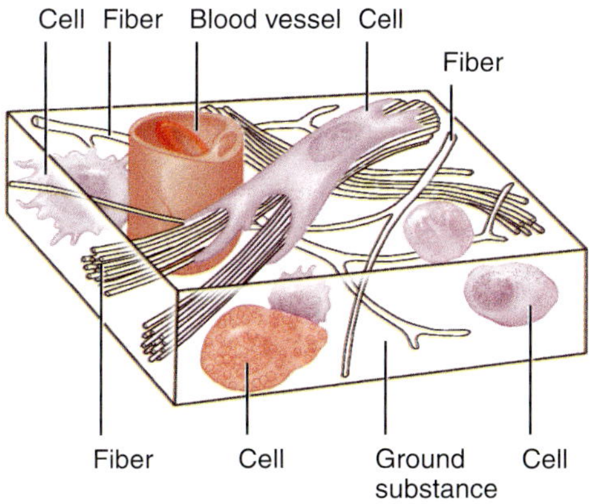

FIGURE 4.3 Connective tissue (areolar).

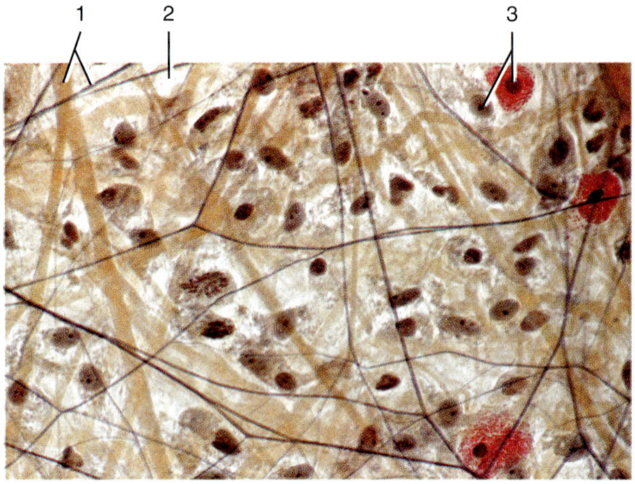

400x, Verhoeff Orange Safrin, human

- fibers
- ground substance
- nuclei of connective tissue cells

1 ____________

2 ____________

3 ____________

FIGURE 4.4 **Areolar connective tissue, mesentery spread.**

DISCUSSION QUESTIONS: CONNECTIVE TISSUE

1 In Figure 4.4, is the extracellular matrix packed with bundles of fibers (very little space between fiber bundles) or does it contain a loose arrangement of fibers?

2 Does the tissue in Figure 4.4 exhibit cellularity compared to epithelial tissue?

C. Muscle Tissue Overview

Muscle tissue contains muscle cells and connective tissue. Thin layers of connective tissue surround muscle cells to protect and support them. Muscle tissue is very cellular with most of the tissue consisting of muscle cells. Muscle cells are elongated cells called **fibers** that contain many microfilaments. These microfilaments, or **myofilaments** as they are called in muscle, cause the muscle cell to shorten when stimulated. This shortening or contraction causes movement. There are three types of muscle tissue—skeletal, cardiac, and smooth—with each type having a distinct appearance. **Skeletal muscle** is the muscle that moves the skeleton. **Cardiac muscle,** found in the wall of the heart, is responsible for forcefully propelling blood through blood vessels. **Smooth muscle** is found in the walls of hollow organs and is responsible for movement of substances through these organs.

Contraction requires a great amount of energy; muscle tissue is highly vascularized to provide the nutrients needed to make ATP for muscle contraction.

Smooth muscle regenerates easily, but skeletal and cardiac muscles do not. When cardiac muscle cells die during a heart attack, they are usually replaced by noncontractile scar tissue.

Skeletal and cardiac muscle cells exhibit **striations** (light and dark bands) due to a regular arrangement of the myofilaments. Skeletal muscle cells are multinucleated, while cardiac muscle cells have one to two nuclei per cell. The striations and size of skeletal and cardiac cells distinguish them from epithelial, connective, and nervous tissue cells. Smooth muscle cells are smaller with tapering ends, uninucleated, and nonstriated.

In this exercise you will observe skeletal muscle tissue. All three muscle tissues will be examined in more detail in the muscle tissue exercise.

ACTIVITY 3 Muscle Tissue

1 Examine and color Figure 4.5, which depicts skeletal muscle tissue. Color a muscle cell and its striations using contrasting colors.

2 Label the photomicrograph of a longitudinal section of skeletal muscle tissue in Figure 4.6.

3 Answer discussion questions with your lab partners.

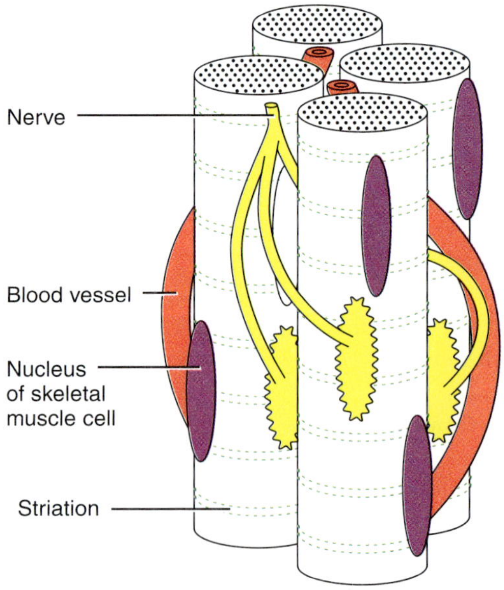

FIGURE 4.5 **Skeletal muscle tissue.**

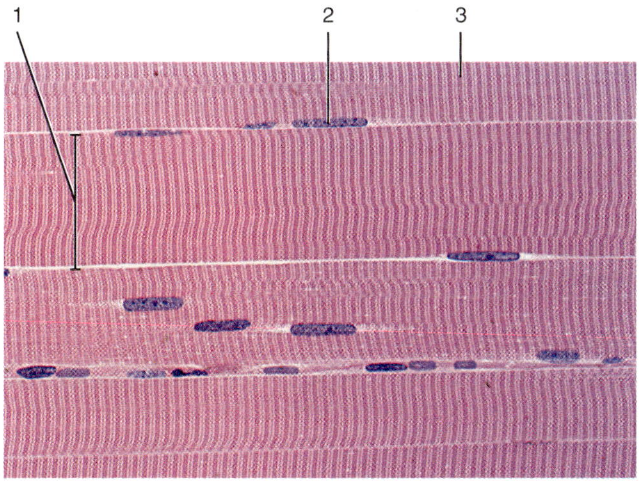

400x, H&E, human

- nucleus of skeletal muscle cell
- striation
- width of muscle cell

1 ____________

2 ____________

3 ____________

FIGURE 4.6 Sectional view of skeletal muscle tissue.

? DISCUSSION QUESTIONS: MUSCLE TISSUE

1 Compare the amount of space between skeletal muscle cells in Figure 4.6 to the amount of space between connective tissue cells in Figure 4.4.

2 Compare the cell size and shape of skeletal muscle cells in Figure 4.6 to the cell size and shape of connective tissue cells in Figure 4.4.

3 What must you do to compare epithelial cell size in Figure 4.2 to skeletal muscle size in Figure 4.6 and connective tissue size in Figure 4.4?

D. Nervous Tissue Overview

Nervous tissue forms the brain, spinal cord, and nerves. Two basic categories of nervous tissue cells are **neurons** and **neuroglial** (*neuro* = nerve; *glia* = glue) **cells.** Neurons receive and send information, whereas neuroglia support the neurons and help them to function. Neurons have one or more processes (cellular extensions) that receive or send information as nerve impulses. **Dendrites** (*dendro* = tree) are processes that receive signals from sensory receptors or other neurons. An **axon** is another type of process that sends signals to other neurons, muscles, or glands. Neurons have only one axon, but may have many dendrites. The main part of the cell where the nucleus is located is called the **cell body.**

There are three structural types of neurons, classified according to the number of processes they have. In this exercise you will observe only **multipolar neurons,** which are neurons with many processes.

Generating nerve impulses requires a tremendous amount of ATP. Nervous tissue is highly vascularized in order to supply the required nutrients. Neurons are not very mitotic and are rarely replaced when the cell body is damaged, whereas neuroglia do divide and replace themselves.

ACTIVITY 4 Nervous Tissue

1 Examine and color Figure 4.7, which depicts nervous tissue. Color the multipolar neuron cell bodies, nuclei, and processes using contrasting colors.

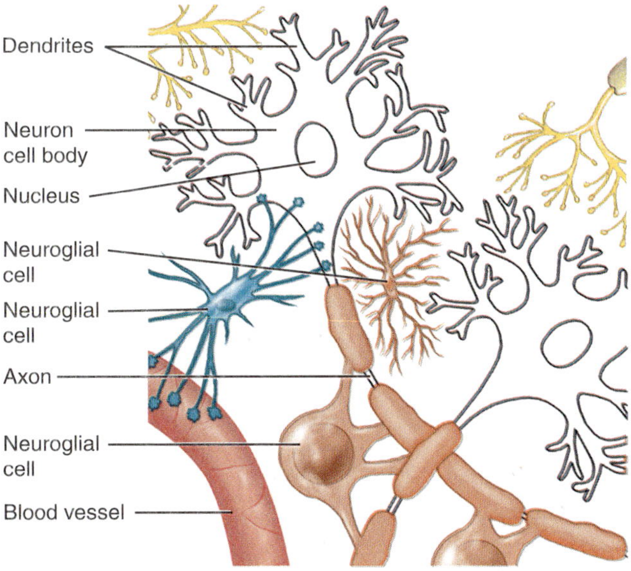

FIGURE 4.7 Nervous tissue.

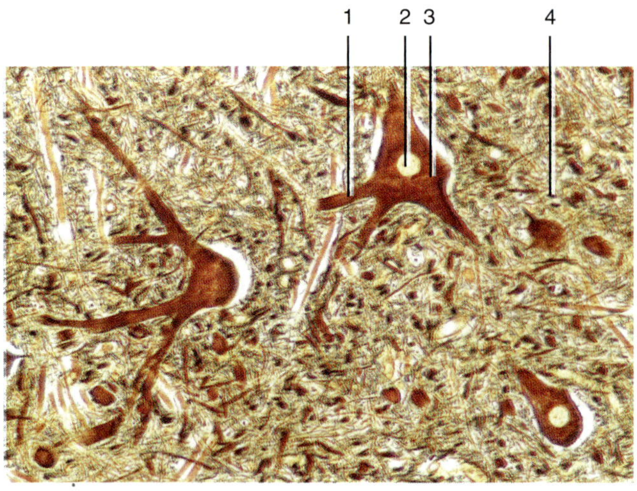

200x, Bielschowski silver, human

- cell body of multipolar neuron — 1 ____________
- neuroglial cell — 2 ____________
- nucleus of multipolar neuron — 3 ____________
- process of multipolar neuron — 4 ____________

FIGURE 4.8 **Sectional view of nervous tissue.**

2 Label the photomicrograph of nervous tissue in Figure 4.8.

3 Answer discussion questions with your lab partners.

DISCUSSION QUESTIONS: NERVOUS TISSUE

1 Compare the size of neuroglial cells to the size of the multipolar neuron.

2 In Figure 4.8, the extracellular space between neuroglial cells and the multipolar neuron cell body is packed with small gold structures. What are they? Remember, nervous tissue is very cellular.

Now that you've reviewed the four primary tissues, specific epithelial and connective tissue types will be studied. Muscle and nervous tissue types will be studied in later exercises.

EPITHELIAL TISSUE TYPES

Epithelial tissues are classified according to cell shape and the number of cell layers (Figure 4.9). If there is only one cell layer, the epithelium is **simple epithelium;** if there are two or more cell layers, the epithelium is **stratified epithelium.**

Epithelial cells have four shapes: squamous, cuboidal, columnar, and transitional. Cell shapes are best seen in side views of the cells (Figure 4.9). **Squamous cells** are the thinnest with a flattened nucleus; **cuboidal cells** are cubelike with a round nucleus in the center of the cell. **Columnar cells** are tall with an oval nucleus close to the base of the cell. **Transitional cells** change shape; they are rounder when the tissue is relaxed and flatten when the tissue is stretched.

When viewed from the **apical surface** (the surface facing free space), all epithelial cells have a similar shape. Their shape enables them to fit closely together like floor tiles to form a lining or barrier.

Simple epithelium provides a selective barrier allowing diffusion, filtration, secretion, and absorption of selected substances. Stratified epithelium is thicker, subject to wear and tear, and forms a protective barrier. Multiple cell layers make the tissue more resistant to damage, thereby preventing pathogens and foreign materials from crossing into underlying tissues.

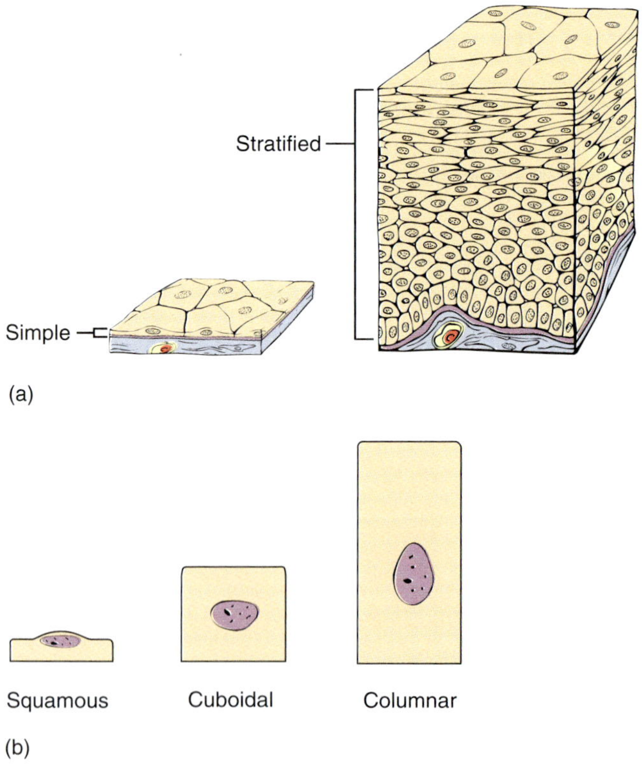

FIGURE 4.9 **Epithelial tissue classification.**

A. Simple Epithelium

1. Simple Squamous Epithelium

This is a very thin cell layer. The short distance between the apical and basal cell surfaces allows for quick passage of material across the cell by diffusion, filtration, or secretion.

Example: Simple squamous epithelium of the peritoneum

The peritoneum is the serous membrane associated with abdominopelvic organs. The parietal and visceral layers of all serous membranes contain epithelial and connective tissues. The epithelial layer is simple squamous epithelium called **mesothelium** that secretes serous fluid into the serosal cavity.

In Activity 5, you will observe epithelium from the surface and from a side view. Epithelial tissues appear similar when viewed from the surface. Notice how the cells fit closely together. Differences in shape are observed when viewing cells from the side.

> **NOTE:** *Observe tissue first with a scanning or low-power objective. Focus first with the coarse focus knob. Before switching to a more powerful objective lens, move the slide so that the area you want to observe is in the center of the field of view. After changing to the more powerful lens, use the fine focus knob only to bring the tissue into focus. Use this procedure with all tissue slides.*

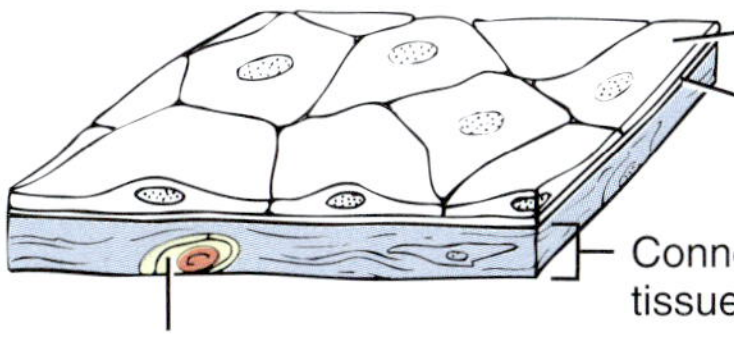

FIGURE 4.10 Simple squamous epithelium.

ACTIVITY 5 Microscopic Examination of Simple Squamous Epithelium

1. Color the simple squamous epithelium and the basement membrane in Figure 4.10 using contrasting colors.
2. Label the photomicrograph in Figure 4.11.
3. Examine a prepared microscope slide showing the surface of epithelial tissue of the peritoneum (or any other epithelial tissue) and identify the structures listed in Figure 4.11.
4. Label Figure 4.12b.
5. Examine a prepared microscope slide showing a side view (sectional view) of simple squamous epithelium (mesothelium) of the peritoneum and identify the structures listed in Figure 4.12b.

Use the survey photomicrograph in Figure 4.12 to help you locate simple squamous epithelium. Survey photomicrographs are provided for all epithelial tissues and some connective tissues in this exercise.

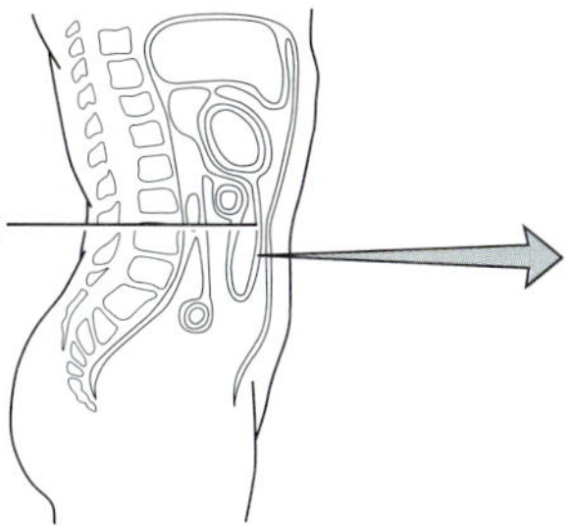

- cell boundary of simple squamous epithelial cell
- cytoplasm of simple squamous epithelial cell
- nucleus of simple squamous epithelial cell

1 ______________________

2 ______________________

3 ______________________

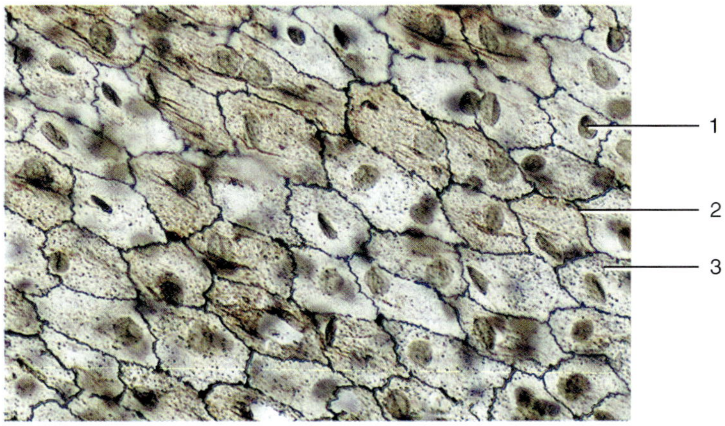

400x, silver, human

FIGURE 4.11 Surface view of simple squamous epithelium of peritoneum.

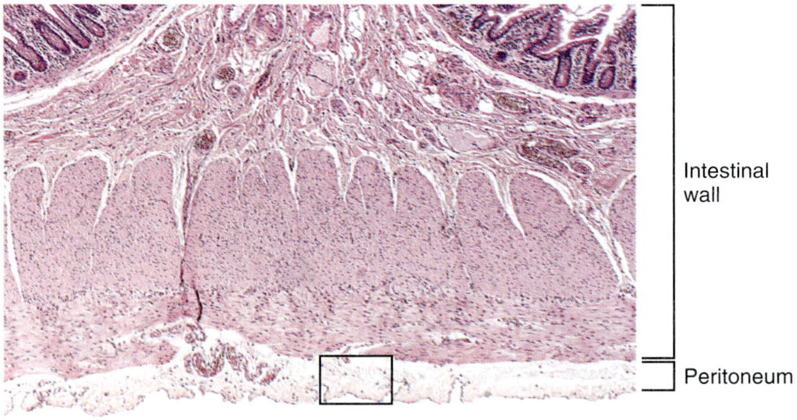

40x

(a) Survey photomicrograph.

- connective tissue
- nucleus of connective tissue cell
- nucleus of simple squamous epithelial cell
- simple squamous epithelium

1 ______________________

2 ______________________

3 ______________________

4 ______________________

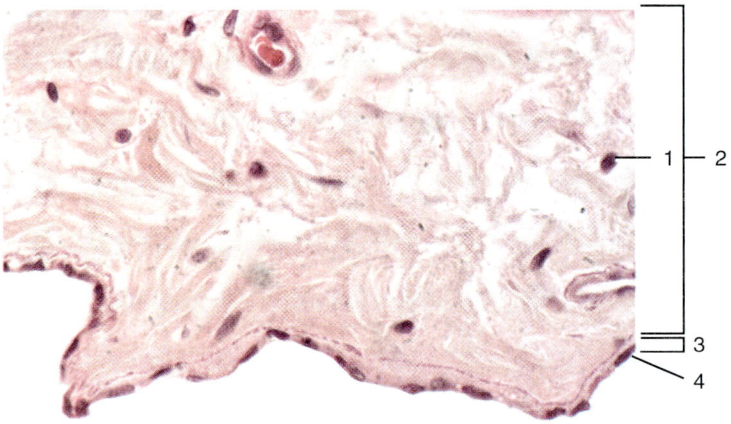

400x, H&E, human

(b) Simple squamous epithelium.

FIGURE 4.12 Sectional view of peritoneum.

2. Simple Cuboidal Epithelium

Simple cuboidal epithelial cells, when viewed from the side, are relatively square with one round nucleus in the middle of the cell. They are involved in absorption and secretion.

Example: Simple cuboidal epithelial cells lining the kidney tubules

Blood is filtered in the kidneys and the filtrate is modified by the kidney tubules to form urine. Part of this tubular system is lined with simple cuboidal epithelium. These cells absorb substances from the filtrate and secrete other substances into the filtrate.

ACTIVITY 6 Microscopic Examination of Simple Cuboidal Epithelium

1 Color the simple cuboidal epithelium and the basement membrane in Figure 4.13 using contrasting colors.

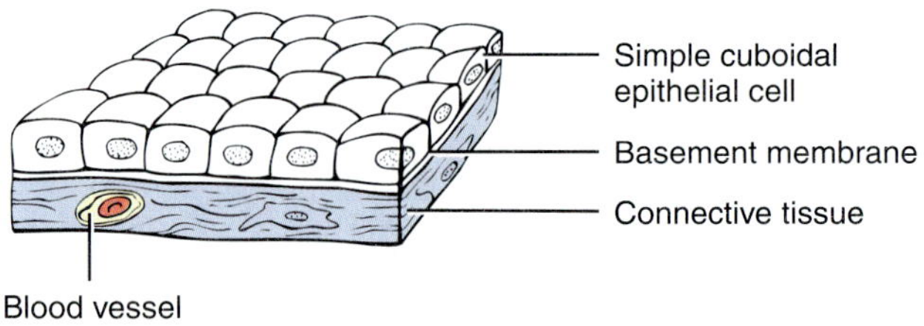

FIGURE 4.13 Simple cuboidal epithelium.

2 Label the photomicrograph in Figure 4.14b. Trace over the cell membrane of a simple cuboidal epithelial cell. Answer the question on the figure.

3 Examine a prepared microscope slide showing sections through kidney tubules and identify the structures listed in Figure 4.14b.

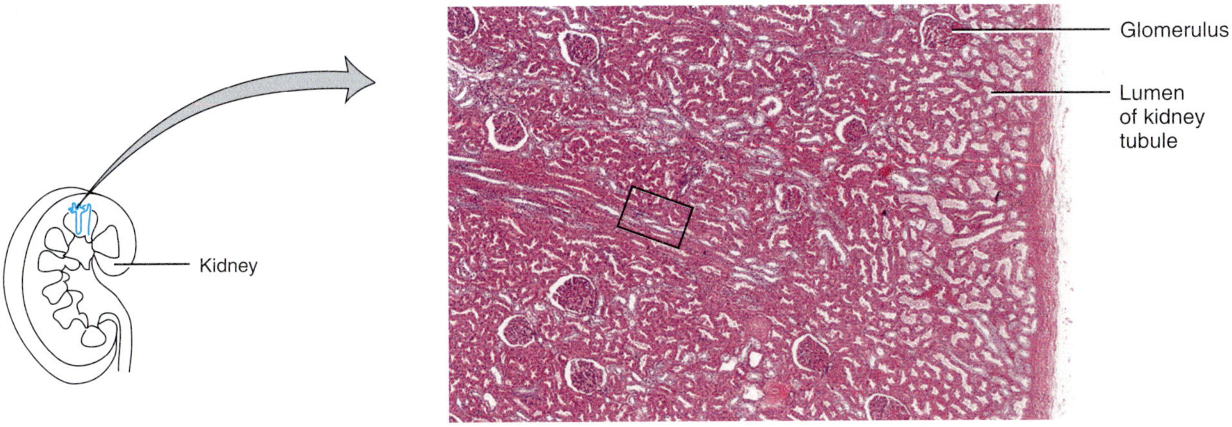

40x (a) Survey photomicrograph.

- apical surface of simple cuboidal epithelial cell
- lumen of kidney tubule
- nucleus of simple cuboidal epithelial cell
- simple cuboidal epithelium

1 ______________________

2 ______________________

3 ______________________

4 ______________________

Question: Explain why some tubule cross-sections are circular and others are oval.

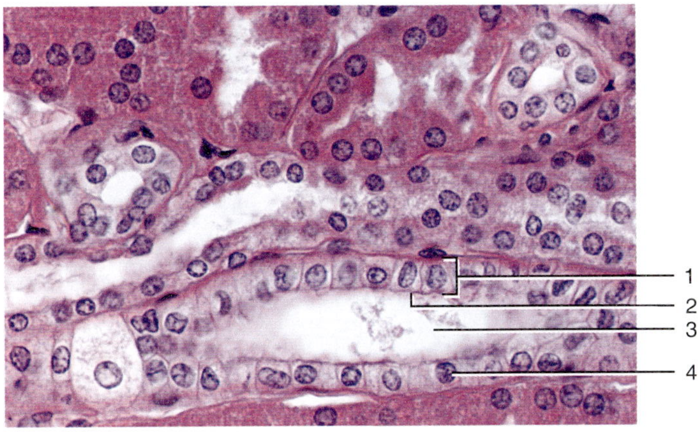

400x, H&E, human (b) Simple cuboidal epithelium.

FIGURE 4.14 **Sectional view of kidney tubules.**

3. Simple Columnar Epithelium

When viewed from the side, simple columnar cells are rectangular with an oval nucleus located near the basal surface of the cell. Simple columnar epithelium also contains goblet cells, which are modified columnar epithelial cells that produce and secrete mucus.

There are two types of simple columnar epithelia, ciliated and nonciliated. Nonciliated simple columnar epithelial cells are involved in secretion and absorption. Ciliated cells use their cilia to move substances over the epithelial surface.

Example: Nonciliated simple columnar epithelium lining the small intestine

The stomach, small intestine, and large intestine are lined with simple columnar epithelium. In the small intestine, these cells secrete digestive juices and absorb nutrients. Goblet cells secrete mucus that covers the epithelial surface, acts as a lubricant, and protects the surface from digestive enzymes. In the small intestine, the apical surface of the simple columnar epithelial cells has **microvilli** (*micro-* = small; *-villi* = shaggy, hairlike) to increase the surface area for absorption.

ACTIVITY 7 Microscopic Examination of Nonciliated Simple Columnar Epithelium

1 Color the simple columnar epithelium and the basement membrane in Figure 4.15 using contrasting colors.

2 Label the photomicrograph in Figure 4.16b. Trace over the plasma membrane of a simple columnar epithelial cell.

3 Examine a prepared microscope slide showing a section through the small intestine and identify the structures listed in Figure 4.16b.

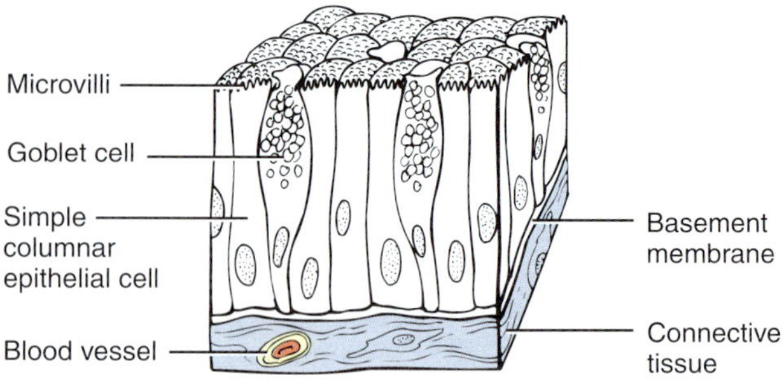

FIGURE 4.15 Simple columnar epithelium.

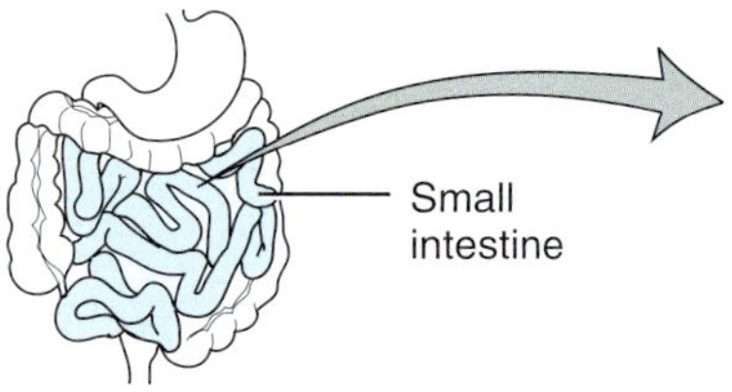

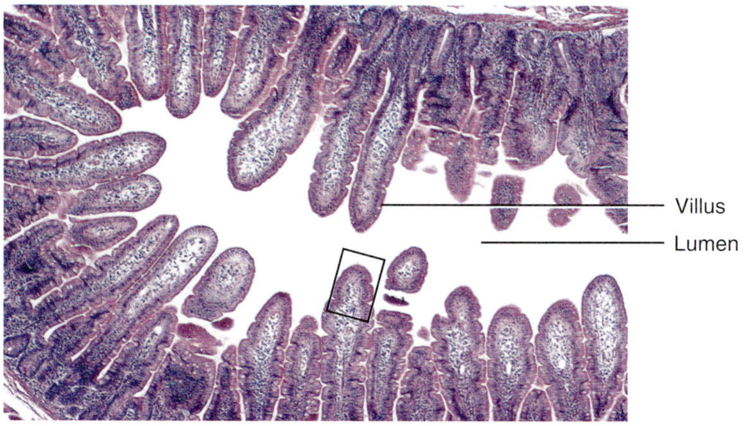

40x

(a) Survey photomicrograph.

- connective tissue
- microvilli on apical surface of simple columnar epithelial cell
- nucleus of simple columnar epithelial cell
- simple columnar epithelium

1 ______________________________

2 ______________________________

3 ______________________________

4 ______________________________

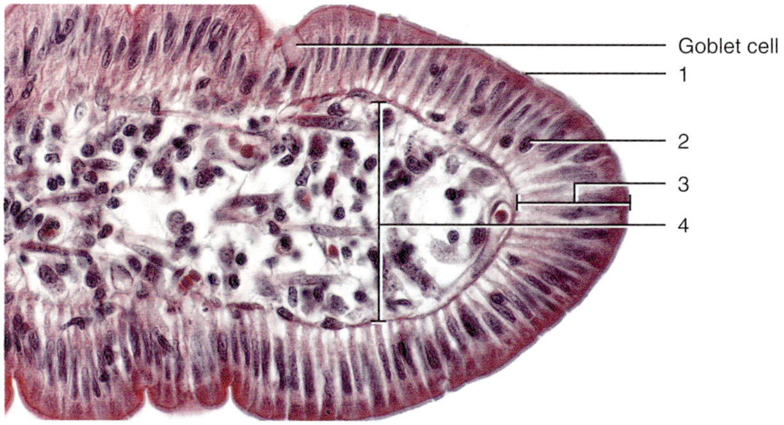

400x, H&E, human

(b) Simple columnar epithelium.

FIGURE 4.16 Sectional view of small intestine.

B. Stratified Epithelium

There are four stratified epithelial tissues: stratified squamous, stratified cuboidal, stratified columnar, and transitional. Stratified squamous and transitional are the most common and are examined below. Consult your textbook for examples of stratified cuboidal and stratified columnar.

1. Stratified Squamous Epithelium

Stratified squamous epithelium contains many cell layers. Cells in the outer layers are flattened or squamous, while the deeper layers contain cuboidal or columnar cells. Multiple cell layers offer protection to underlying tissues. Stratified squamous epithelium is located in areas subjected to friction and abrasion.

The two types of stratified squamous epithelium are nonkeratinized and keratinized (*keratin* = horn, tough). **Nonkeratinized stratified squamous epithelium** is moist and lines body cavities that are subjected to friction. **Keratinized stratified squamous epithelium** has a dry outer surface and is only found on the surface of skin. A photomicrograph and description of this tissue is located in the integumentary exercise.

Example: Nonkeratinized stratified squamous epithelium lining the esophagus

Observe the cell shape of the basal layers. They are cuboidal or columnar and become progessively flattened as they move toward the surface. The shape of the cells in the apical layer is squamous. Observe the nuclei in these cells. Although these cells are far from the basal surface, they receive enough nutrients to remain viable. This epithelial lining protects the underlying tissues from damage as food and liquids pass through the esophagus to the stomach.

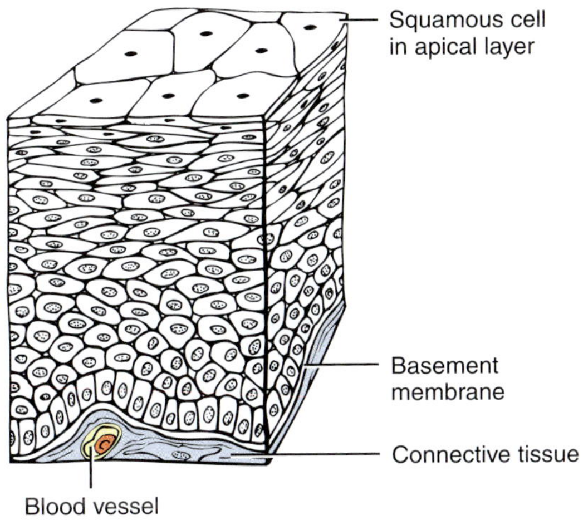

FIGURE 4.17 Nonkeratinized stratified squamous epithelium.

ACTIVITY 8 Microscopic Examination of Nonkeratinized Stratified Squamous Epithelium

1. Color the nonkeratinized stratified epithelium and the basement membrane in Figure 4.17 using contrasting colors.
2. Label the photomicrograph in Figure 4.18b. Trace over the plasma membrane of a squamous epithelial cell in the apical cell layer.
3. Examine a prepared microscope slide showing a section through the esophagus and identify the structures listed in Figure 4.18b.

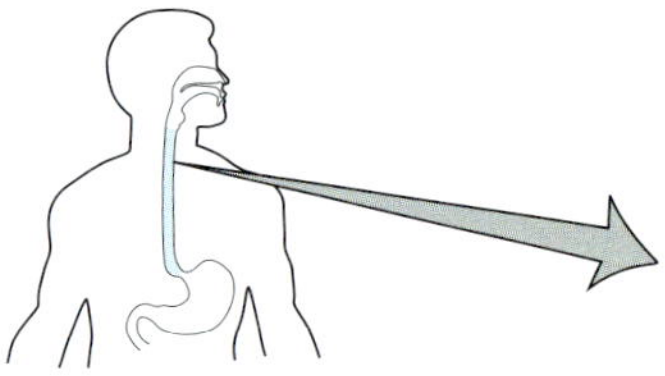

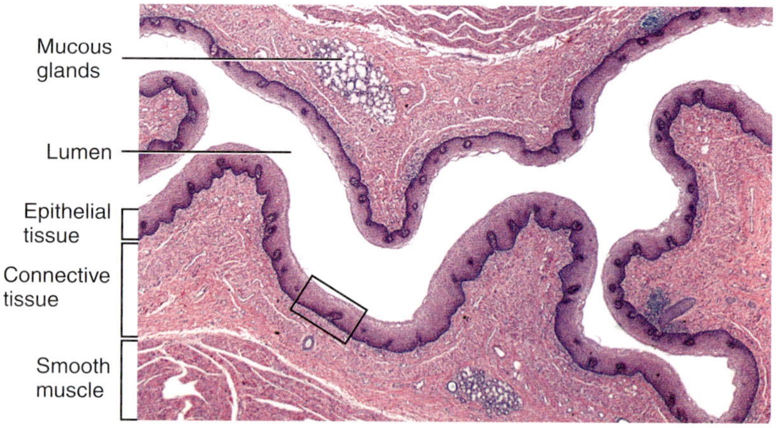

40x

(a) Survey photomicrograph.

- connective tissue
- nucleus of epithelial cell in basal layer of epithelium
- nucleus of squamous epithelial cell
- stratified squamous epithelium

1 ______________________

2 ______________________

3 ______________________

4 ______________________

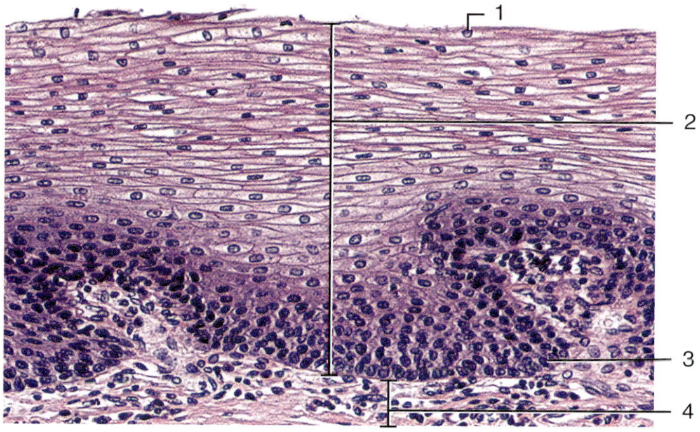

200x, H&E, human

(b) Nonkeratinized stratified squamous epithelium.

FIGURE 4.18 **Sectional view of esophagus.**

2. Transitional Epithelium

Transitional epithelial cells change shape as the tissue is stretched or distended. When the tissue is relaxed, the cells in the apical layer are plump and rounded. As the tissue distends, the apical layer of cells becomes flatter and the number of cell layers decreases. This tissue is found lining the bladder and portions of the ureter and urethra.

Example: Transitional epithelium of relaxed urinary bladder

The thick epithelial layer protects underlying tissues from urine and the distensible outer cells allow the bladder to increase in size as it fills with urine.

ACTIVITY 9 Microscopic Examination of Transitional Epithelium

1. Color the relaxed transitional epithelium and the basement membrane in Figure 4.19 using contrasting colors.
2. Label the photomicrograph in Figure 4.20b. Trace over the plasma membrane of a transitional epithelial cell in the apical cell layer.
3. Examine a prepared microscope slide showing a section through a relaxed urinary bladder and identify the structures listed in Figure 4.20b.

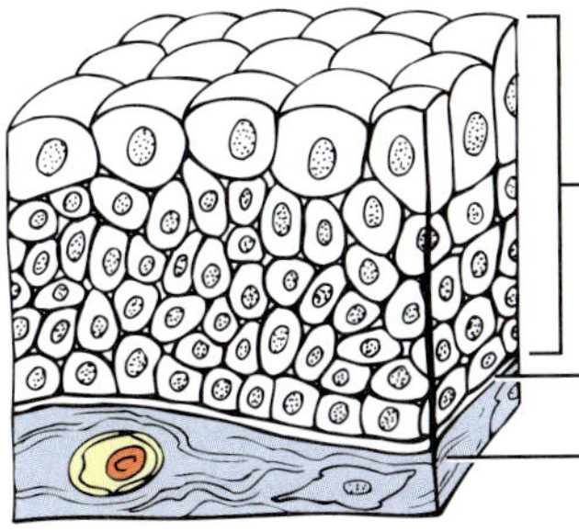

FIGURE 4.19 **Relaxed transitional epithelium.**

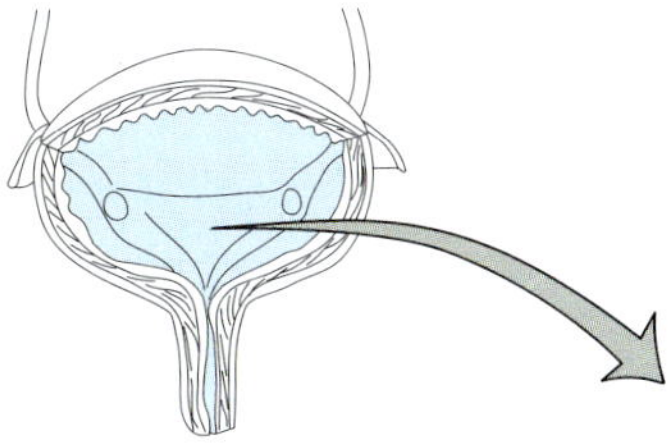

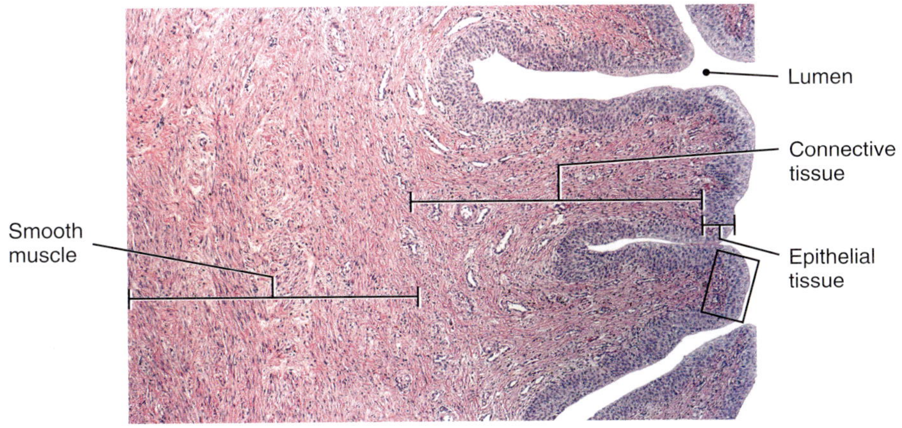

40x

(a) Survey photomicrograph.

- connective tissue
- nucleus of transitional epithelial cell in apical layer
- nucleus of transitional epithelial cell in basal layer
- transitional epithelium

1 ______________________________

2 ______________________________

3 ______________________________

4 ______________________________

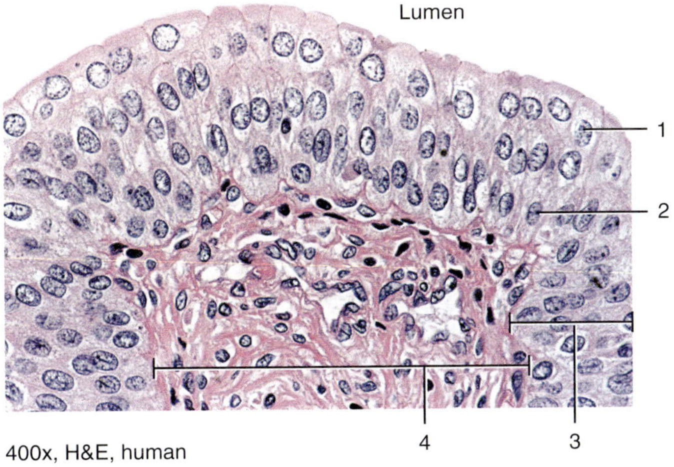

400x, H&E, human

(b) Transitional epithelium.

FIGURE 4.20 **Sectional view of a relaxed urinary bladder.**

C. Pseudostratified Columnar Epithelium

Pseudostratified (*pseudo-* = false) **columnar epithelium** is only one cell layer thick because all the cells touch the basement membrane, although not all reach the apical surface. Therefore, there are cells of different shapes and heights, and their nuclei are at different levels. This gives the illusion of several different layers of cells. The tallest cells are narrow where they touch the basement membrane, but have a columnar shape toward the outer surface, while the basal cells do not reach the apical surface.

There are two types of pseudostratified columnar epithelia, ciliated and nonciliated. **Ciliated pseudostratified columnar epithelium** has cilia on the apical surface of the columnar cells, and goblet cells that extend to the apical surface. **Nonciliated pseudostratified columnar epithelium** does not have cilia or goblet cells. We will observe only ciliated pseudostratified columnar epithelium.

Example: Pseudostratified ciliated columnar epithelium of the trachea

Pseudostratified ciliated columnar epithelium of the trachea secretes mucus that traps dust and pathogens. Cilia move the mucus away from the lungs toward the throat, protecting the lungs from dust and pathogens.

ACTIVITY 10 Microscopic Examination of Pseudostratified Columnar Epithelium

1. Color the ciliated columnar, basal and goblet cells of the pseudostratified ciliated columnar epithelium in Figure 4.21 contrasting colors.
2. Label the photomicrograph in Figure 4.22b.
3. Examine a prepared microscope slide showing a section through the trachea and identify the structures listed in Figure 4.22b.

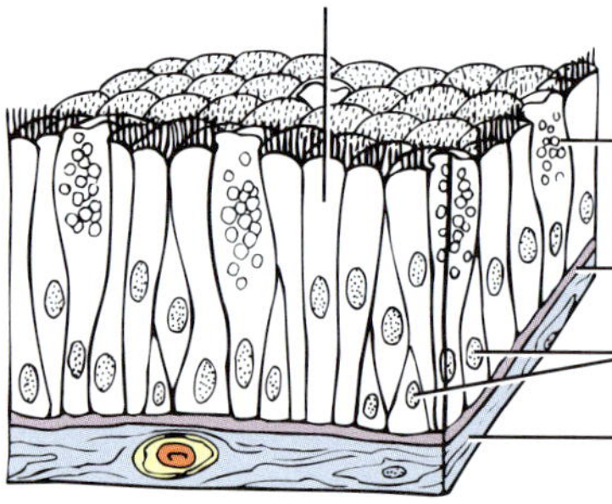

FIGURE 4.21 Pseudostratified ciliated columnar epithelium.

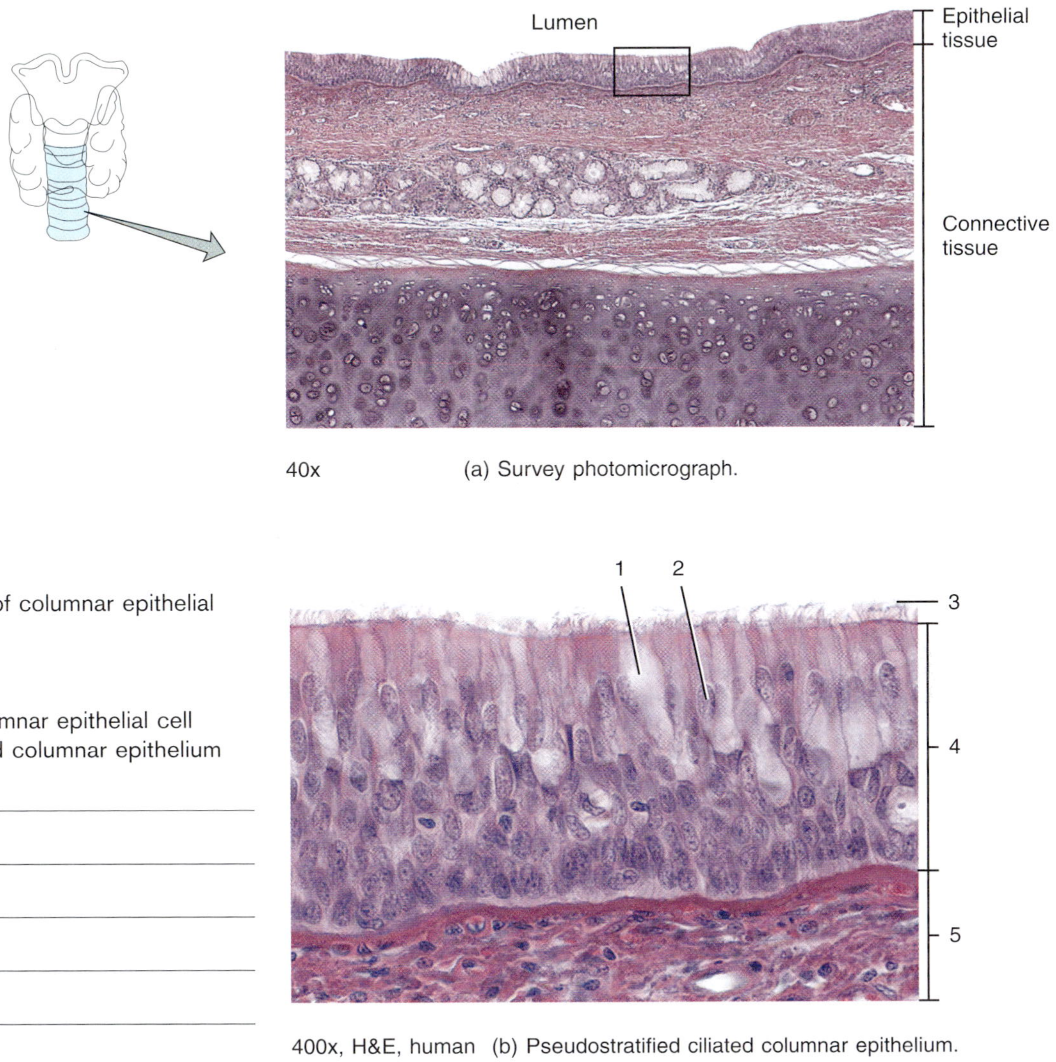

- cilia on apical surface of columnar epithelial cell
- connective tissue
- goblet cell
- nucleus of ciliated columnar epithelial cell
- pseudostratified ciliated columnar epithelium

1 ______________________________

2 ______________________________

3 ______________________________

4 ______________________________

5 ______________________________

FIGURE 4.22 **Sectional view of the trachea.**

CONNECTIVE TISSUE TYPES

All mature connective tissues are derived from mesenchyme, a connective tissue present in the embryo and fetus. Mature connective tissues include loose connective tissue, dense connective tissue, cartilage, bone, and blood. The connective tissue types have different connective tissue cells forming the extracellular matrix. The extracellular matrix of **loose and dense connective tissues** is formed by **fibroblasts** (*blast* = early, developing stage); the extracellular matrix of **cartilage** is formed by **chondroblasts** (*chondro-* = cartilage) and maintained by **chondrocytes;** and the extracellular matrix of **bone** is formed by **osteoblasts** (*osteo-* = bone) and maintained by **osteocytes. Blood** was considered a connective tissue by early histologists because it connected tissues by transporting substances from one to another. **Plasma** is the extracellular matrix in which blood cells and platelets are suspended; however, it is not made by these cells.

Other types of cells found in connective tissue are white blood cells, macrophages, mast cells, and adipose cells. Connective tissue function is determined by the properties of the extracellular matrix components, fibers, and ground substance. The three major types of fibers are **collagen fibers** (provide strength), **elastin fibers** (provide strength and elasticity), and **reticular fibers** (fine, branching collagen fibers that provide a netlike framework). The number and type of fibers present contribute to the strength, elasticity, and structure of the extracellular matrix. The **ground substance** may be fluid, semifluid, gelatinous, or hard. It secures the connective tissue cells and fibers in the extracellular matrix and is the medium through which interstitial fluid diffuses between blood and cells and through which macrophages and white blood cells move.

A. Loose Connective Tissue

In **loose connective tissue,** the fibers in the extracellular matrix are loosely arranged. Collagen, elastic, and reticular fibers in this tissue provide strength, elasticity, and support. The ground substance is semifluid (viscous), but interstitial fluid can easily diffuse through it. Fibroblasts and adipocytes (lipid-storing cells) permanently reside in the tissue. Other cells, such as macrophages, mast cells, and white blood cells, enter the connective tissue from blood and are involved in body defenses.

Loose connective tissue includes areolar, reticular, and adipose tissues.

1. Areolar Connective Tissue

Areolar connective tissue is the most abundant connective tissue. It contains all three fiber types, fibroblasts, a variety of cells involved in body defenses, and a viscous ground substance. The extracellular matrix of areolar connective tissue holds excess fluid that leaks out of capillaries.

Spread preparations of mesentery (thin sheets of peritoneum that support the intestine) exhibit different types of fibers and cells. However, different fiber and cell types are not easily distinguished in other tissue sections containing areolar connective tissue underlying covering and lining epithelium or surrounding glandular epithelium.

Example: Areolar connective tissue spread of mesentery

Areolar connective tissue fibers support the mesothelial layers of mesentery and interstitial fluid within the extracellular matrix is used by the mesothelial cells to produce serous fluid. White blood cells, macrophages, and plasma cells in areolar connective tissue play an important role in fighting infection.

Example: Areolar connective tissue in mammary glands

Areolar connective tissue supports the glandular epithelium. Fluid and nutrients are filtered across capillaries, diffused through the alveolar connective tissue, and are used by the glandular epithelium to make milk. Plasma cells within the areolar connective tissue produce antibodies that are taken up by the glandular epithelial cells and become a component of milk.

ACTIVITY 11 Microscopic Examination of Areolar Connective Tissue

1 Color the collagen and reticular fibers in the areolar connective tissue in Figure 4.23 contrasting colors.

2 Label the photomicrograph of an areolar connective tissue spread in Figure 4.24. Note that collagen and elastic fibers stain differently and that collagen fibers are thicker than elastic fibers. Reticular fibers are present but are not observable with this stain. Mast cells stain orange while fibroblasts, macrophages, and white blood cells all stain various shades of gray.

3 Examine a prepared microscope slide of an areolar connective tissue spread preparation and identify the structures listed in Figure 4.24.

4 Label the photomicrograph of areolar connective tissue in the mammary glands in Figure 4.25b. Note that the different fiber and cell types cannot be distinguished.

5 Examine a prepared microscope slide with a tissue section of mammary gland, intestine, or skin. Locate the areolar connective tissue and identify the structures listed in Figure 4.25b.

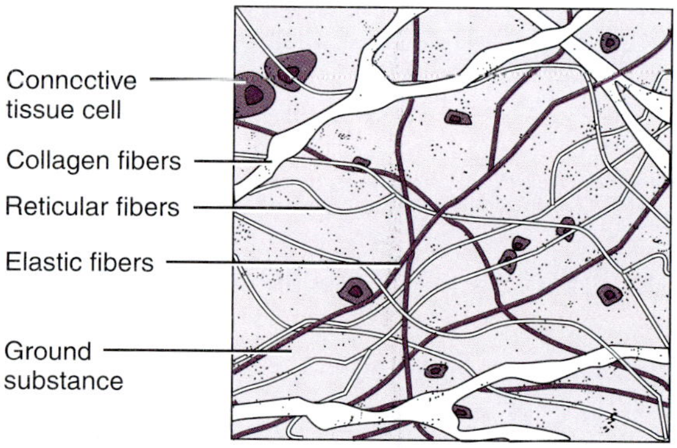

FIGURE 4.23 Areolar connective tissue.

- collagen fiber
- connective tissue cells (fibroblasts or lymphocytes)
- elastic fiber
- mast cell

1 ______________________

2 ______________________

3 ______________________

4 ______________________

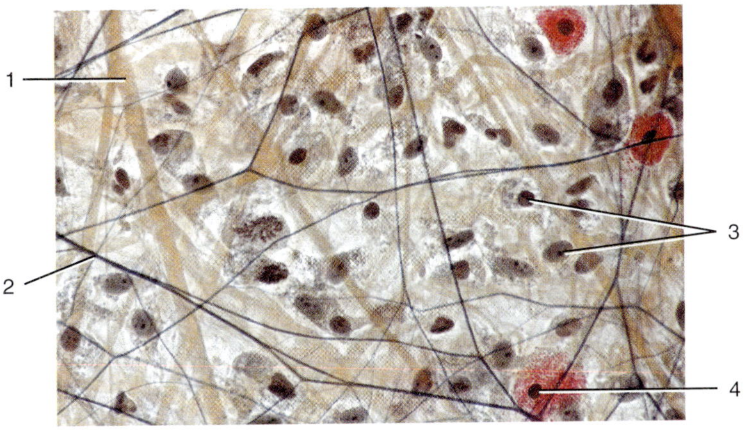

400x, Verhoeff Orange Safrin, human

FIGURE 4.24 Areolar connective tissue spread of mesentery.

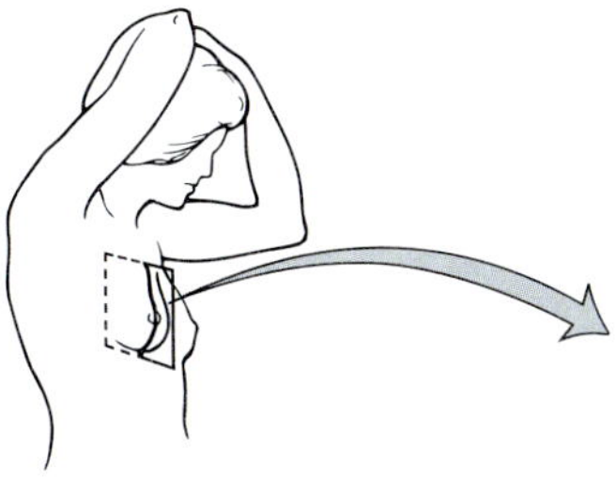

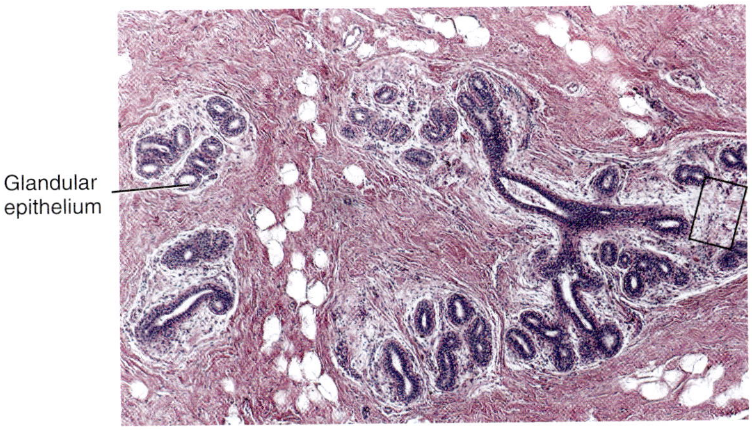

40x

(a) Survey photomicrograph.

- connective tissue cell
- fiber

1 ______________________

2 ______________________

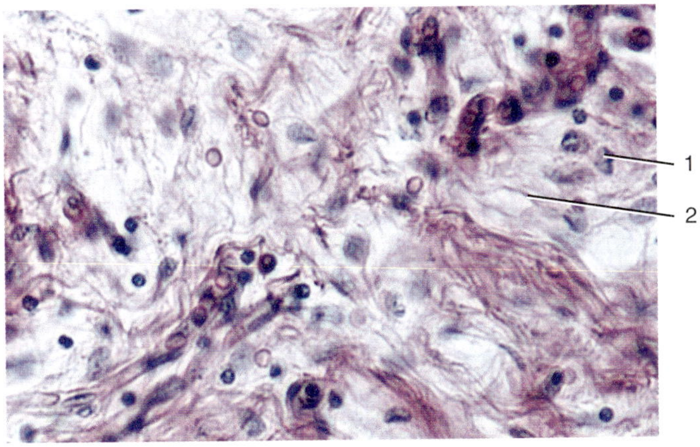

400x, H&E, human

(b) Areolar connective tissue.

FIGURE 4.25 Sectional view of mammary gland.

2. Reticular Connective Tissue

Reticular (*reticulo-* = netlike) **fibers** are the dominant fiber type in **reticular connective tissue. Reticular cells** synthesize the reticular fibers and ground substance. Reticular cells are actually fibroblasts, but they synthesize more reticular fibers than collagen fibers. Reticular fibers form an internal framework or stroma within nonmuscular organs.

Example: Lymph node

In the lymph node, reticular connective tissue provides a support structure (stroma) for macrophages and white blood cells that are involved in body defenses. Macrophages attach themselves to the reticular fibers while white blood cells are located in the spaces between the fibers.

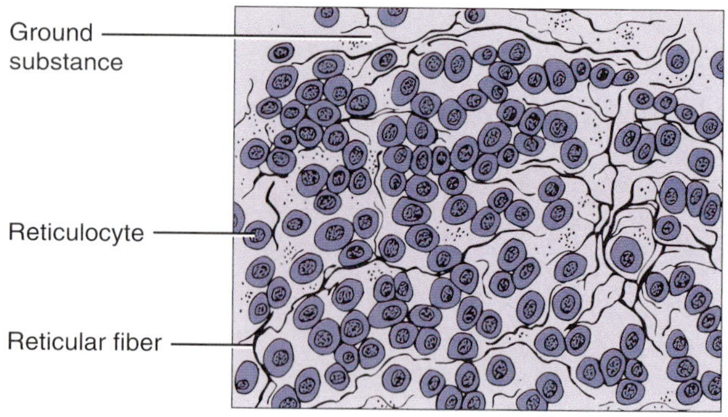

FIGURE 4.26 Reticular connective tissue.

ACTIVITY 12 Microscopic Examination of Reticular Tissue

1. Examine the reticular tissue in Figure 4.26.
2. Label the photomicrograph in Figure 4.27.
3. Examine a prepared microscope slide of reticular connective tissue and identify the structures listed in Figure 4.27.

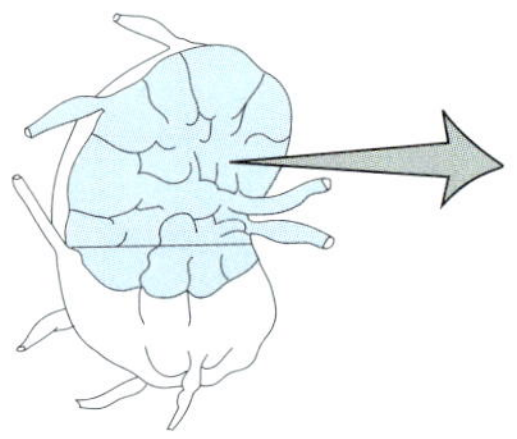

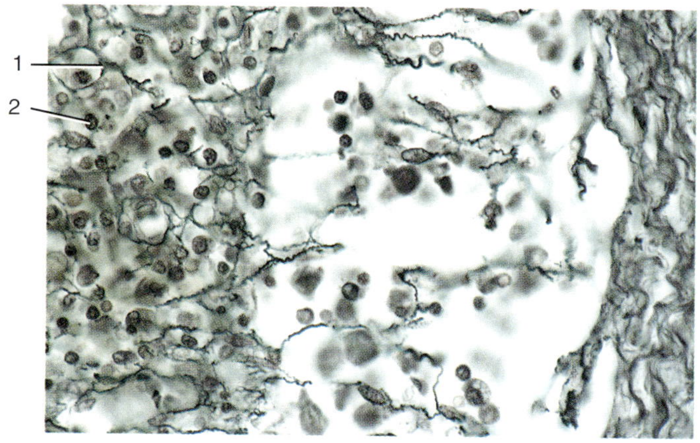

400x, human

- reticular cell
- reticular fiber

1 ______________________

2 ______________________

FIGURE 4.27 Sectional view of reticular tissue of the lymph node.

3. Adipose Tissue

Adipose (*adipo-* = pertaining to fat) **tissue,** like areolar connective tissue, contains fibroblasts, fibers, ground substance, and adipose cells. However, adipose tissue has a greater number of adipose cells or **adipocytes** and much less extracellular matrix. Adipocytes are specialized connective tissue cells that store lipid. The lipid within the cell occupies most of the cell volume and pushes cytoplasm and organelles to the periphery. Some slides do not have the lipid stained, or the lipid has been removed during tissue preparation. In those slides, the nucleus and cytoplasm are stained, and the space inside the cell normally occupied by lipid appears "empty."

Example: Adipose tissue surrounding the heart

Besides providing storage for energy-rich lipids, adipose tissue cushions and insulates the organs it surrounds.

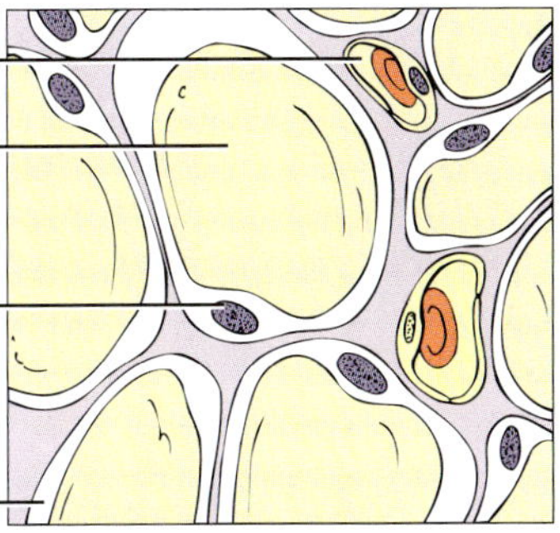

FIGURE 4.28 **Adipose connective tissue.**

ACTIVITY 13 Microscopic Examination of Adipose Tissue

1. Color the cytoplasm of an adipocyte in Figure 4.28.
2. Label the photomicrograph in Figure 4.29. Trace over the plasma membrane of an adipocyte.
3. Examine a prepared microscope slide showing adipose tissue and identify the structures listed in Figure 4.29.

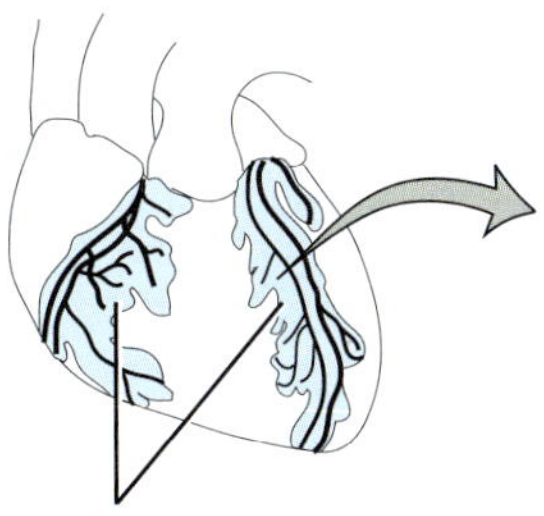

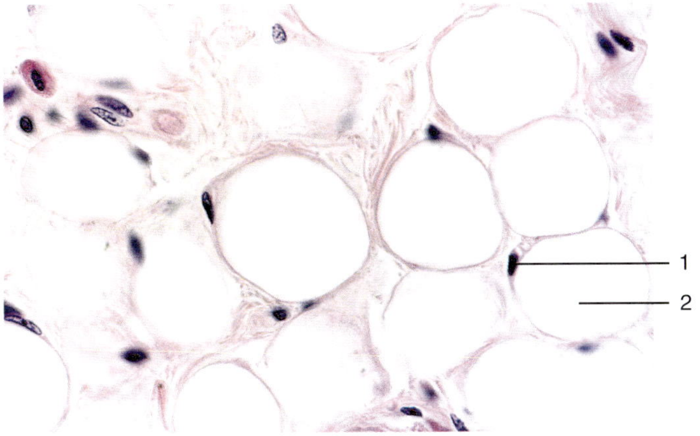

400x, H&E, human

- lipid storage area
- nucleus of adipocyte

1 ______________________

2 ______________________

FIGURE 4.29 **Sectional view of adipose tissue.**

B. Dense Connective Tissue

The extracellular matrix of dense connective tissue is packed with fibers and contains very little ground substance and few fibroblasts. There are three types of dense connective tissue: dense regular, dense irregular, and elastic connective tissue.

1. Dense Regular Connective Tissue

The extracellular matrix of **dense regular connective tissue** is packed with parallel bundles of collagen fibers that run in the direction of the pulling forces applied to the tissue. Fibroblasts are squeezed between the bundles, and the cytoplasm extends between and around collagen bundles. Fibroblasts secrete collagen fibers and ground substance. Collagen fibers give unstained tissue a silvery white appearance, which is why this tissue is often called white fibrous tissue.

Example: Dense regular connective tissue forming tendons

Collagen fibers are very strong and provide resistance to pulling forces while providing flexibility.

ACTIVITY 14 Microscopic Examination of Dense Regular Connective Tissue

1 Color fibroblasts in the dense regular connective tissue in Figure 4.30.

2 Label the photomicrograph in Figure 4.31. The collagen fibers are not silvery white because the tissue has been stained.

3 Examine a prepared microscope slide showing dense regular connective tissue and identify the structures listed in Figure 4.31.

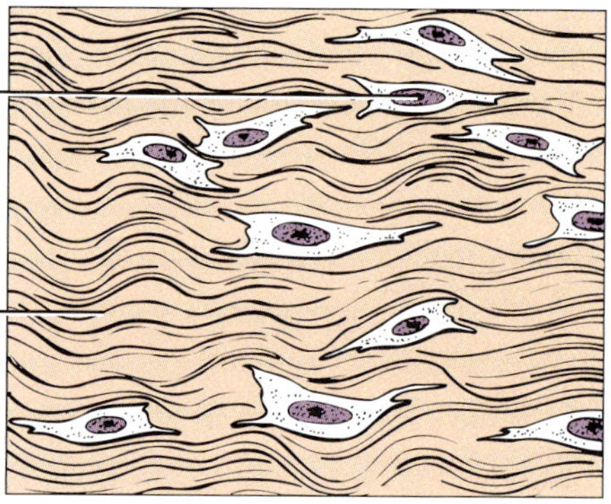

FIGURE 4.30 Dense regular connective tissue.

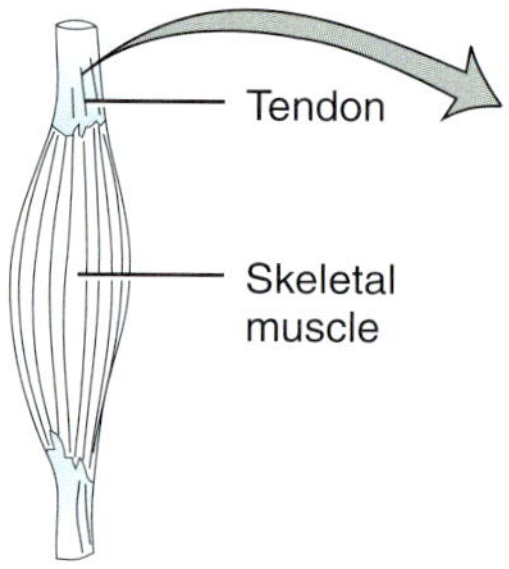

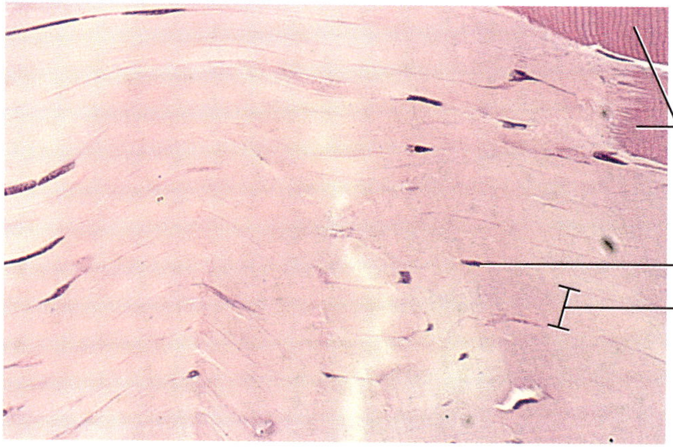

400x, H&E, human

- collagen fiber bundle
- fibroblast

1 ______________________

2 ______________________

FIGURE 4.31 Sectional view of dense regular connective tissue forming tendons.

2. Dense Irregular Connective Tissue

Dense irregular connective tissue, like dense regular connective tissue, has little ground substance and few fibroblasts. The extracellular space is also packed with bundles of collagen fibers with fibroblasts squeezed between these bundles. In dense irregular connective tissue, however, the bundles of collagen fibers are irregularly arranged. This reflects the direction of the pulling forces to which this tissue is exposed, usually from many different directions.

Example: Dense irregular connective tissue in the dermis of skin

Within the dermis of the skin there is a layer of dense irregular connective tissue. As the skin is stretched from different directions during movement or weight gain, the irregularly arranged collagen fibers in the dense irregular connective tissue prevent the skin from being pulled apart.

ACTIVITY 15 Microscopic Examination of Dense Irregular Connective Tissue

1. Color the fibroblasts in the dense irregular connective tissue in Figure 4.32.
2. Label the photomicrograph in Figure 4.33.
3. Examine a prepared microscope slide showing dense irregular connective tissue and identify the structures listed in Figure 4.33.

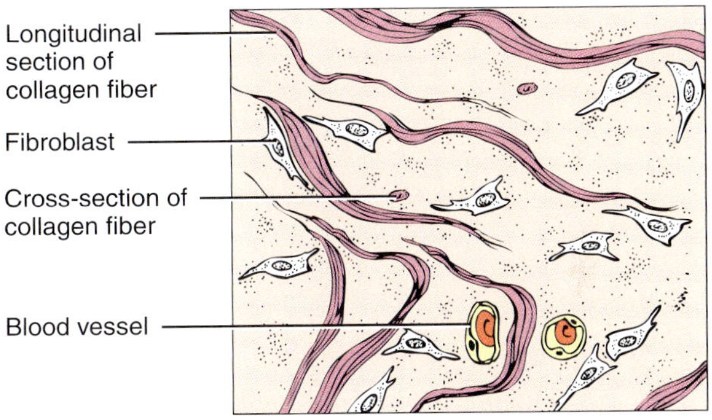

FIGURE 4.32 Dense irregular connective tissue.

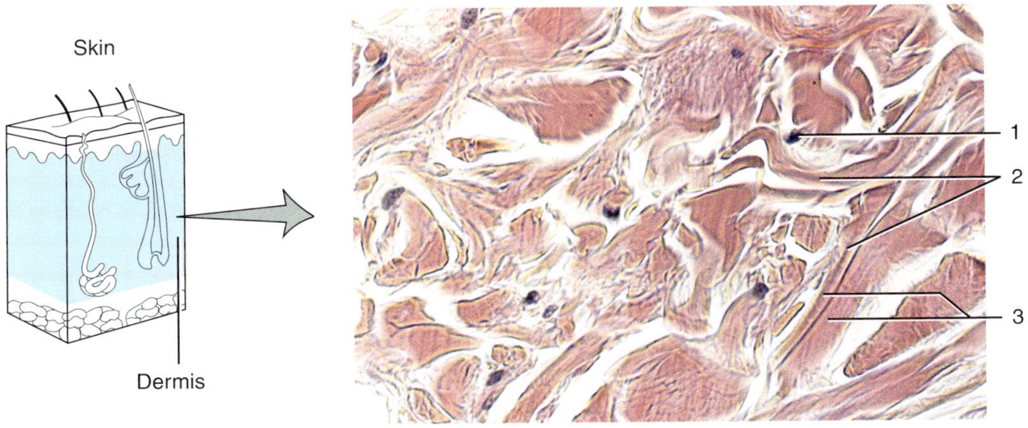

400x, H&E, human

- collagen fiber bundles running in different directions
- fibroblast
- parallel collagen fiber bundles

1 ______________________

2 ______________________

3 ______________________

FIGURE 4.33 Sectional view of dense irregular connective tissue in skin.

3. Elastic Connective Tissue

Elastic fibers are the predominant fiber type in elastic tissue and fibroblasts are found in the spaces between elastic fibers. Elastic fibers allow the tissue to be stretched and then regain its original size and shape (recoil).

Example: Elastic tissue in the aorta

The heart pumps blood into the aorta with great force. The force of the blood stretches the wall of the aorta, and when the heart relaxes, the recoil of the elastic tissue helps to force blood through the blood vessels. The large arteries near the heart, like the aorta, are called elastic arteries.

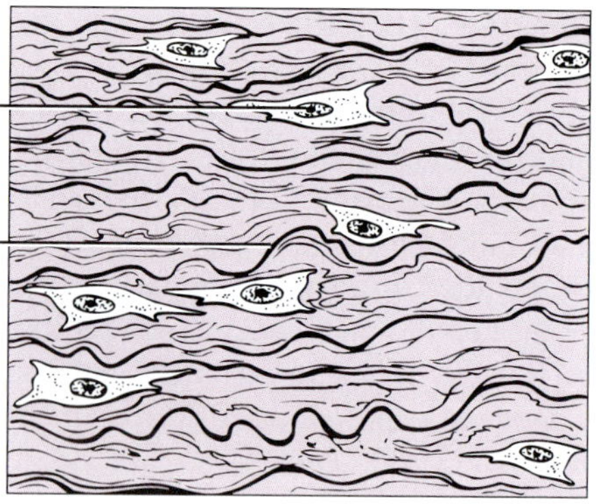

FIGURE 4.34 Elastic connective tissue.

ACTIVITY 16 Microscopic Examination of Elastic Connective Tissue

1. Color the fibroblasts in the elastic connective tissue in Figure 4.34.
2. Label the photomicrograph in Figure 4.35.
3. Examine a prepared microscope slide showing elastic connective tissue and identify the structures listed in Figure 4.35.

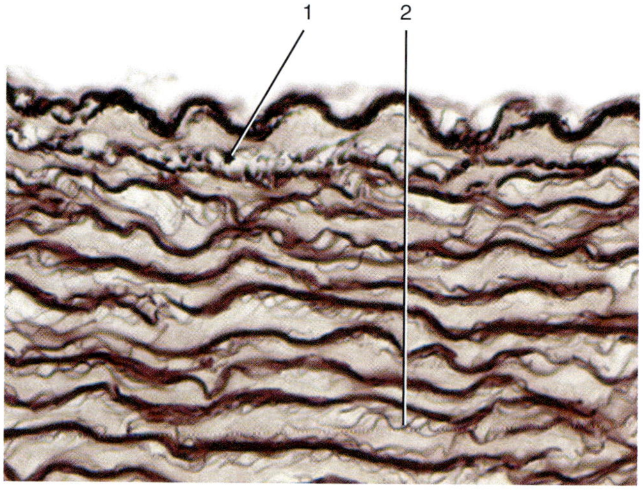

400x, human

- elastic fiber
- fibroblast

1 ______________________

2 ______________________

FIGURE 4.35 Sectional view of elastic connective tissue in the wall of the aorta.

C. Cartilage

Cartilage is a specialized form of connective tissue. Its extracellular matrix consists of collagen and elastic fibers embedded in a gelatinous ground substance. Collagen fibers give the tissue its strength and the ground substance (containing chondroitin sulfate) binds water to form a gel, giving cartilage resiliency. **Chondroblasts** (*chondro-* = cartilage), which secrete the fibers and ground substance, become isolated in spaces called **lacunae** (little lakes) and transform into **chondrocytes.** Since the tissue is avascular, the chondrocytes receive their nutrients through diffusion from adjacent vascular tissues.

There are three types of cartilage: **hyaline** (*hyalos* = glass), **elastic,** and **fibrous.** These cartilage types differ in the amount and kinds of fibers and ground substance molecules present in their extracellular matrix. Hyaline cartilage is the most common cartilage in the body and is examined in this exercise. The three types of cartilage are examined in detail in the skeletal tissue exercise.

Example: Hyaline cartilage in the trachea

The trachea contains incomplete rings of hyaline cartilage that keep the lumen of the trachea open at all times. Therefore, during inspiration and expiration the body does not have to work to open the airways for air flow.

ACTIVITY 17 Microscopic Examination of Hyaline Cartilage

1. Color the chondrocytes and lacuna in the hyaline cartilage in Figure 4.36 using contrasting colors.
2. Label the photomicrograph in Figure 4.37b. Trace over the plasma membrane of a chondrocyte. Collagen fibers cannot be distinguished from the ground substance in this preparation.
3. Examine a prepared microscope slide showing hyaline cartilage and identify the structures listed in Figure 4.37b.

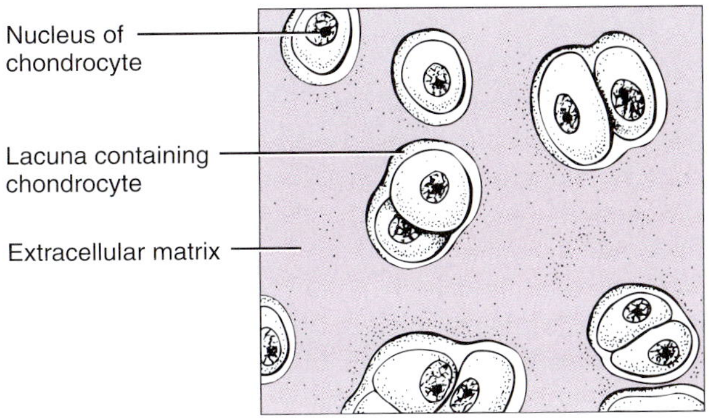

FIGURE 4.36 **Hyaline cartilage.**

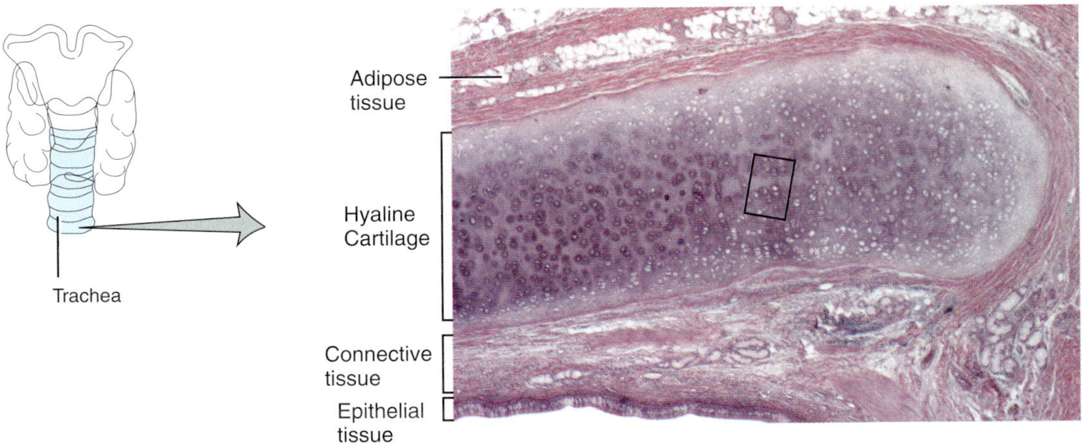

40x

(a) Survey photomicrograph.

- extracellular matrix
- lacuna (la-KOO-na)
- nucleus of chondrocyte

1 ______________________________

2 ______________________________

3 ______________________________

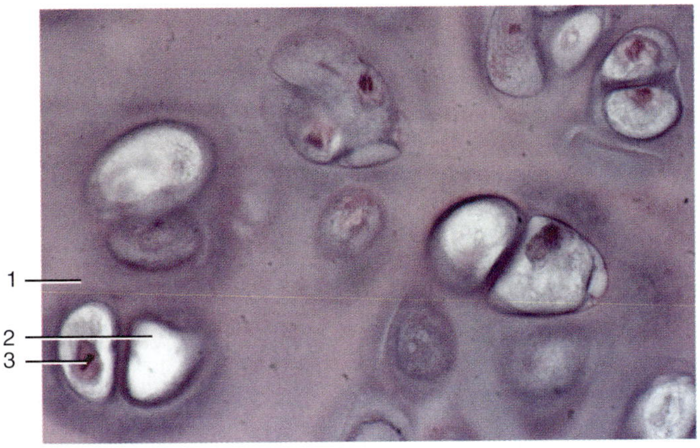

400x, H&E, human

(b) Hyaline cartilage.

FIGURE 4.37 **Sectional view of hyaline cartilage in the wall of the trachea.**

D. Bone

Bone is the hardest of the connective tissues. It protects body organs and provides support for organs and skeletal muscles. The extracellular matrix is organized in layers called **lamellae** and consists of collagen fibers, ground substance, and inorganic salts. Inorganic salts, especially calcium salts that are deposited onto the ground substance, give bone its hardness; collagen fibers provide strength and flexibility. **Osteocytes** (mature bone cells) are trapped in spaces called **lacunae.** Small canals called **canaliculi** are two-way canals that connect lacunae to larger canals that contain blood vessels. Nutrients diffuse from a blood vessel through the canaliculi to the osteocytes, and waste materials diffuse back to a blood vessel for removal.

The two types of bone tissue are **compact bone** and **spongy bone.** The extracellular matrix of compact bone is organized into repeating structural units called **osteons.** In the center of each osteon is a large central canal. Spongy bone does not have osteons. The structure of compact and spongy bone is discussed in detail later in the bone tissue exercise.

Example: Dried compact bone

The hard extracellular matrix enables bones such as the femur to support the weight of the body while standing and to act as levers allowing movement. Other bones such as those of the skull provide protection to body organs.

ACTIVITY 18 Microscopic Examination of Bone

1 Color a lamella in the dried compact bone tissue in Figure 4.38.

2 Label the photomicrograph in Figure 4.39b. Collagen fibers cannot be distinguished in the calcified extracellular matrix of bone. Osteocytes also cannot be observed in dried bone because the cells of dried bone were destroyed during tissue preparation. Lacunae and canaliculi are stained dark and can be easily observed.

3 Examine a prepared microscope slide showing dried compact bone and identify the structures listed in Figure 4.39b.

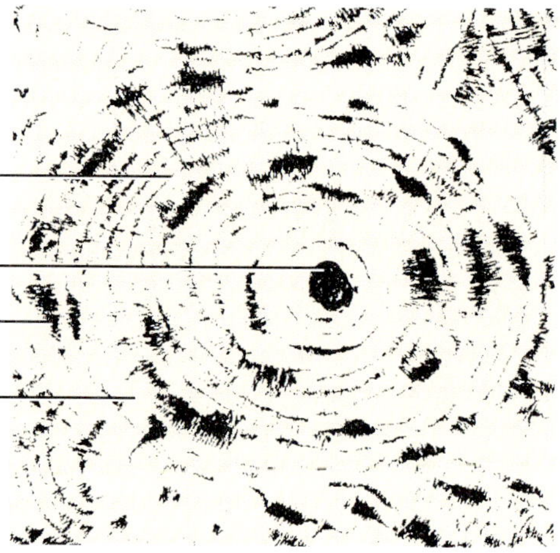

FIGURE 4.38 Dried compact bone.

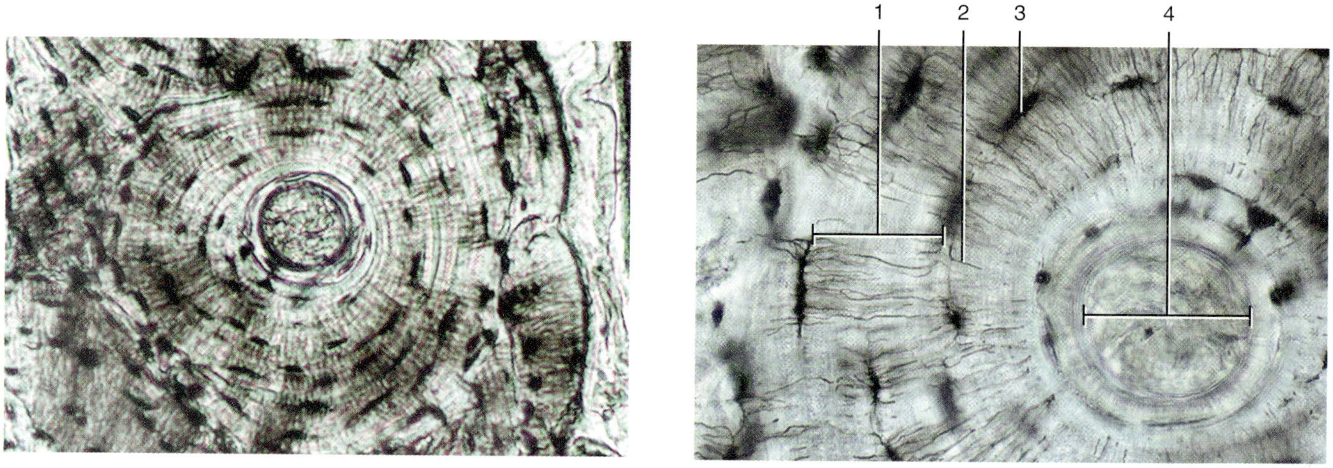

100x (a) Osteon of compact bone.

400x, unstained, human (b) Section of osteon.

- canaliculus
- central canal
- lamella
- lacuna

1 ____________________

2 ____________________

3 ____________________

4 ____________________

FIGURE 4.39 Sectional view of dried compact bone.

E. Blood

Blood is considered a connective tissue because it provides a transport system that connects different body tissues. Nutrients and chemical messengers are transported to all body tissues by blood, and wastes are transported from tissues to excretory organs via the blood. Blood is composed of red blood cells, white blood cells, platelets, and plasma. **Plasma** is the extracellular matrix with fibers that are observed only during blood clotting. Red blood cells obtain their red color from hemoglobin, and the mature cells do not contain a nucleus (anucleate). White blood cells, which appear white or clear on unstained slides, are nucleated. There are five different types of white blood cells and each stains differently. Platelets, anucleate fragments of cells that are much smaller than red blood cells, are derived from large cells in bone marrow.

ACTIVITY 19 Microscopic Examination of Blood

1 Color the nucleus and cytoplasm of the white blood cells in Figure 4.40 with contrasting colors.

2 Label the photomicrograph in Figure 4.41b.

3 Examine a prepared microscope slide showing a blood smear and identify the structures listed in Figure 4.41b.

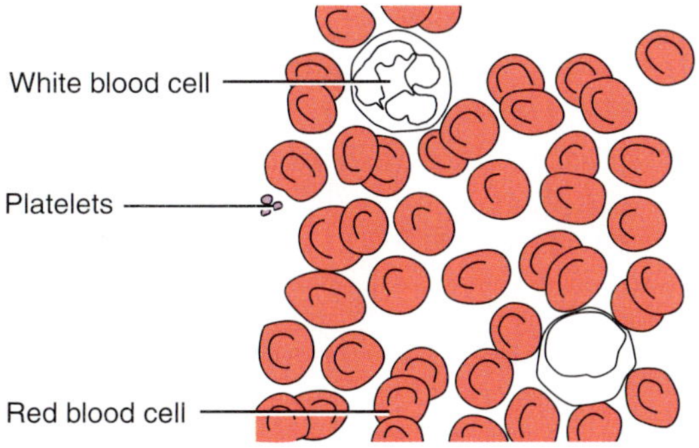

FIGURE 4.40 Blood.

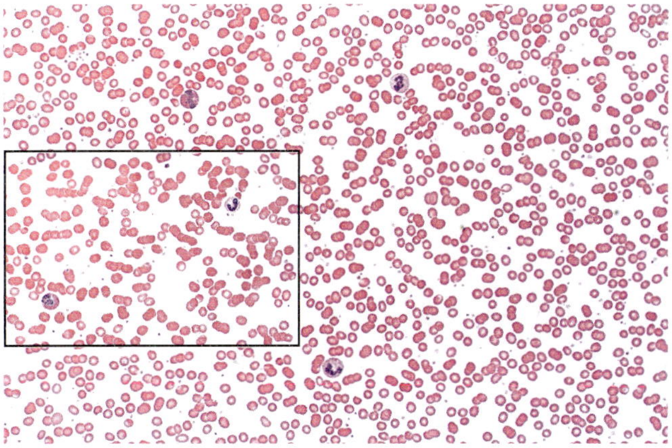

175x

(a) Survey photomicrograph.

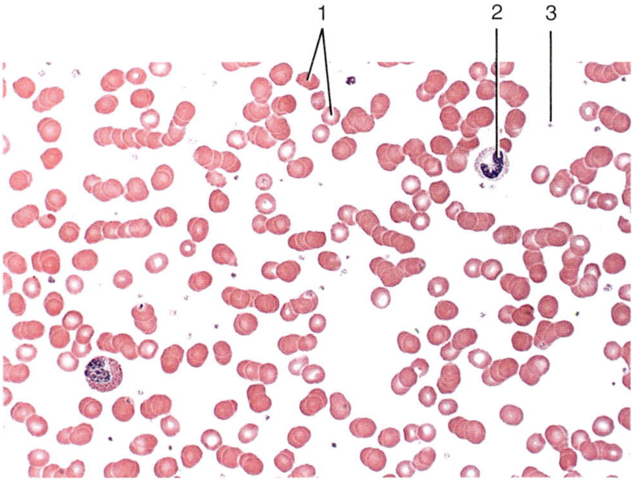

(b) Blood cells.

- nucleus of white blood cell
- platelet
- red blood cells

1 ______________

2 ______________

3 ______________

FIGURE 4.41 Blood smear.

BODY MEMBRANES

The body contains synovial and epithelial membranes. These membranes cover or line body structures or cavities. **Synovial membranes** are examined in the articulations exercise. These membranes line synovial joint cavities and produce synovial fluid that lubricates the joints.

Epithelial membranes are layers of epithelial tissue that are supported by underlying connective tissue. The body contains three types of epithelial membranes: mucous, serous, and cutaneous membranes. **Mucous membranes** are wet or moist membranes that line body cavities opening to the exterior of the body, and are found lining part of the urinary tract and the digestive, respiratory, and reproductive tracts. Although mucous glands are found in some mucous membranes, not all mucous membranes are moistened by secretions of mucus (mucus = noun; mucous = adjective). The epithelial layer of the mucous membranes varies, but the underlying connective tissue layer, **lamina propria** (*propria* = one's own), is areolar connective tissue.

Serous membranes are moist membranes that line the ventral body cavities. They produce serous fluid and are composed of simple squamous epithelium (mesothelium) over areolar connective tissue.

The **cutaneous membrane** is the dry membrane that forms the skin and is composed of stratified squamous epithelium and a thick connective tissue layer. The cutaneous membrane or integument will be examined in detail in the integumentary system exercise.

ACTIVITY 20 Body Membranes

1 Examine the serous membrane in Figure 4.12.

2 Examine the mucous membranes in Figures 4.16, 4.18, 4.20, and 4.22.

Name ______________________ Date ______________ Section ________________

EXERCISE 4

REVIEWING YOUR KNOWLEDGE

A. Primary Tissue Structure and Function

Match tissue characteristic to the primary tissue type. A characteristic could describe more than one primary tissue.

a. epithelial tissue
b. connective tissue
c. muscle tissue
d. nervous tissue

____________ **1.** Cells contain processes that receive and generate electrical signals to communicate with other cells.

____________ **2.** Most types of this tissue regenerate easily.

____________ **3.** All types of this primary tissue are avascular.

____________ **4.** Cells of this tissue form glands.

____________ **5.** Has elongated cells that shorten and cause movement.

____________ **6.** Tissue contains more extracellular matrix than cells.

____________ **7.** Cells form a barrier that controls passage of molecules.

____________ **8.** Some cell types contain striations.

____________ **9.** Primary tissue type(s) that exhibit(s) cellularity.

____________ **10.** Primary tissue type(s) that is (are) vascular.

____________ **11.** Properties of cells determine function of tissue.

____________ **12.** Properties of extracellular matrix determine function of tissue.

B. Identification of the Four Primary Tissue Types

Identify primary tissue type in Figure 4.42.

1 ______________________

2 ______________________

3 ______________________

4 ______________________

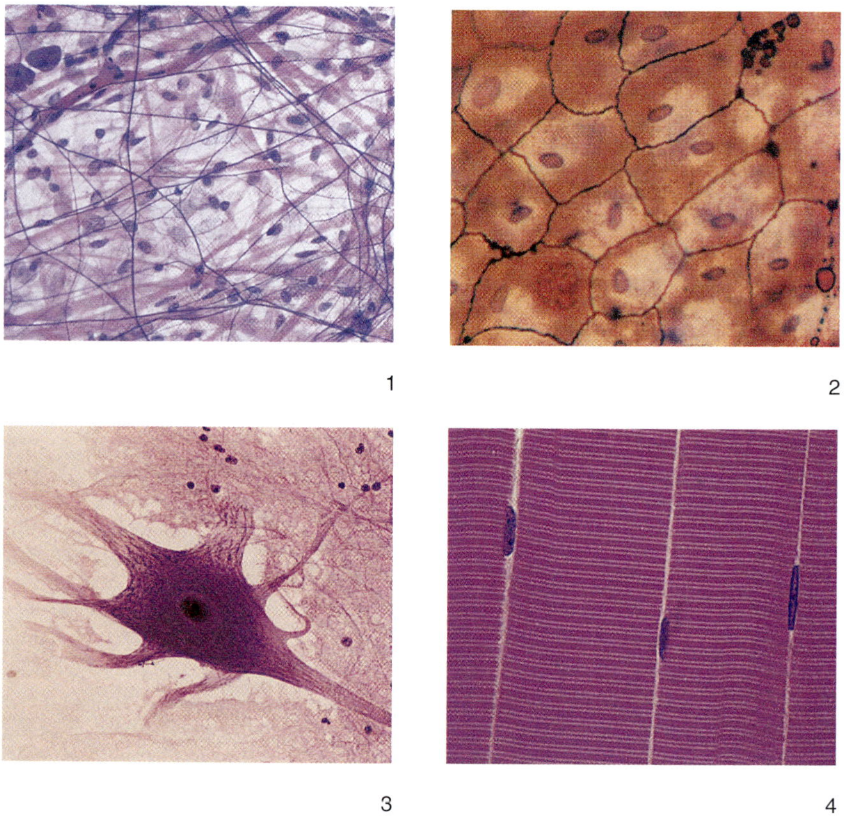

FIGURE 4.42 **Photomicrographs of primary tissues.**

C. Epithelial Tissues

Match function to an epithelial tissue type. An epithelial tissue type could have more than one function.

a. absorption
b. diffusion
c. distensible
d. filtration
e. movement of substances over the epithelial surface
f. protects underlying tissues in areas subjected to abrasion
g. secretion

__________ **1.** Stratified squamous epithelium lining the mouth.

__________ **2.** Simple squamous epithelium forming air sacs of the lung.

__________ **3.** Simple cuboidal epithelium forming kidney tubules.

__________ **4.** Ciliated pseudostratified epithelium lining the nasal cavities.

__________ **5.** Simple squamous epithelium forming mesothelium of serous membranes.

__________ **6.** Nonciliated simple columnar epithelium lining the stomach.

__________ **7.** Transitional epithelium lining the ureters.

D. Connective Tissues

Match each connective tissue type to its function.

a. areolar connective tissue
b. reticular connective tissue
c. adipose connective tissue
d. dense regular connective tissue
e. dense irregular connective tissue
f. elastic connective tissue
g. hyaline cartilage
h. bone
i. blood

___________ **1.** Connective tissue that contains elastic fibers and is found in the lung. This tissue allows the lungs to inflate during inhalation and return to their original shape after exhaling.

___________ **2.** Connective tissue packed with parallel bundles of collagen fibers and is found in tendons. This tissue resists pulling forces applied by muscles.

___________ **3.** Connective tissue with a gelatinous matrix containing collagen fibers. This tissue is found in the tracheal wall; it provides support and prevents the trachea from collapsing.

___________ **4.** Connective tissue found under covering and lining epithelium. Its extracellular matrix contains a loose arrangement of fibers and its viscous ground substance facilitates the flow of interstitial fluid containing nutrients to epithelial tissues. It also cushions and supports epithelial tissues.

___________ **5.** Connective tissue that forms a framework in the spleen, bone marrow, and lymph nodes. It contains finely branching collagen fibers.

___________ **6.** Connective tissue that is packed with bundles of collagen fibers running in different directions. It is found in skin and allows skin to resist pulling forces from many different directions.

___________ **7.** Fluid extracellular matrix used to transport substances throughout the body.

___________ **8.** Connective tissue that contains a large number of lipid-storing cells. It is found throughout the body, cushions and insulates organs, and stores lipids for future energy needs.

___________ **9.** Connective tissue with hardest extracellular matrix. Involved in protection and support.

___________ **10.** Fibroblasts produce extracellular matrix.

___________ **11.** Osteoblasts produce extracellular matrix.

___________ **12.** Chondroblasts produce extracellular matrix.

___________ **13.** Fibers not present unless injury occurs. Extracellular matrix not produced by cells present in this tissue.

Match each fiber type to its properties.

a. collagen fibers   b. elastic fibers   c. reticular fibers

____ **14.** Fine branching fibers with high tensile strength.

____ **15.** Thicker fibers with high tensile strength (resists pulling forces).

____ **16.** Is resilient (can return to original shape after stretching).

E. Epithelial Membranes

Match the epithelial membrane to the correct statement.

a. cutaneous membrane
b. mucous membrane
c. serous membrane

____ **1.** Moist membranes that line body cavities that are open to the exterior.

____ **2.** Dry membrane.

____ **3.** Membrane composed of simple squamous epithelium over areolar connective tissue.

____ **4.** Membrane that lines the digestive tract.

____ **5.** Membrane covering the soles of the feet.

____ **6.** Membrane that lines the respiratory tract.

____ **7.** Membrane that lines the urinary and reproductive tracts.

____ **8.** Membrane forming pericardium and pleura.

F. Tissue Identification

Identify the indicated epithelial and connective tissue types in Figure 4.43.

1. ______________________

2. ______________________

3. ______________________

4. ______________________

5. ______________________

6. ______________________

7. ______________________

8. ______________________

9. ______________________

10. ______________________

11. ______________________

12. ______________________

13. ______________________

14. ______________________

15. ______________________

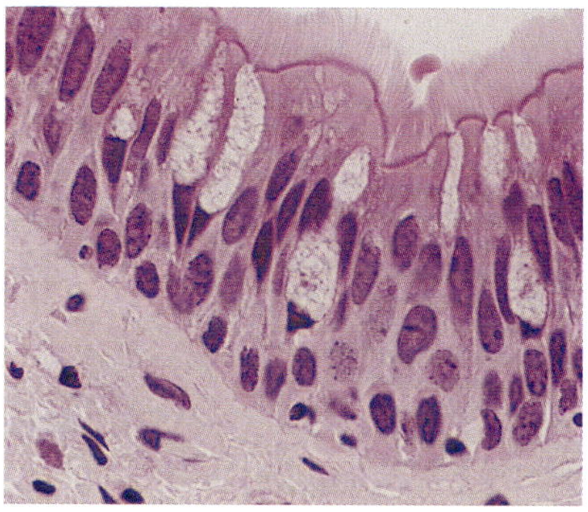

1

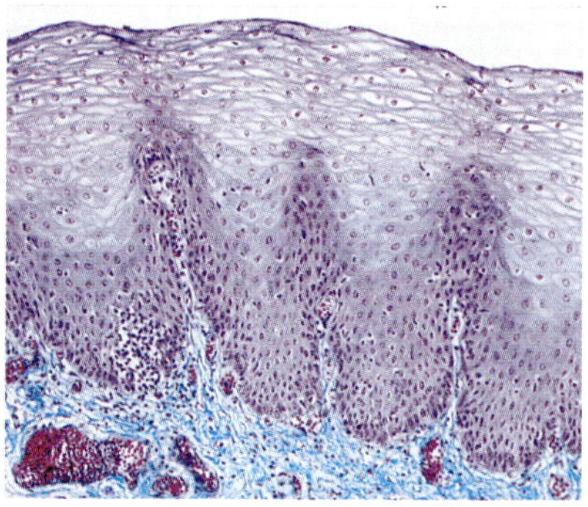

2

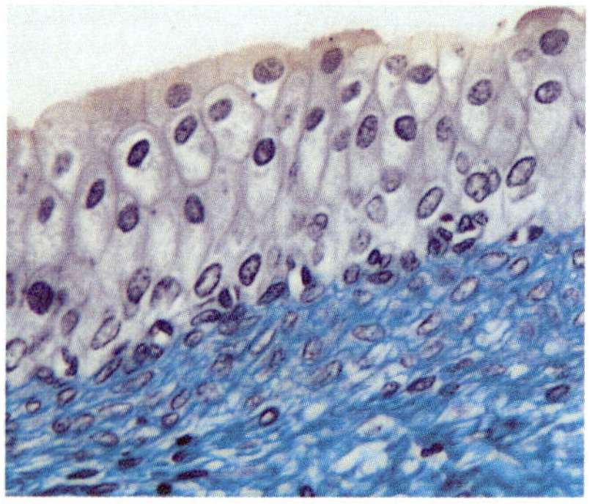

3

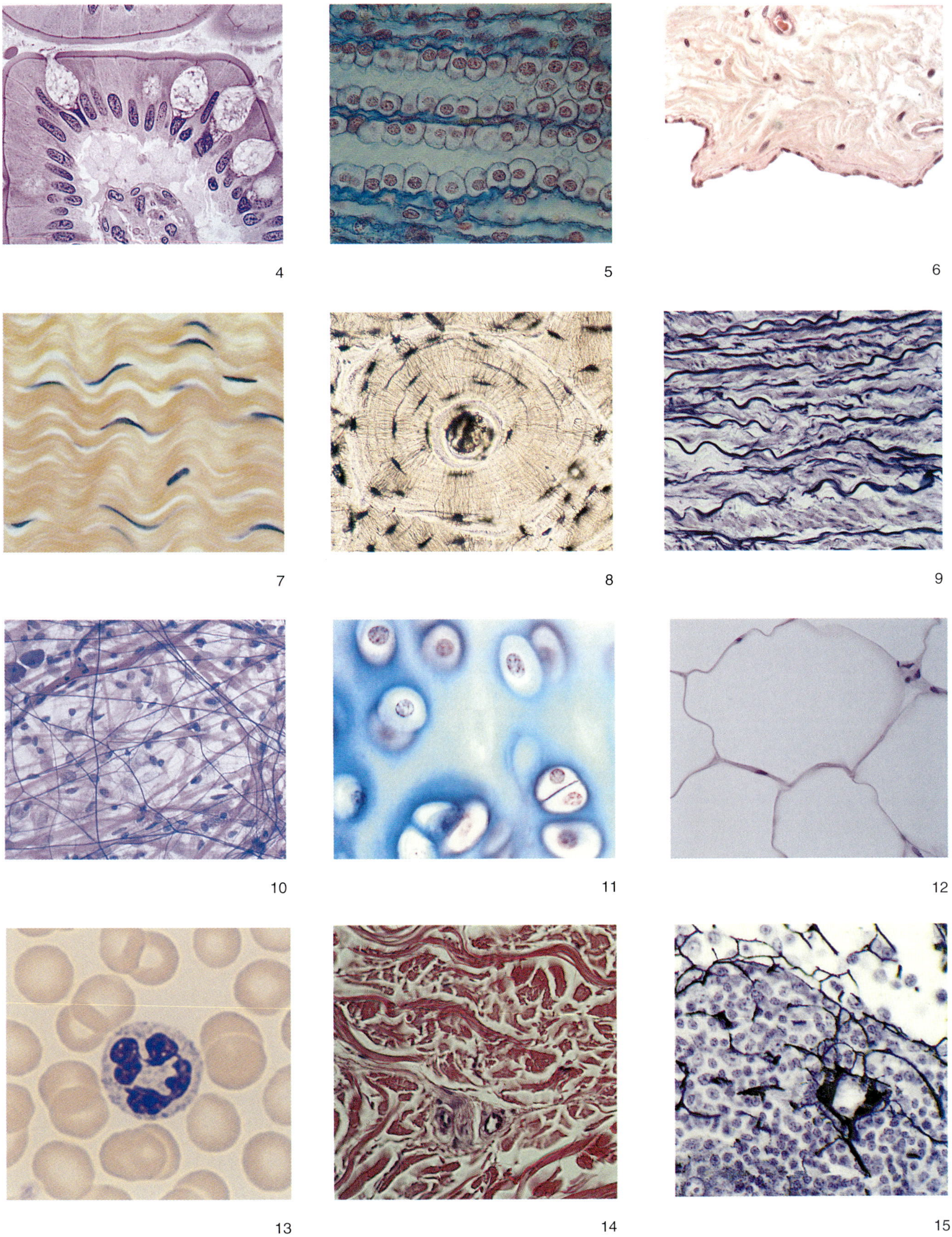

FIGURE 4.43 Identification of epithelial and connective tissue types.

Name ______________________ Date ______________ Section ______________

EXERCISE 4

USING YOUR KNOWLEDGE

A. Genetic Diseases and Tissue Function

Each of the following diseases is due to a gene mutation and the production of an abnormal protein. Look up the diseases in your textbook or another resource. For each disease (1) identify the abnormal protein and (2) state how the abnormal protein affects the function of the tissue.

Marfan's syndrome and connective tissue

1. Abnormal protein:

2. The effect of the abnormal protein on tissue function:

Hemophilia A and blood

3. Abnormal protein:

4. The effect of the abnormal protein on tissue function:

B. Nutritional Deficiencies and Tissue Function

Nutritional deficiencies interfere with cell metabolism and tissue structure. Look up rickets in your textbook or another resource and (1) describe how rickets affects the extracellular matrix of bone and (2) describe how this change in extracellular matrix causes the symptoms of rickets.

Rickets and bone

5. Affect on extracellular matrix:

6. Extracellular matrix changes and symptoms:

C. Tissues Forming Organs

Name the tissue types that form the wall of each organ in questions 7–10. Use your textbook as a reference and list the tissues in order from lumen to outer surface.

7. esophagus ____

____

8. small intestine ____

____

9. trachea ____

____

10. ureter ____

____

EXERCISE 5

THE INTEGUMENTARY SYSTEM

OUTLINE

OBJECTIVES

After completing this exercise, you should be able to:

- Name the functions of the integumentary system
- Identify the layers of the epidermis and dermis, and the hypodermis on materials supplied by your instructor
- Identify the accessory structures of the skin on materials supplied by your instructor
- Describe the function of the epidermal accessory structures

MATERIALS

- integumentary system model or chart
- microscope slides: thick skin, thin skin with hair
- compound microscopes and lens paper
- colored pencils
- 1 cm × 1 cm squares of bond paper (4 per student)
- Betadine-soaked cotton swabs
- surgical tape

The **integumentary system** (*inte-* = whole; *-gument* = body covering) consists of the skin, hair, nails, sweat and sebaceous glands, and associated muscle and nervous tissue. This system protects the body from dehydration, infection, abrasion, toxic compounds, and UV radiation. It contains sensory receptors for tactile sensations, temperature, and pain. It plays an important role in vitamin D synthesis and body temperature regulation, and minor roles in excretion and absorption.

A. Major Divisions of the Skin

The skin has two major divisions: the epidermis and the dermis. The **epidermis** (*epi* = above), the outer layer of the skin, is composed of epithelial tissue. The **dermis** is the connective tissue layer that is firmly attached to the epidermis by a basement membrane, supports the epidermis, and connects it to the underlying hypodermis. Although it is not a part of the integumentary system, the **hypodermis** (*hypo* = below) or **subcutaneous layer** (subQ) is located below the skin and is usually discussed with the skin. The hypodermis is a major storage site for adipose tissue.

1. Epidermis

The epidermis is **keratinized stratified squamous epithelium.** This is a very thick epithelial layer in comparison with other epithelial layers of the body. Keratinization is a process that results in tough, waterproof, dead cells in the superficial layer of the epithelium.

Four types of cells are found in the epidermis: keratinocytes, melanocytes, Langerhans cells, and Merkel cells. **Keratinocytes** (*keratino* = hornlike; *cytes* = cells) comprise 90% of the cells of the epidermis and produce keratin, a fibrous protein, and undergo keratinization. **Melanocytes** (*melano* = black) comprise 8% of the epidermal cells and produce and secrete the pigment melanin. **Langerhan cells** are immune system cells which attack pathogens that enter the skin. **Merkel** cells are the least abundant cell type and are only found in the deepest layer of the epidermis. These cells function as touch receptors and are associated with sensory neurons.

The layers of the epidermis are in order from deepest to most superficial: stratum basale, stratum spinosum, stratum granulosum, stratum lucidum and stratum corneum. The **stratum basale** (*strata* = layers; *basa-* = base) layer, a single row of cells, contains the most dividing cells. As new cells are formed, the older cells are pushed toward the surface. Melanocytes, Langerhans cells, and Merkel cells are also found within this layer.

The **stratum spinosum** (*spinos-* = thornlike) layer contains 8–10 rows of cells, mainly keratinocytes. In prepared slides, cells in this layer have thornlike projections caused by the tissue preparation process.

Granules are observed in the **stratum granulosum** (*granulos-* = little grains). This layer contains three to five rows of flattened keratinocytes that are beginning to die. No dividing cells are present in this layer or in more superficial layers.

The **stratum lucidum** (*lucid-* = clear) layer contains three to five rows of flat, dead keratinocytes. This layer is translucent in specimens of fresh skin; but, in prepared slides, it may be clear or stained.

The outermost layer, the **stratum corneum** (*corne-* = hard or hooflike) is a very thick layer containing 25–30 rows of dead, squamous-shaped keratinocytes. This layer is tough and water-repellent. These cells continually slough off and are replaced by cells in the adjacent layer.

The epidermis differs in thickness in thin and thick skin. Thick skin is found on the palms of the hands and the soles of the feet and has all five strata. Thin skin, which covers the rest of the body, is missing the stratum lucidum layer.

2. Dermis

The dermis consists of two regions, the papillary (*papilla* = nipples) region and the reticular (*reticul-* = netlike) region. The **papillary region** is a thin layer of areolar connective tissue that is deep to the stratum basale of the epidermis. **Dermal papillae** are fingerlike projections of the papillary region that extend into the epidermis. In the palms, fingers, soles, and toes, the dermal papillae cause genetically determined whorls in the epidermis called **epidermal ridges** that increase surface area, friction, and grip. Sweat glands deposit their secretions onto these ridges, resulting in fingerprints when these ridges touch surfaces. The **reticular layer** is the deeper and thicker region of the dermis. It is composed mainly of dense irregular connective tissue whose collagen fibers provide the skin with strength and whose elastic fibers provide elasticity, and some adipose tissue.

The dermis is highly vascularized, allowing nutrients to diffuse from the dermis into the epidermis. Hair follicles, sweat glands, and sebaceous glands—that are all derived from epithelial tissue—are found in the dermis. Nerves and lymphatic vessels are also found in this layer.

ACTIVITY 1 Major Divisions of the Skin

1 Label the skin structures in Figure 5.1.

2 Label the layers of the epidermis in thick skin in Figure 5.2.

3 Identify the skin structures in Figures 5.1 and 5.2 on a model or chart.

4 Pronounce the terms as you point to them.

5 Examine a microscope slide of thick skin.
- Using the scanning or low power objective, identify the structures in Figure 5.1.
- Using the high power objective, identify the layers of the epidermis in Fig. 5.2. Observe the different cell shapes in the apical and basal layers of the stratified squamous epithelium that forms the epidermis.
- Observe the areolar connective tissue in the papillary layer of the dermis, the dense irregular connective tissue in the reticular layer of dermis, and the adipose tissue in the hypodermis.

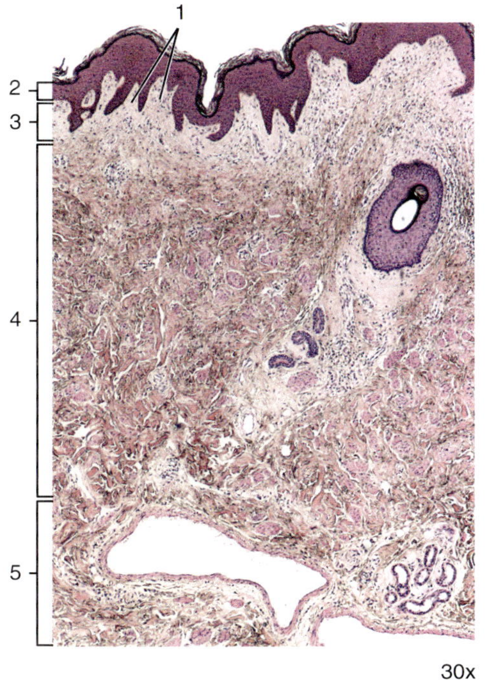

- epidermis (epi-i-DERM-is)
- dermal papillae (puh-PILL-ee)
- hypodermis
- papillary layer (PAP-il-lary) of dermis
- reticular layer of dermis

1 ______________________

2 ______________________

3 ______________________

4 ______________________

5 ______________________

FIGURE 5.1 **Photomicrograph of the skin.**

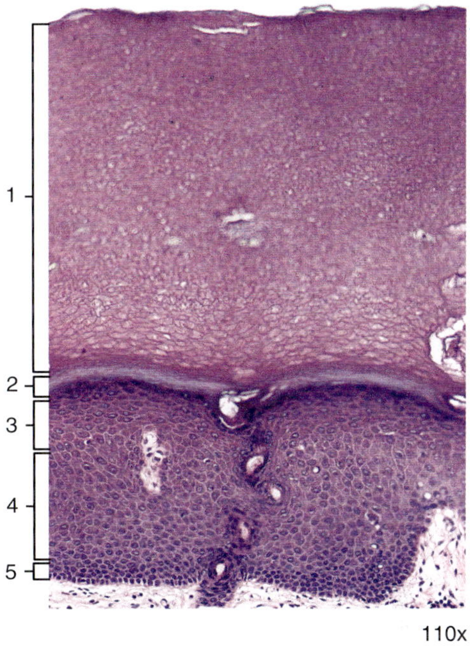

- stratum basale (bay-SAL)
- stratum corneum (kor-NEE-um)
- stratum granulosum (gran-you-LOW-sum)
- stratum lucidum (LOU-sih-dum)
- stratum spinosum (spy-NO-sum)

1 ______________________

2 ______________________

3 ______________________

4 ______________________

5 ______________________

FIGURE 5.2 **Photomicrograph of the epidermal layers in thick skin.**

B. Accessory Structures of the Skin

The accessory structures of the skin include hairs, hair follicles, nails, sweat glands, sebaceous glands, ceruminous glands, and mammary glands. All of these are derived from epithelial tissues, but are located in connective tissue.

1. Sudoriferous and Sebaceous Glands

Sudoriferous glands (*sudori* = sweat; *-ferous* = bearing) or sweat glands are located in the dermis and secrete a watery substance that is important in body temperature regulation and excretion. There are two types of sudoriferous glands: eccrine glands and apocrine glands. **Eccrine glands** (*eccrine* = sweating outwardly) are the most common type of sudoriferous gland and are found on most areas of the body. Ducts from the eccrine glands deposit their secretions, called sweat, on the epithelial surface. Sweat is composed mainly of water, salts, and nitrogen-containing wastes. **Apocrine glands,** which do not become active until after puberty, are found only in the axilla, genital areas, and pigmented area around the nipples (areolae). Apocrine glands produce a secretion similar in composition to sweat, but it is more viscous and contains lipids and proteins. This secretion, which is deposited on the distal end of the hair root, is odorless until broken down by bacteria.

Ceruminous glands and mammary glands are modified suderiferous glands. **Ceruminous glands** (*ceri-* = wax) are found in the ear canal and secrete a waxy substance called cerumen that prevents foreign substances (including insects) from entering the auditory canal. **Mammary glands** are found in the breasts and synthesize and secrete milk after appropriate hormonal stimulation. **Sebaceous glands** (*sebace-* = greasy) or oil glands are found surrounding hair follicles and deposit sebum, an oily substance that lubricates the skin and hair, onto the hair shaft.

2. Hair and Hair Follicles

Hairs, which help protect and insulate, are found all over the body with the exception of the palms, soles, lips, and parts of the external genitalia. Hair consists of dead, keratinized epithelial cells and has two sections: the **shaft,** which is located in the epidermis and projects from the skin surface, and the **root,** which is embedded in the dermal layers of the skin. The **hair follicle,** which is located in the dermis and surrounds the hair root, is formed from epidermal layers that project into the dermis. The expanded base of the hair follicle, the **hair bulb,** contains the papilla of the hair and the matrix. The **papilla** of the hair is a projection of connective tissue into the hair follicle and contains blood vessels that provide nutrients to the dividing cells of the matrix. The **matrix,** which is derived from the stratum basale layer of the epidermis, forms new hair cells that are added to the base of the hair root. Surrounding the hair follicle is a **connective tissue sheath** comprised of dermal tissue.

Attached to the connective tissue sheath around the hair follicle is a bundle of smooth muscle cells called the **arrector pili** (*arrect* = to raise) muscle. Contraction of the arrector pili muscle moves the hair from its normal angle to a 90° angle (perpendicular) with skin surface, elevating the skin surrounding the hair shaft and causing goosebumps. Arrector pili muscles contract in response to stress (including cold temperature).

Examination of the hair in cross-section shows three layers: the cuticle (outer layer), the cortex (middle layer), and the medulla (inner layer). The **cuticle,** the layer of hair that we see, is a thin layer of dead, flattened, keratinized cells that overlap each other like shingles on a roof. Split ends occur when the free ends of these cells are pulled away from each other. Cells in the **cortex** and **medulla** contain pigment granules that give hair its color. The shape of hair in cross-section indicates whether the hair is curly, wavy, or straight. Curly hair is flat in cross-section, wavy hair is oval, and straight hair is round.

ACTIVITY 2 Hair, Hair Follicles, Sebaceous Glands, and Sudoriferous Glands

1. Label the diagram of the skin and accessory structures in Figure 5.3.
2. Point to the structures on a model or chart of the integumentary system.
3. Pronounce the names of the structures as you point to them.
4. Label the photomicrograph in Figure 5.4.
5. Examine a slide of hairy skin, and identify the structures in Figure 5.4.
6. Examine different types of hair (curly, wavy, straight) with the compound microscope.
   - Using a scalpel, cut a strand of curly, wavy, or straight hair.
   - Hold the hair perpendicular to the stage to observe the cross-section with the 4x objective lens.
   - Describe its cross-sectional shape.
   - Hold the hair parallel to the stage to observe the cuticle of the hair shaft with the 4x objective lens.
   - If someone is willing to donate hair with "split ends," compare the cuticle of a hair with split ends with undamaged hair.

- apocrine sweat gland
- arrector pili muscle
- eccrine sweat gland
- hair bulb
- hair follicle
- hair root
- hair shaft
- papilla of hair
- sebaceous gland

1 ______________________

2 ______________________

3 ______________________

4 ______________________

5 ______________________

6 ______________________

7 ______________________

8 ______________________

9 ______________________

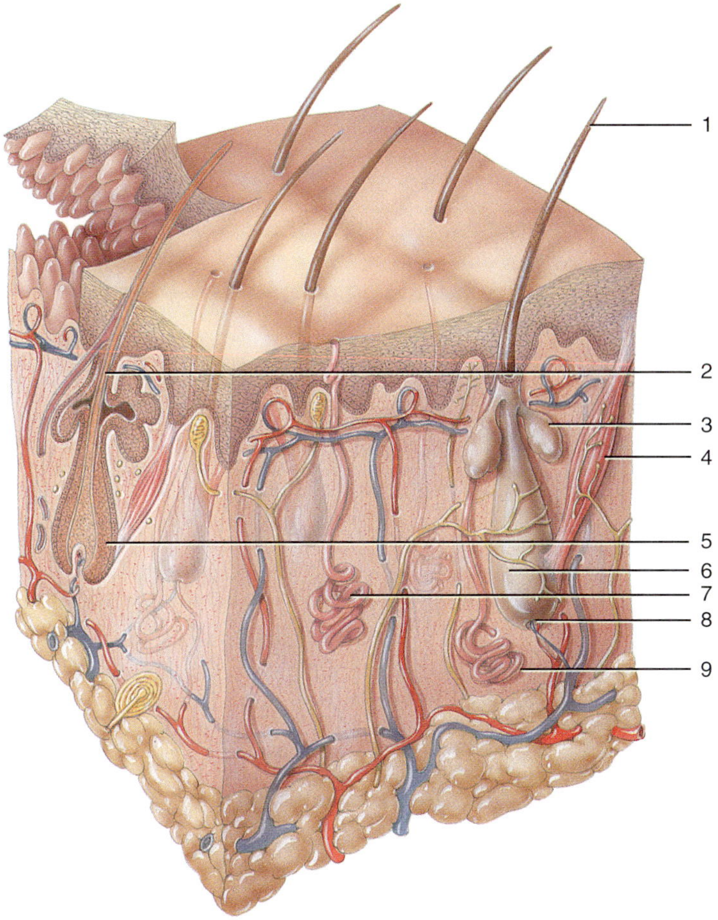

FIGURE 5.3 Diagram of the skin and accessory structures.

- hair bulbs
- hair follicle
- hair root
- papilla of hair
- sebaceous gland

1 ______________________

2 ______________________

3 ______________________

4 ______________________

5 ______________________

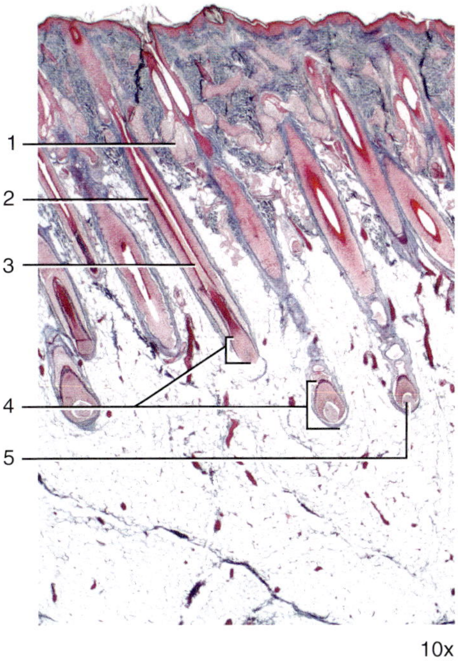

FIGURE 5.4 Photomicrograph of the skin and accessory structures.

TABLE 5.1 Eccrine Sweat Gland Density

BODY AREA	ECCRINE SWEAT GLAND DENSITY (No. of Glands/cm²) Individual Value	Class Average
Forehead		
Right anterior forearm		
Right palm		
Right anterior leg		

7 Compare concentration of sweat glands in different areas of the body.
- Obtain 4 squares of bond paper (each square 1 cm × 1 cm), a Betadine-soaked cotton swab, and tape.
- Find areas on your forehead, right anterior forearm, right palm, and right anterior leg that do not have large crease lines.
- For each location, apply Betadine to an area slightly larger than the paper square.
- Securely tape a paper square over the Betadine-covered area at each location.
- After 20 minutes, remove the tape and paper squares, and count the blue-black dots on each square. Each blue-black dot is an active sweat gland.
- Record the number of dots per cm^2 in Table 5.1.
- Pool the class data, calculate the average eccrine gland density, and record the value in Table 5.1.

8 Answer the discussion questions with your lab partners.

DISCUSSION QUESTIONS: ECCRINE GLAND DENSITY

1 Which body area had the highest density of eccrine glands and which had the lowest?

2 Compare eccrine gland density with the amount of sweat that appears on these body areas during exercise or nervousness.

3. Nails

Nails, which are found on the distal ends of the digits, assist in grabbing and manipulating objects, and protect the digits. The nail consists of a nail body, a free edge, and a root. The **nail body** is the part of the nail that is visible, the **free edge** extends beyond the digit, and the **root** is underneath the skinfold at the proximal end of the nail body. The **lunula** (*lunula* = little moon) is the crescent-shaped area of the nail body distal to the nail root. The **cuticle** or **eponychium** (*epi-* = above; *-onych* = nail) is the thickened epithelial tissue along the proximal border of the nail body. The **hyponychium** (*hypo-* = below) is deep to the free edge and forms the nail bed. The **nail matrix** is the epithelial tissue within the nail root that divides to produce new cells that are added to the nail body as it grows.

ACTIVITY 3 Nail Structure

1 Identify the nail structures on the diagram in Figure 5.5.

2 Identify nail structures on your own nails.

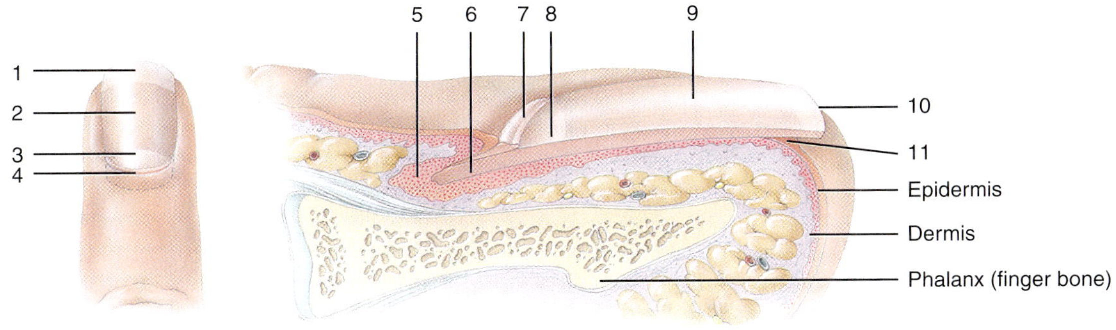

(a) Dorsal view

(b) Sagittal section through finger

(a) Dorsal view
- eponychium
- free edge
- lunula
- nail body

1 ______________________________

2 ______________________________

3 ______________________________

4 ______________________________

(b) Sagittal section through finger
- eponychium
- free edge
- hyponychium
- lunula
- nail root
- nail body
- nail matrix

5 ______________________________

6 ______________________________

7 ______________________________

8 ______________________________

9 ______________________________

10 ______________________________

11 ______________________________

FIGURE 5.5 **Nail structures.**

Name ______________________ Date ______________ Section ______________

EXERCISE 5

REVIEWING YOUR KNOWLEDGE

A. Identification of Skin Layers and Accessory Structures

Label the skin layers and accessory structures in Figure 5.6.

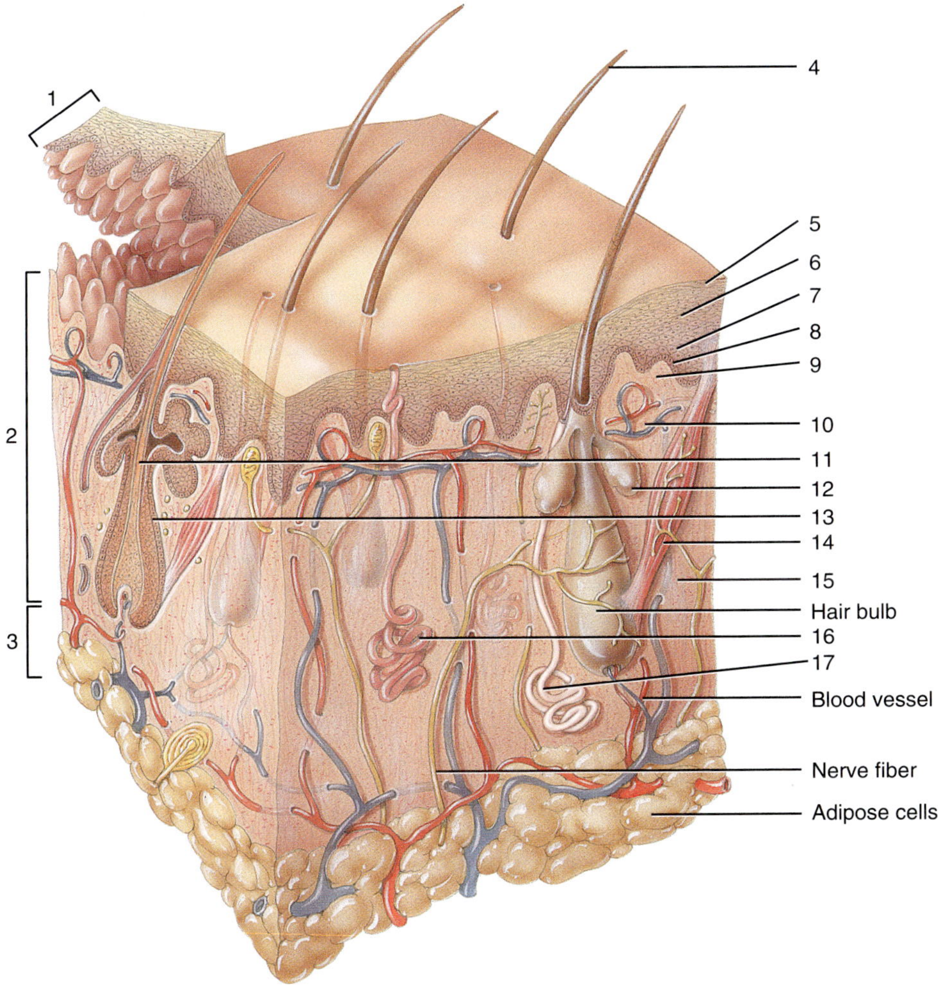

1. ______________________
2. ______________________
3. ______________________
4. ______________________
5. ______________________
6. ______________________
7. ______________________
8. ______________________
9. ______________________
10. ______________________
11. ______________________
12. ______________________
13. ______________________
14. ______________________
15. ______________________
16. ______________________
17. ______________________

FIGURE 5.6 Skin layers and accessory structures.

B. Skin Layers

Choose the skin layer or structure that fits the description.

a. dermal papillae
b. papillary layer
c. reticular layer
d. stratum basale
e. stratum corneum
f. stratum granulosum
g. stratum lucidum
h. stratum spinosum

____ **1.** Layer of epidermis where there is the most rapid cell division

____ **2.** Tough, water-repellent epidermal layer; contains dead squamous-shaped cells

____ **3.** Areolar connective tissue layer beneath basement membrane

____ **4.** Projections of dermis that causes epidermal ridges

____ **5.** Translucent layer found in thick skin, absent in thin skin

____ **6.** Appears to have thornlike projections in prepared slides

____ **7.** Thick dermal layer containing dense irregular connective tissue

____ **8.** Epidermal layer containing visible granules

C. Cells of the Epidermis

Choose the epidermal cell(s) that fits the description. Cells may be used more than once.

a. keratinocytes
b. Langerhans cells
c. melanocytes
d. Merkel cells

__________ **1.** Defends skin against microbes

__________ **2.** Produces keratin

__________ **3.** Produces the pigment melanin that shields cell nuclei from UV radiation

__________ **4.** Associated with sensory neuron and functions in sensation of touch

D. Accessory Structures of the Skin

Select the choice that best fits the description.

a. apocrine sweat gland
b. arrector pili muscle
c. cuticle
d. eccrine sweat gland
e. free edge
f. hair bulb
g. hair follicle
h. hair root
i. hair shaft
j. hyponychium
k. lunula
l. nail body
m. nail root
n. papilla of hair
o. sebaceous gland

____ **1.** Sudoriferous glands located in axillary and genital areas; become active after puberty

____ **2.** Connective tissue projection; provides blood supply for hair matrix

____ **3.** Secures nail to digit

____ **4.** Epithelial layer that surrounds hair root

____ **5.** Secretes sebum onto hair and skin

____ **6.** Part of nail that overlies nail bed

____ **7.** Part of nail that extends beyond digit

____ **8.** Part of hair that contains the matrix

____ **9.** Sudoriferous glands that deposit sweat onto epidermal ridges causing fingerprints

____ **10.** Part of hair in epidermis and extending beyond skin surface

____ **11.** Moves hair shaft perpendicular to skin; causes goosebumps

____ **12.** Thickened epithelial tissue at proximal end of nail body

____ **13.** Crescent-shaped area of nail body near cuticle

____ **14.** Part of hair within dermis

____ **15.** Part of nail within skin

4. Orbit of Eye

The orbit of the eye is a mosaic of six different bones, three cranial bones (frontal, sphenoid, and ethmoid) and three facial bones (maxilla, zygomatic, and lacrimal).

ACTIVITY 3 Orbit of Eye

1 Label the bones forming the orbit of eye on Figure 7.7.
2 Pronounce each term as you point to it on a skull.

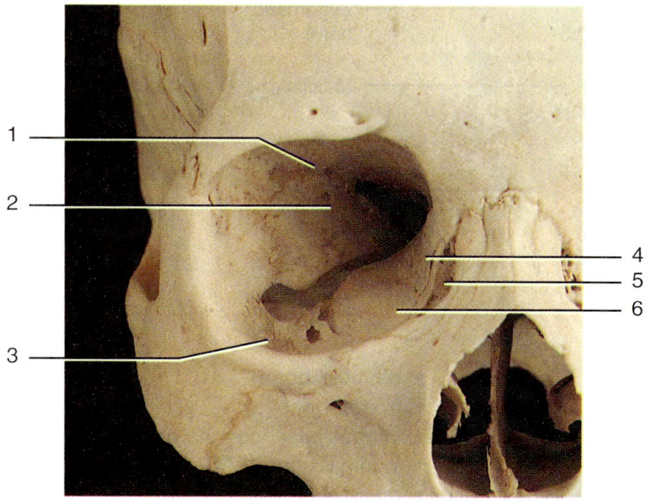

- ethmoid bone
- frontal bone
- lacrimal bone
- maxilla
- sphenoid bone
- zygomatic bone

1 ______________________
2 ______________________
3 ______________________
4 ______________________
5 ______________________
6 ______________________

FIGURE 7.7 Orbit of eye.

TABLE 7.1 Bone Markings

MARKING	DESCRIPTION	PURPOSE
DEPRESSIONS OR OPENINGS		
1. Fissure (FISH-er)	Narrow slit or cleft in a bone	Opening for blood vessels and nerves
2. Foramen (for-AY-men)	Opening or hole	Opening for blood vessels and nerves
3. Fossa (FOS-sa)	Shallow depression	Muscle attachment or articulation (joint)
4. Meatus (me-AY-tus)	Tubelike opening	Tubular passageway for blood vessels and nerves
PROCESSES		
5. Condyle (CON-dile)	Smooth, rounded articular process	Articulation
6. Ramus (RAY-mus)	A small branch	Articulation

5. Selected Bone Surface Markings of the Skull

Bones of the skull are not totally smooth on the exterior, but have bumps, depressions, grooves, holes, and projections. Bone markings have specific names and distinct purposes and are classified according to their function. Several bone markings found on the skull are listed in Table 7.1 along with their descriptions and functions. Selected bones and their markings are listed below.

Cranial Bones: Selected Bone Surface Markings

1. *Frontal bone* (1)
   - **supraorbital foramina** (*supra-* = above; *orbit* = wheel rut; *foram-* = opening) – openings located above the orbit of the eye for supraorbital nerve and artery
   - **supraorbital ridges or margins** – thickening of frontal bone superior to orbit of eye
2. *Temporal bone* (2) – Each temporal bone has one of each structure listed below:
   - **external auditory meatus** (*meatus* = passageway) – tubelike openings for the ear canal
   - **mastoid process** (*mastoid* = breastlike) – rounded projection posterior to external auditory meatus; attachment for muscles
   - **styloid process** (*stylo-* = point) – long, thin projection on inferior skull surface; attachment for muscles and ligaments of tongue and neck
   - **zygomatic process** – projection that articulates with the zygomatic bone
   - **mandibular fossa** – depression for articulation with condylar process (mandibular condyle)
   - **foramen lacerum** (*lacerare* = torn or lacerated) – jagged opening filled with cartilage in a living person
   - **carotid foramen (canal)** – foramen for carotid artery
   - **jugular foramen** (*jugular* = throat) – foramen for jugular vein
   - **stylomastoid foramen** – opening for an artery and cranial nerve VII (facial)
   - **internal auditory meatus** – opening for cranial nerve VIII (vestibulocochlear)
3. *Occipital bone* (1)
   - **foramen magnum** (*magnum* = large) – opening connecting lower brain to spinal cord
   - **hypoglossal foramina** – two openings for cranial nerve XII (hypoglossal)
   - **occipital condyles** – two rounded processes that articulate with the atlas (C1)
4. *Ethmoid bone* (1)
   - **cribriform plates** (*cribr-* = sieve) – one on either side of crista galli; form roof of nasal cavity
   - **crista galli** (*crist-* = crest; *galli* = rooster) – projection for attachment of membranes covering brain
   - **olfactory foramina** (*olfact-* = smell) – tiny holes in cribriform plates for cranial nerve I (olfactory)
   - **perpendicular plate** – forms superior part of nasal septum
   - **middle nasal conchae** – scroll-like projections on each lateral wall of nasal cavity
   - **superior nasal conchae** – scroll-like projections on each lateral wall of nasal cavity
5. *Sphenoid bone* (1)
   - **foramina ovale** (*ovale* = oval) – openings for mandibular branch of cranial nerve V (trigeminal)
   - **foramina rotundum** – two openings for maxillary branch of cranial nerve V
   - **optic foramina** – openings for cranial nerve II (optic)
   - **greater and lesser wings** – form anterior and lateral floor of cranium
   - **sella turcica** (*sella* = saddle; *turcica* = Turkish) – bony projection that surrounds pituitary gland
   - **inferior orbital fissures** – openings for blood vessels and nerves
   - **superior orbital fissures** (*fissure* = cleft) – openings for blood vessels and nerves

Facial Bones: Selected Bone Surface Markings

1. *Maxillae* (2)
   - **alveoli** (*alve-* = socket) – teeth sockets
   - **palatine process** – two fused processes that form the anterior part of hard palate
2. *Mandible* (1)
   - **alveoli** – teeth sockets
   - **body** – curved, anterior portion
   - **mental foramina** (*menta* = chin) – two openings in chin for nerves and blood vessels
   - **rami** – two small, branchlike processes; one on either side of the mandible
   - **condylar processes (mandibular condyles)** – two rounded processes on rami that articulate with temporal bone at the mandibular fossa

ACTIVITY 4 Bone Surface Markings

1 Label the bone markings listed below on Figures 7.8, 7.9, 7.10, and 7.11.

2 Identify these structures on an articulated skull (and a Beauchene skull, if available).

3 Pronounce the terms as you point to them on a skull.

4 Using two rounded coffee stirrers, poke each stirrer into an orbit of the eye and through an optic foramen. Observe the straws in the superior view of the cranial floor and notice that the straws cross above the sella turcica. This simulates the crossing of the optic nerves called the optic chiasma.

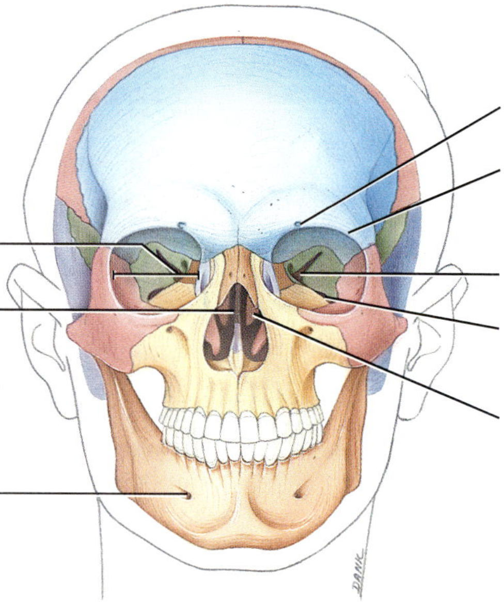

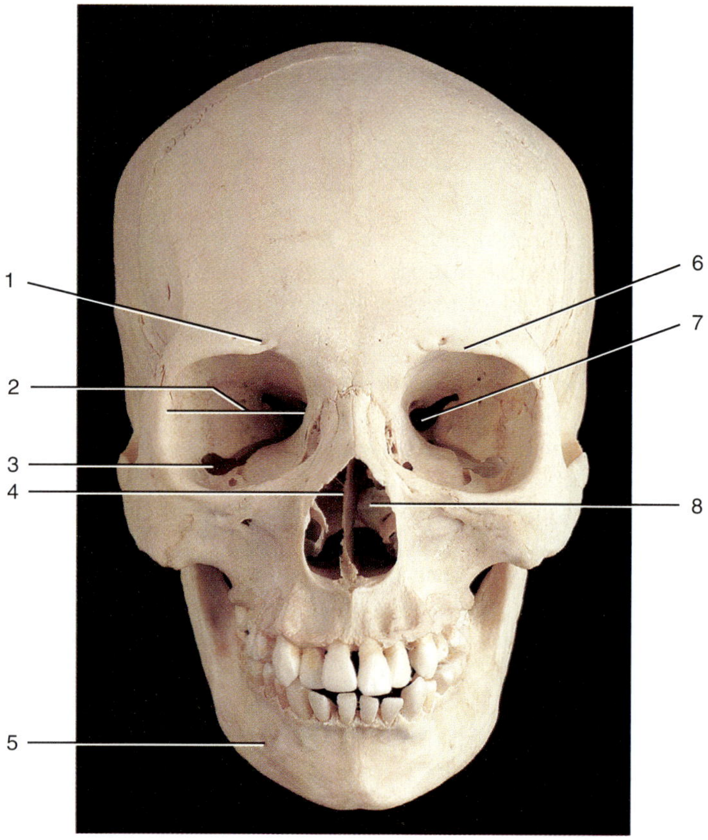

- inferior orbital fissure
- mental foramen
- middle nasal concha
- orbit of eye
- perpendicular plate of ethmoid
- superior orbital fissure
- supraorbital foramen (supra-OR-bi-tal)
- supraorbital margin

1 ______________________

2 ______________________

3 ______________________

4 ______________________

5 ______________________

6 ______________________

7 ______________________

8 ______________________

FIGURE 7.8 Anterior view of skull.

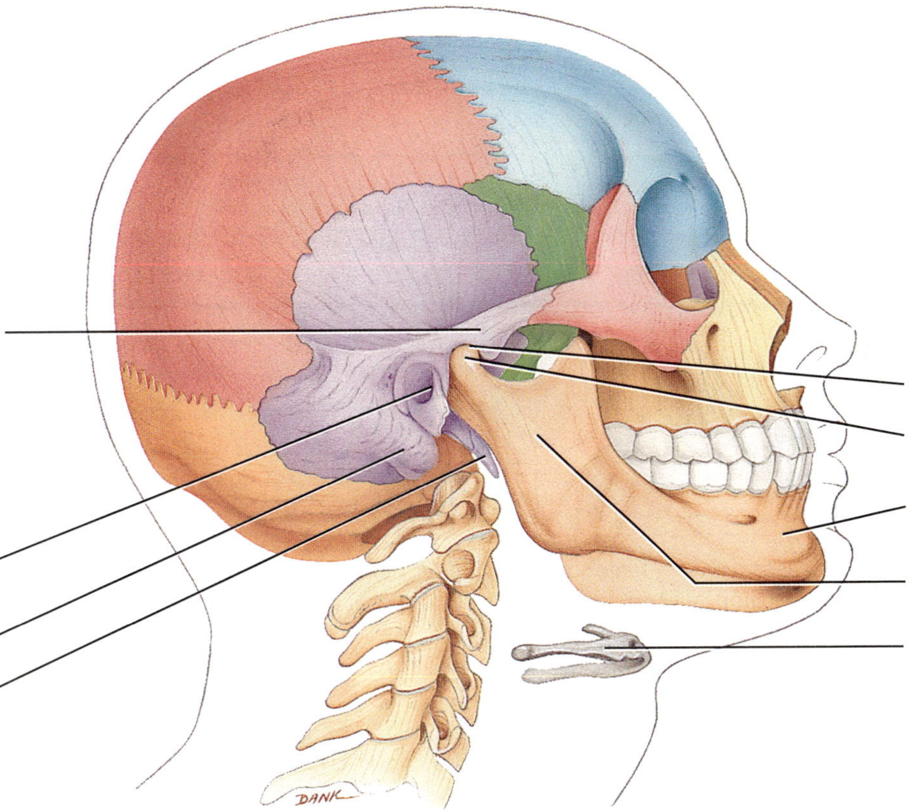

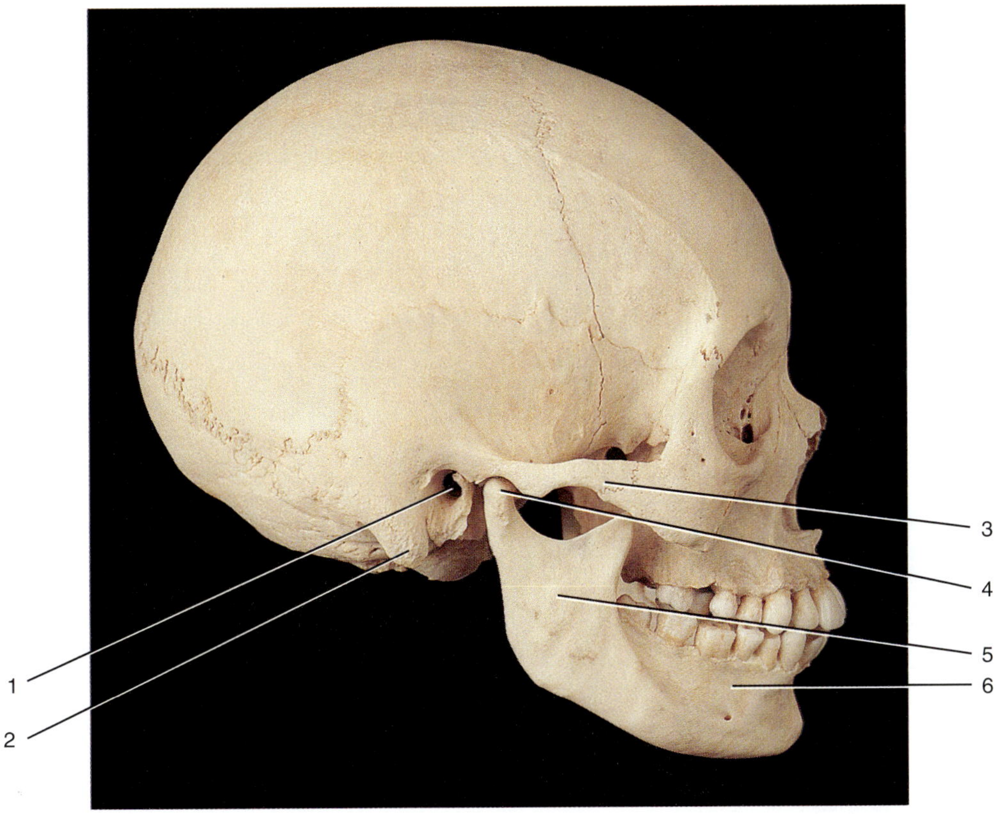

- body of mandible
- condylar process (CON-dih-lur) (mandibular condyle)
- external auditory meatus
- mastoid process (MAS-toid)
- ramus of mandible
- zygomatic process of temporal bone

1 ______________

2 ______________

3 ______________

4 ______________

5 ______________

6 ______________

FIGURE 7.9 Lateral view of skull.

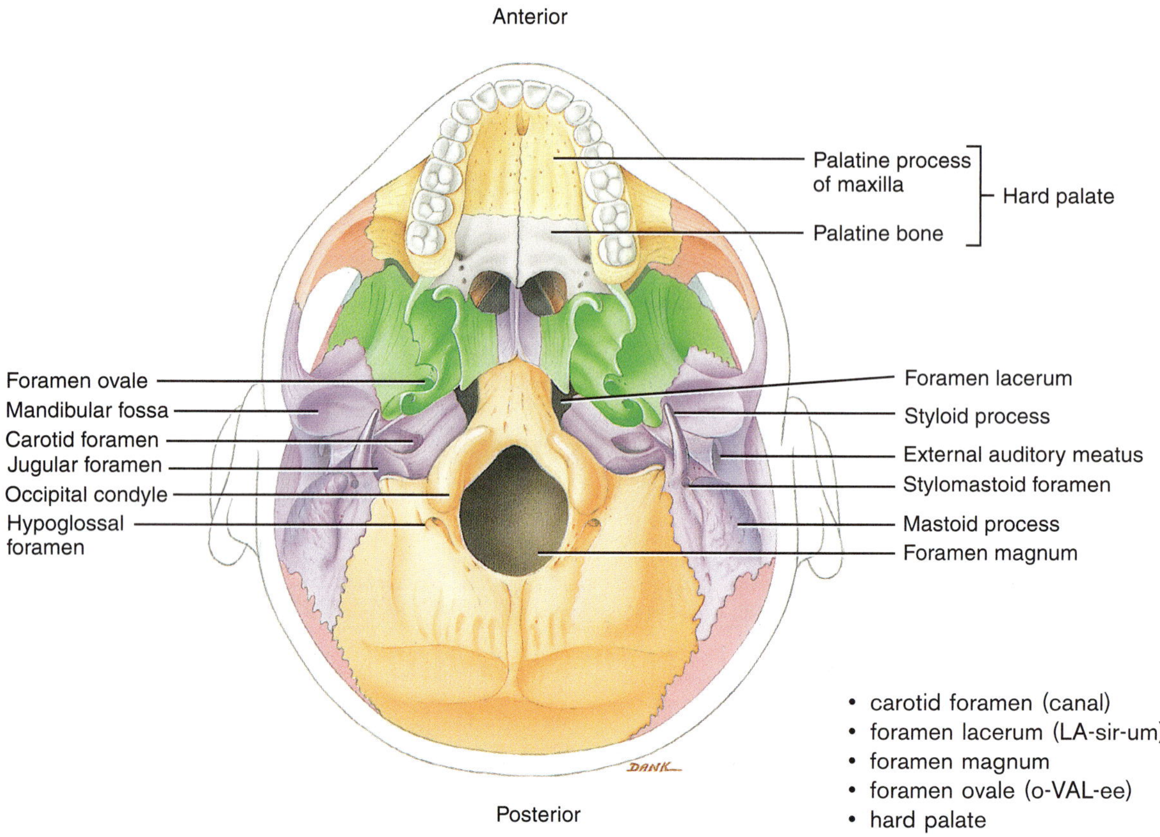

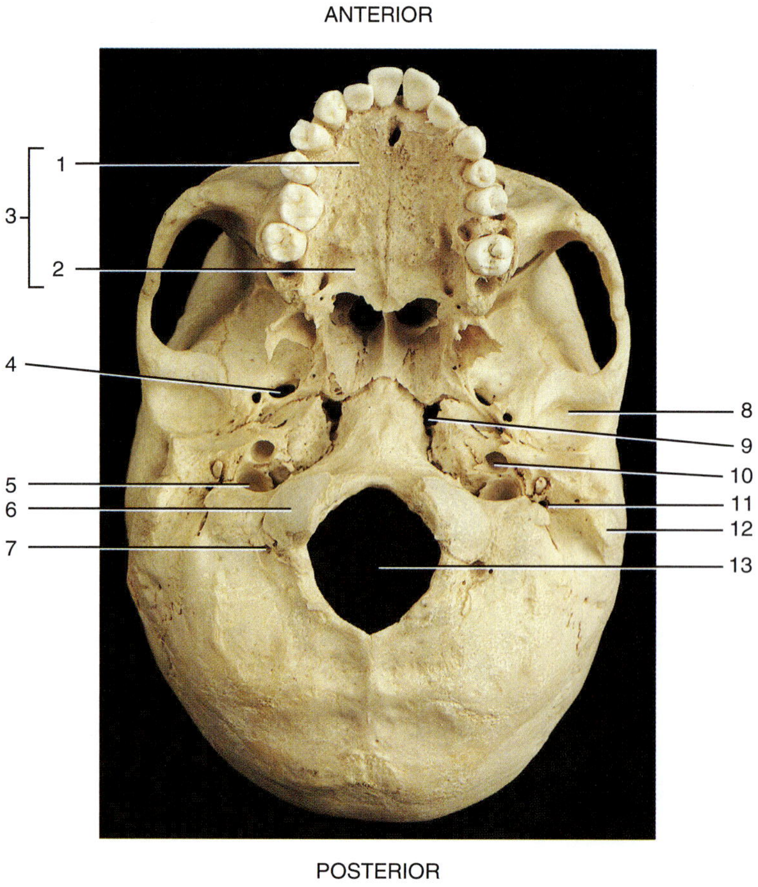

- carotid foramen (canal)
- foramen lacerum (LA-sir-um)
- foramen magnum
- foramen ovale (o-VAL-ee)
- hard palate
- hypoglossal foramen
- jugular foramen (JUG-u-lar)
- mandibular fossa
- mastoid process
- occipital condyle (ox-CI-pi-tal)
- palatine bone
- palatine process of maxilla
- stylomastoid foramen (sty-lo-MAS-toid)

1 ______________________

2 ______________________

3 ______________________

4 ______________________

5 ______________________

6 ______________________

7 ______________________

8 ______________________

9 ______________________

10 ______________________

11 ______________________

12 ______________________

13 ______________________

FIGURE 7.10 Inferior view of skull.

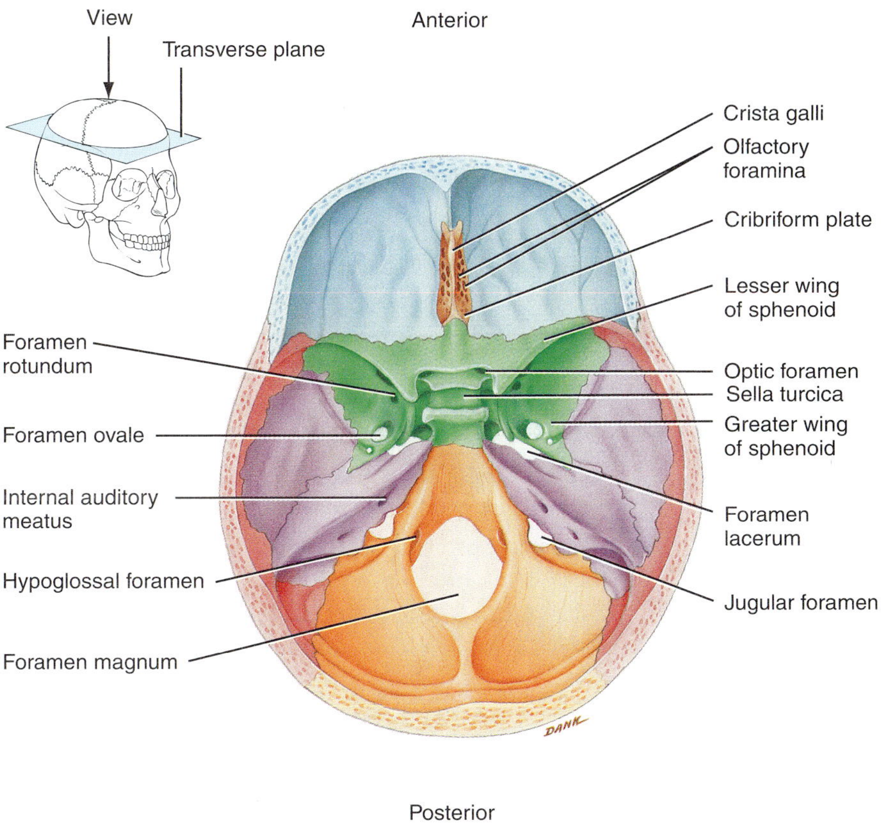

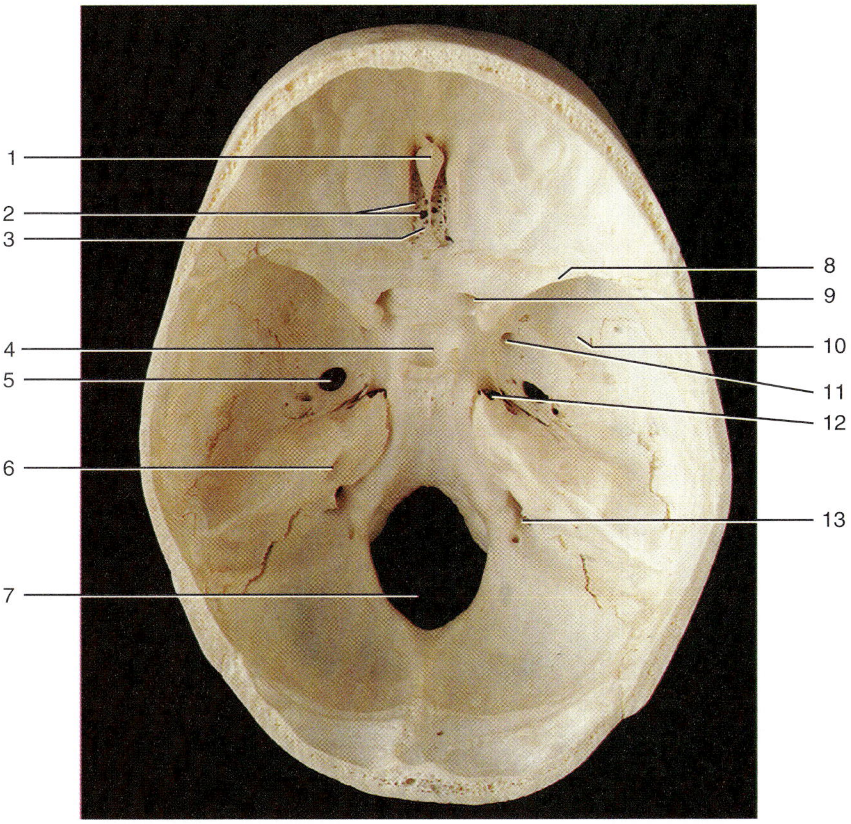

- cribriform plate of ethmoid (CRIB-ri-form)
- crista galli of ethmoid (CRIS-ta GAL-li)
- foramen lacerum
- foramen magnum
- foramen ovale
- foramen rotundum
- greater wing of sphenoid
- internal auditory meatus
- lesser wing of sphenoid
- jugular foramen
- olfactory foramina of ethmoid (OL-fac-to-ry for-AY-mi-na)
- optic foramen
- sella turcica (SEL-la TUR-si-ca)

1 ______________________

2 ______________________

3 ______________________

4 ______________________

5 ______________________

6 ______________________

7 ______________________

8 ______________________

9 ______________________

10 ______________________

11 ______________________

12 ______________________

13 ______________________

FIGURE 7.11 Superior view of floor of cranium.

6. Paranasal Sinuses

Paranasal (*para-* = next to; *nasal* = nose) **sinuses** (*sinu-* = hollow) are cavities lined with mucous membranes that are located near and have openings into the nasal cavities. The four paranasal sinuses, the **ethmoidal, frontal, maxillary,** and **sphenoidal,** are named for their locations in bones of the same name.

ACTIVITY 5 Paranasal Sinuses

Label the four paranasal sinuses in Figure 7.12.

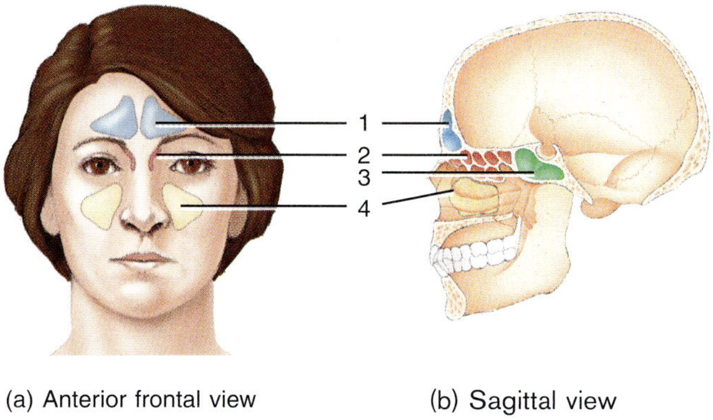

- ethmoidal sinus
- frontal sinus
- maxillary sinus
- sphenoidal sinus

1 ______________________

2 ______________________

3 ______________________

4 ______________________

FIGURE 7.12 Paranasal sinuses.

7. Nasal Septum

The **nasal septum** (*saeptum* = wall or partition) is comprised of bone and cartilage. The inferior bone is the **vomer,** and the **perpendicular plate** of the **ethmoid** bone is superior. The **septal cartilage** is anterior to the two bones.

ACTIVITY 6 Nasal Septum

1 Label the bones and cartilage of the nasal septum in Figure 7.13.

2 Identify these structures on an articulated skull (and a Beauchene skull, if available).

3 Palpate your nasal septum to find the junction of the nasal bones and nasal cartilage.

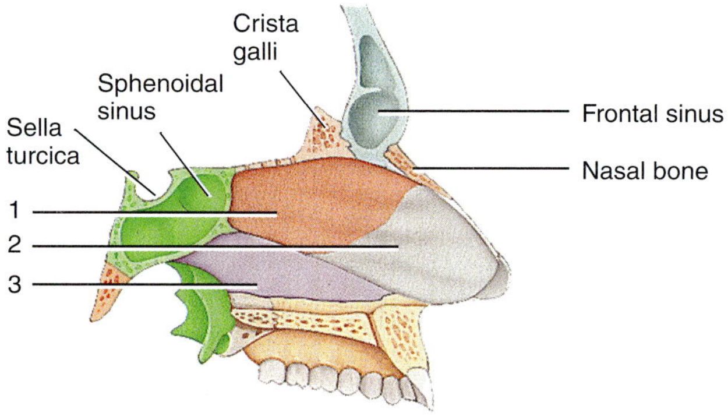

- perpendicular plate of ethmoid
- septal cartilage
- vomer

1 ______________________

2 ______________________

3 ______________________

FIGURE 7.13 Nasal septum.

8. Hard Palate

The **hard palate,** or roof of the mouth, is formed by the fusion of four bones: two **palatine processes of the maxillary bones** and two **palatine bones.** Approximately three-fourths of the hard palate is composed of the palatine processes of the maxillary bones and one-fourth is the palatine bones.

> **CLINICAL NOTE:** *A **cleft palate** is a common congenital malformation of the hard palate. This defect is the result of bones of the palate failing to fuse along the midline during embryonic development. The cleft can be partial or complete.*

ACTIVITY 7 Hard Palate

1. Identify the bones of the hard palate in Figure 7.10.
2. Locate these bones on a skull.

9. Fetal Skull

The fetal skull is not completely ossified, but has membranous sections composed of fibrous connective tissue called **fontanels** (*fontaine* = fountain) or "soft spots." Fontanels are membrane templates that are present at birth and eventually ossify. Fontanels allow the cranial bones to compress during the journey through the birth canal, and also allow for future growth of the brain. At birth, the physician or midwife can tell how the baby is presenting itself in the birth canal by palpating the fontanel. If the fontanel is a diamond shape, the baby is presenting the frontal bone first and is face down. If the fontanel is triangular in shape, the baby is presenting the occipital bone and is face up.

ACTIVITY 8 Fetal Skull and Major Fontanels

1. Label the fontanels in Figure 7.14(a) and (b).
2. Identify the fontanels on a fetal skull (if available).
3. Compare the location of the fontanels and sutures in the fetal skull with adult sutures.

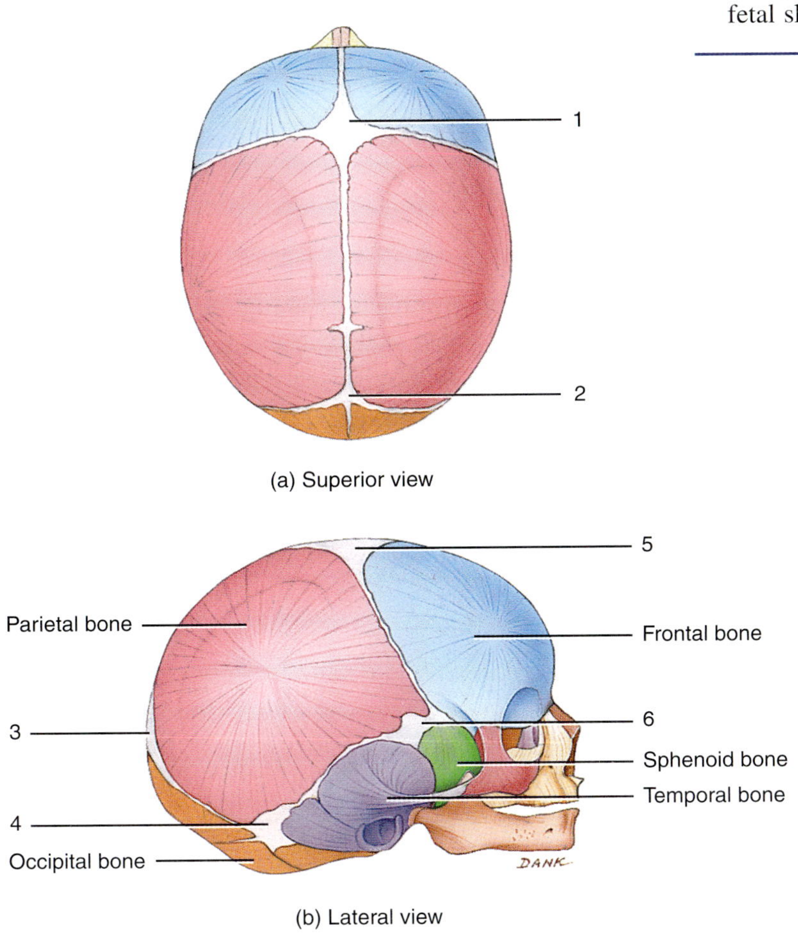

(a) Superior View
- anterior (frontal) fontanel
- posterior (occipital) fontanel

1 ______________________

2 ______________________

(b) Lateral View
- anterior (frontal) fontanel (fon-ta-NEL)
- anterolateral (sphenoidal) fontanel
- posterior (occipital) fontanel
- posterolateral (mastoid) fontanel

3 ______________________

4 ______________________

5 ______________________

6 ______________________

FIGURE 7.14 Major fontanels of the fetal skull.

C. Hyoid Bone

The hyoid bone is not attached to the axial skeleton, but is included with the axial skeleton because of its midline location and proximity to the mandible and vertebral column. This bone is U-shaped and has the distinction of not articulating with any other bones. It is secured in place by ligaments and muscles, including many muscles of the tongue and neck. It is located in the anterior neck region between the mandible and larynx. (This is the bone that is crushed during strangulation.)

ACTIVITY 9 Hyoid Bone

1. Locate the hyoid bone in Figure 7.9.
2. Identify the hyoid bone on an articulated skeleton and with a disarticulated skeleton.
3. Palpate your hyoid bone by placing the thumb and middle finger of one hand on either side of the neck about one inch inferior to the mandible. This bone can be moved laterally from side to side.

D. Vertebral Column

The vertebral column protects the spinal cord and provides attachment points for back muscles. The curved **vertebral column** (backbone or spine) is a flexible structure that can be bent, twisted, and rotated, especially in the cervical region. The vertebral column consists of **cervical** (*cervic-* = neck), **thoracic** (*thorac-* = chest), and **lumbar** (*lumb-* = loin) **vertebrae** in addition to the **sacrum** (*sacer* = sacred) and **coccyx** (cuckoo's beak). The sacrum consists of five vertebrae that are fused in the adult. The coccyx (tailbone) is usually composed of four small, fused vertebrae. A baby has 33 individual vertebrae and the adult has 26 due to fusion of the sacral and coccygeal vertebrae. The vertebral column articulates with the skull superiorly, the ribs laterally, and the pelvis inferiorly.

1. Regions and Normal Curvatures of the Vertebral Column

The five regions of the vertebral column and number of vertebrae in the adult from superior to inferior, are: **cervical** (7), **thoracic** (12), **lumbar** (5), **sacral** (1), and **coccygeal** (1). To remember the number of vertebrae in the first three groups, students say they eat "breakfast at 7, lunch at 12, and dinner at 5." There are four normal spinal curvatures that correspond with the regions of the spinal column: **cervical, thoracic, lumbar,** and **sacral** (pelvic) **curvatures.** A newborn has a single primary spinal curve that will become the thoracic curve and sacral curve, also known as kyphotic curvatures. Two secondary curves, the cervical and lumbar, develop several months later and are also known as lordotic curves. The cervical curve develops when the baby can hold the head erect. The lumbar curve develops when the baby can stand.

ACTIVITY 10 The Vertebral Column

1. Label the five regions of the vertebral column in Figure 7.15.
2. Label the four normal spinal curvatures in Figure 7.15.
3. Identify the five regions on an articulated skeleton or vertebral column model.
4. Identify the four spinal curvatures on an articulated skeleton or vertebral column.
5. Pronounce the terms as you point to them on a skeleton or vertebral column.

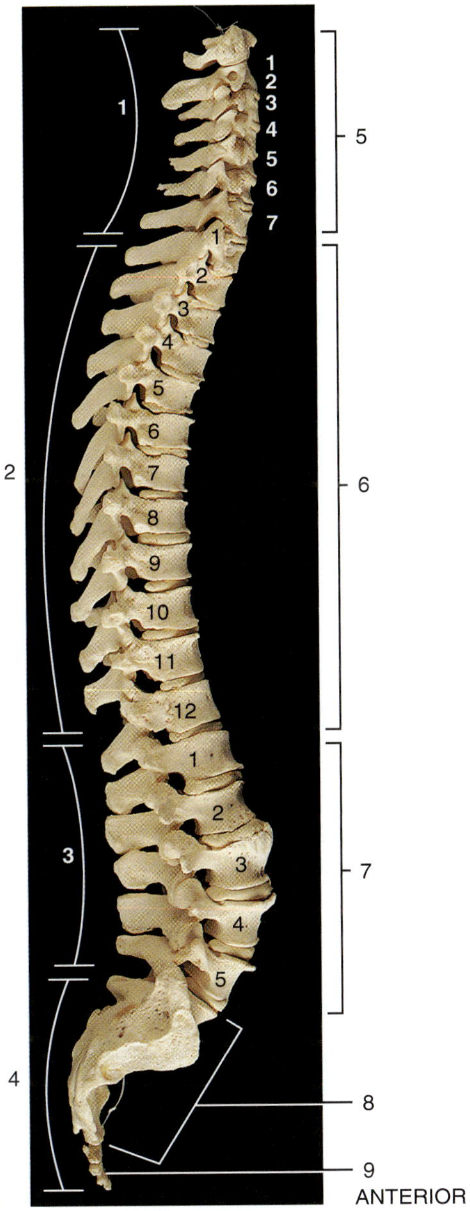

1 ____________________

2 ____________________

3 ____________________

4 ____________________

5 ____________________

6 ____________________

7 ____________________

8 ____________________

9 ____________________

- cervical curve
- cervical vertebrae (VER-te-bray)
- coccyx (COCK-six)
- lumbar curve
- lumbar vertebrae
- sacral curve
- sacrum (SAY-crum)
- thoracic curve
- thoracic vertebrae

FIGURE 7.15 Normal spinal curvatures of the vertebral column.

2. Parts of a Typical Vertebra

The cervical, thoracic, and lumbar vertebrae have similar as well as different structures. The similarities are studied in this activity, and the differences will be studied in Activity 12.

- **body** – located anteriorly; is the largest part of the vertebra
- **pedicle** (*pediculus* = little foot) – attached to and extends posteriorly on either side of the body
- **transverse process** – extends laterally from each pedicle
- **lamina** (*lamin-* = plate) – connects transverse processes to the spinous process
- **spinous process** – projects posteriorly from fused lamina
- **vertebral arch** – formed by the fusion of pedicles and laminas.
- **vertebral foramen** – large opening formed by the vertebral arch that protects the spinal cord
- **superior** and **inferior articular processes** (with **facets**) – extend from the vertebra at the junction of the pedicle and lamina to articulate with a superior and inferior vertebra respectively.

ACTIVITY 11 Parts of a Typical Vertebra

1 Locate the parts of a vertebra shown in Figure 7.16.

2 Identify the parts on a disarticulated thoracic vertebra.

3 Pronounce the terms as you point to them on the vertebra.

4 Palpate the spinous processes of your vertebral column.

3. Comparison of Cervical, Thoracic, and Lumbar Vertebrae

The first two of the seven cervical vertebrae look different from the others. The **atlas** is C_1 and is named for the mythical Greek god who held up the world on his shoulders. The large **superior articular facets** of the atlas articulate with the **occipital condyles** of the skull and allow the head to move up and down in a nodding motion. The **axis,** C_2, has a superior toothlike protuberance called the **dens** (*dens* = tooth in Latin) or **odontoid process** (*odous* = tooth in Greek). The dens extends superiorly into the vertebral foramen of the atlas and allows the atlas to pivot laterally in a "no" type motion. Some head traumas push the head onto the vertebral column and the dens is shoved into the medulla oblongata (brain stem). This is the cause of

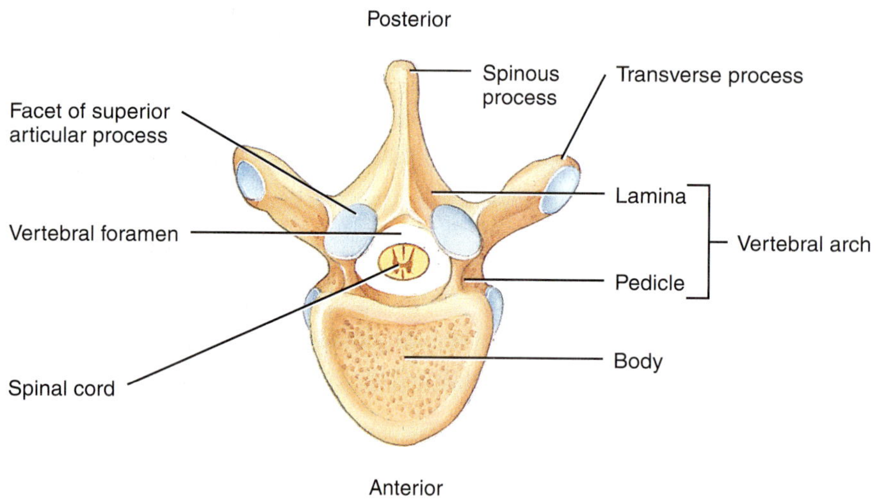

FIGURE 7.16 **Parts of a typical vertebra.**

death in such head injuries. The easiest way to distinguish any **cervical vertebra** is by its three foramina (plural)—a **vertebral foramen** plus two **transverse foramina.** The transverse foramina, found only in cervical vertebrae, allow passage of the vertebral arteries, veins, and sympathetic nerves to and from the brain. Since the cervical vertebrae do not carry much weight, they are lightweight and have small bodies. C_3 through C_6 have bifurcated (forked) spinous processes. A **whiplash,** which occurs in some rear-ended auto accidents, causes partial or complete dislocation of the cervical vertebrae.

A **thoracic vertebra** has a medium-sized body and a long, narrow spinous process that commonly slants inferiorly at a sharp angle. Thoracic vertebrae also have facets (*facette* = little face) on the transverse processes and demifacets (*demi-* = half) on the bodies, both of which articulate with ribs.

Lumbar vertebrae have the largest bodies to support more weight and thick, hatchet-shaped spinous processes that extend horizontally.

Intervertebral discs can be found between the bodies of vertebrae from C_2 to the sacrum. As you recall, they are made of fibrocartilage to give strength, permit movement, and absorb shock. The outer portion of the disc called the **annulus fibrosus** (*annulus* = ringlike) consists of tough fibrocartilage. The inner part, the **nucleus pulposus** (*pulposus* = pulplike), is soft and pulpy. A *herniated* or *slipped disc* occurs when the fibrocartilage of the annulus is stressed and torn or cracked. In this situation, the inner pulplike center protrudes outward and causes pressure on the spinal cord or a spinal nerve. A *laminectomy* (removal of the lamina and sometimes spinous process of the vertebra) relieves the pressure.

Intervertebral foramina are formed when vertebrae are stacked on one another. Spinal nerves exit the vertebral column through these foramina.

ACTIVITY 12 Comparison of Cervical, Thoracic, and Lumbar Vertebrae

1. Identify the specific parts of an atlas, axis, and cervical vertebra in Figure 7.17(a), (b), and (c).
2. Identify the specific parts of a thoracic vertebra in Figure 7.18(a) and (b) and a lumbar vertebra in Figure 7.19(a) and (b).
3. Pronounce each term as you point to it.
4. Using disarticulated vertebrae, place all three types side by side and note their differences. Mix them up and identify each type of vertebra with a partner.
5. Identify the parts of articulated vertebrae in Figure 7.20(a) and a herniated disc in Figure 7.20(b).

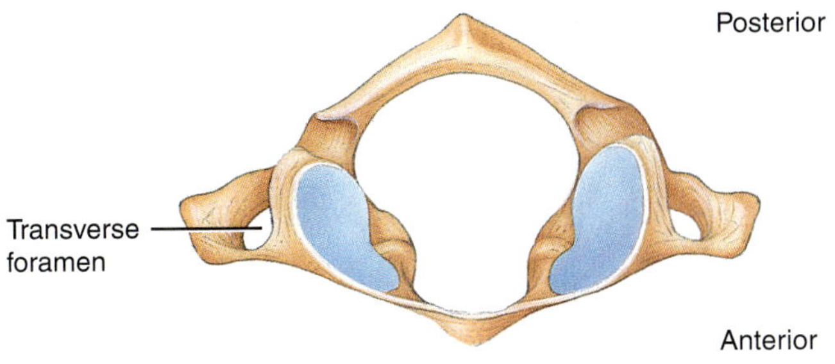

(a) Superior view of the atlas (C1)

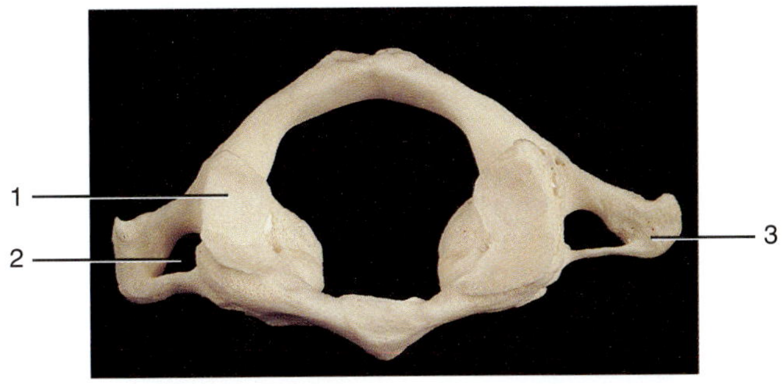

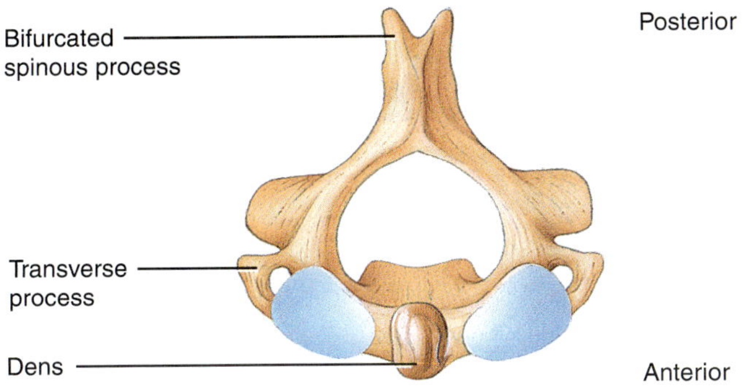

(b) Superior view of the axis (C2)

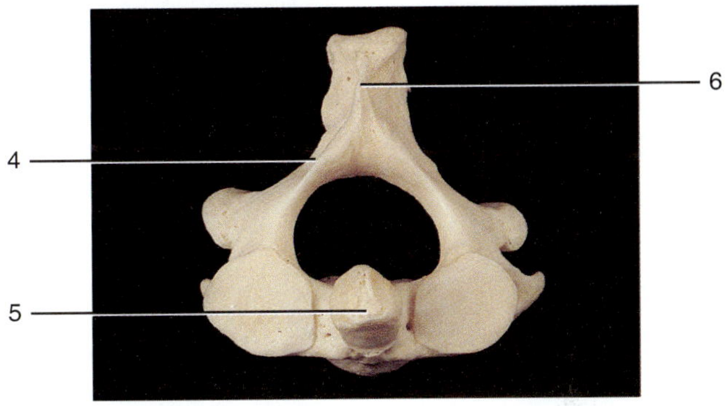

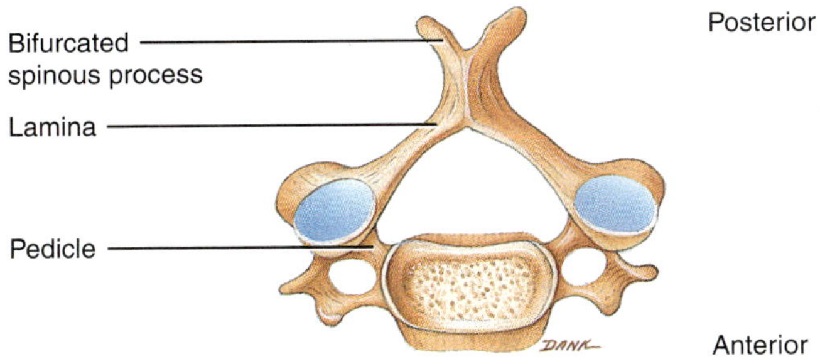

(c) Superior view of a typical cervical vertebra (C3)

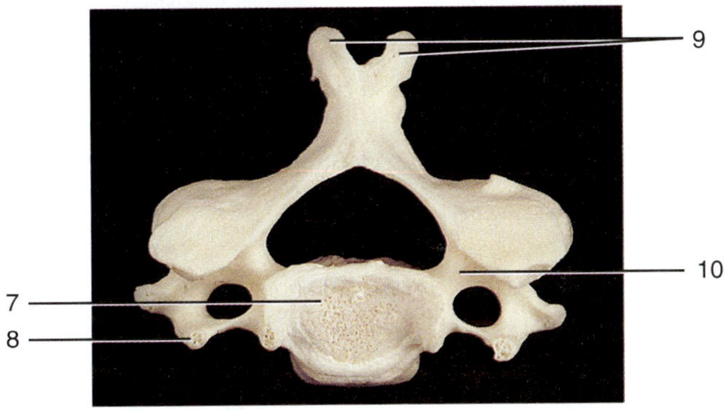

(a) Atlas
- superior articular facet
- transverse foramen
- transverse process

(b) Axis (Note: The transverse foramen cannot be seen in this photo.)
- dens or odontoid process
- lamina
- spinous process

1 ______________
2 ______________
3 ______________
4 ______________
5 ______________
6 ______________

(c) Typical cervical vertebra
- bifurcated spinous process
- body
- pedicle
- transverse process

7 ______________
8 ______________
9 ______________
10 ______________

FIGURE 7.17 **Cervical vertebrae.**

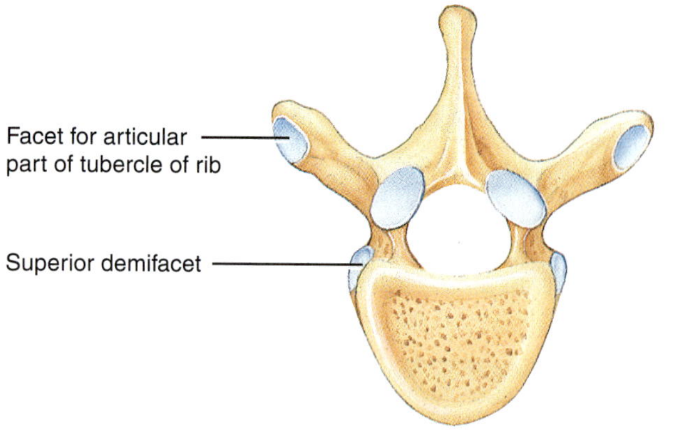

(a) Superior view

POSTERIOR

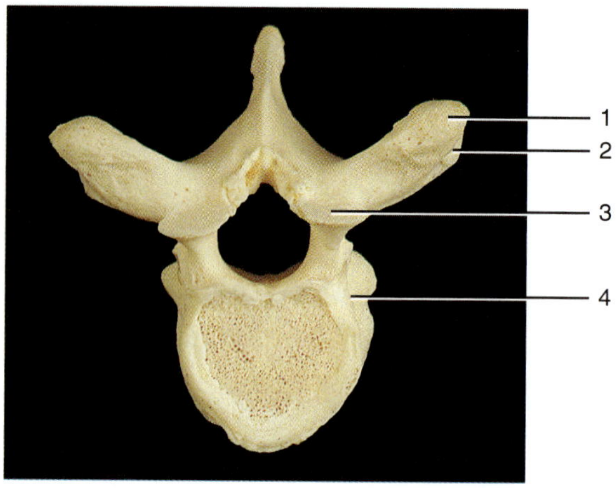

ANTERIOR

(a) Superior view

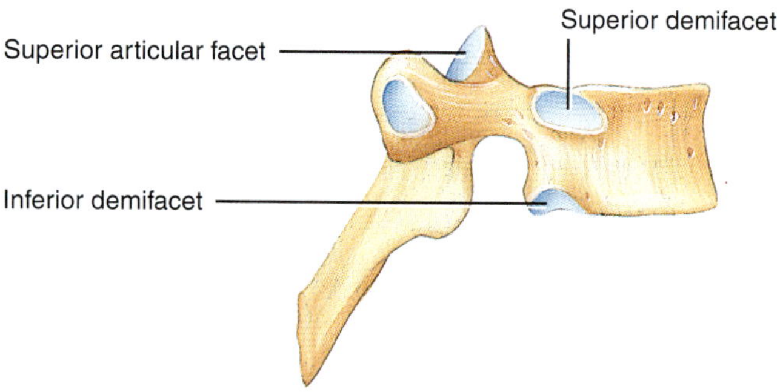

(b) Right lateral view

SUPERIOR

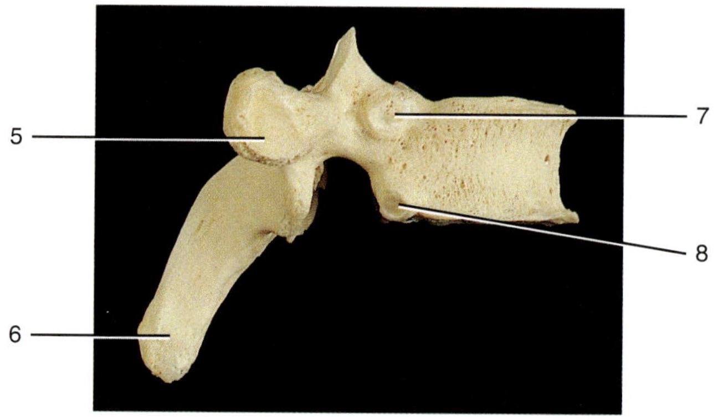

POSTERIOR ANTERIOR

(b) Right lateral view

(a) Superior view
- facet for articular part of tubercle of rib
- superior articular facet
- superior demifacet
- transverse process

(b) Right lateral view
- facet for articular part of tubercle of rib
- inferior demifacet
- slanted spinous process
- superior demifacet

1 ______________________

2 ______________________

3 ______________________

4 ______________________

5 ______________________

6 ______________________

7 ______________________

8 ______________________

FIGURE 7.18 **Thoracic vertebrae.**

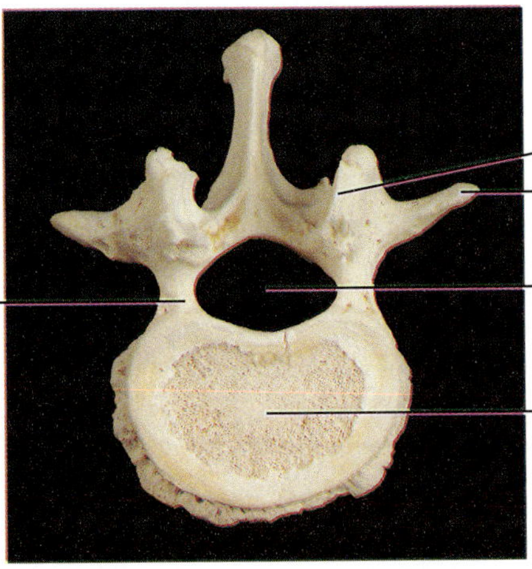

(a) Superior view

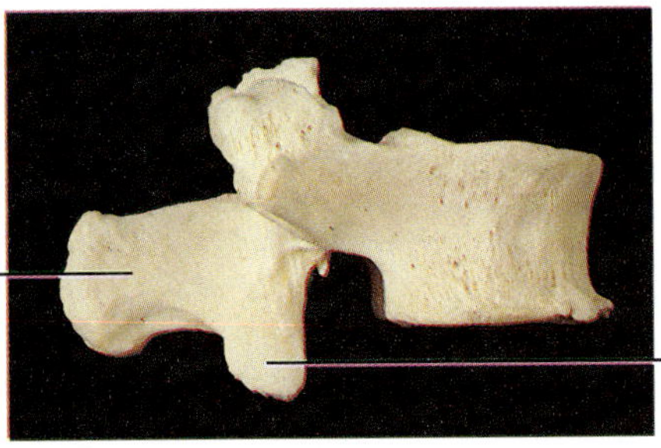

(b) Right lateral view

(a) Superior view
- body
- pedicle
- superior articular process
- transverse process
- vertebral foramen

1 ______________________

2 ______________________

3 ______________________

4 ______________________

5 ______________________

(b) Right lateral view
- hatchet-shaped spinous process
- inferior articular facet

6 ______________________

7 ______________________

FIGURE 7.19 **Lumbar vertebrae.**

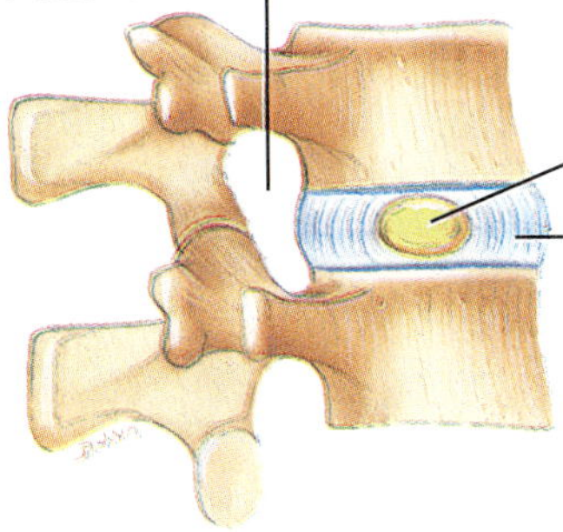

(a) Right lateral view of articulated vertebrae with intervertebral disc

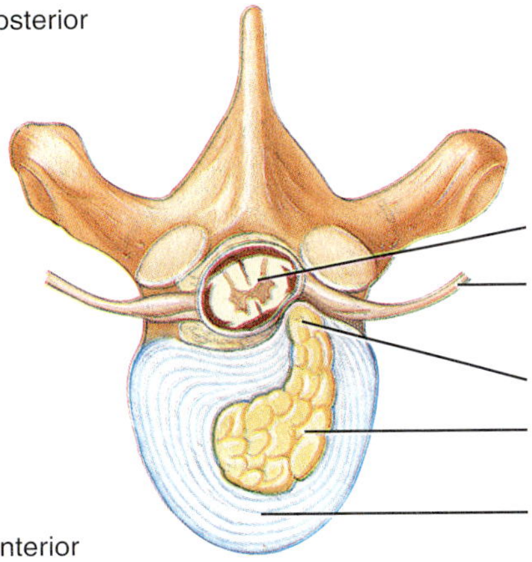

(b) Superior view of herniated disc

(a) Articulated vertebrae
- annulus fibrosus
- intervertebral disc
- intervertebral foramen
- nucleus pulposus

1 ______________________

2 ______________________

3 ______________________

4 ______________________

(b) Herniated disc
- annulus fibrosus
- herniation
- nucleus pulposus

5 ______________________

6 ______________________

7 ______________________

FIGURE 7.20 **Vertebrae.**

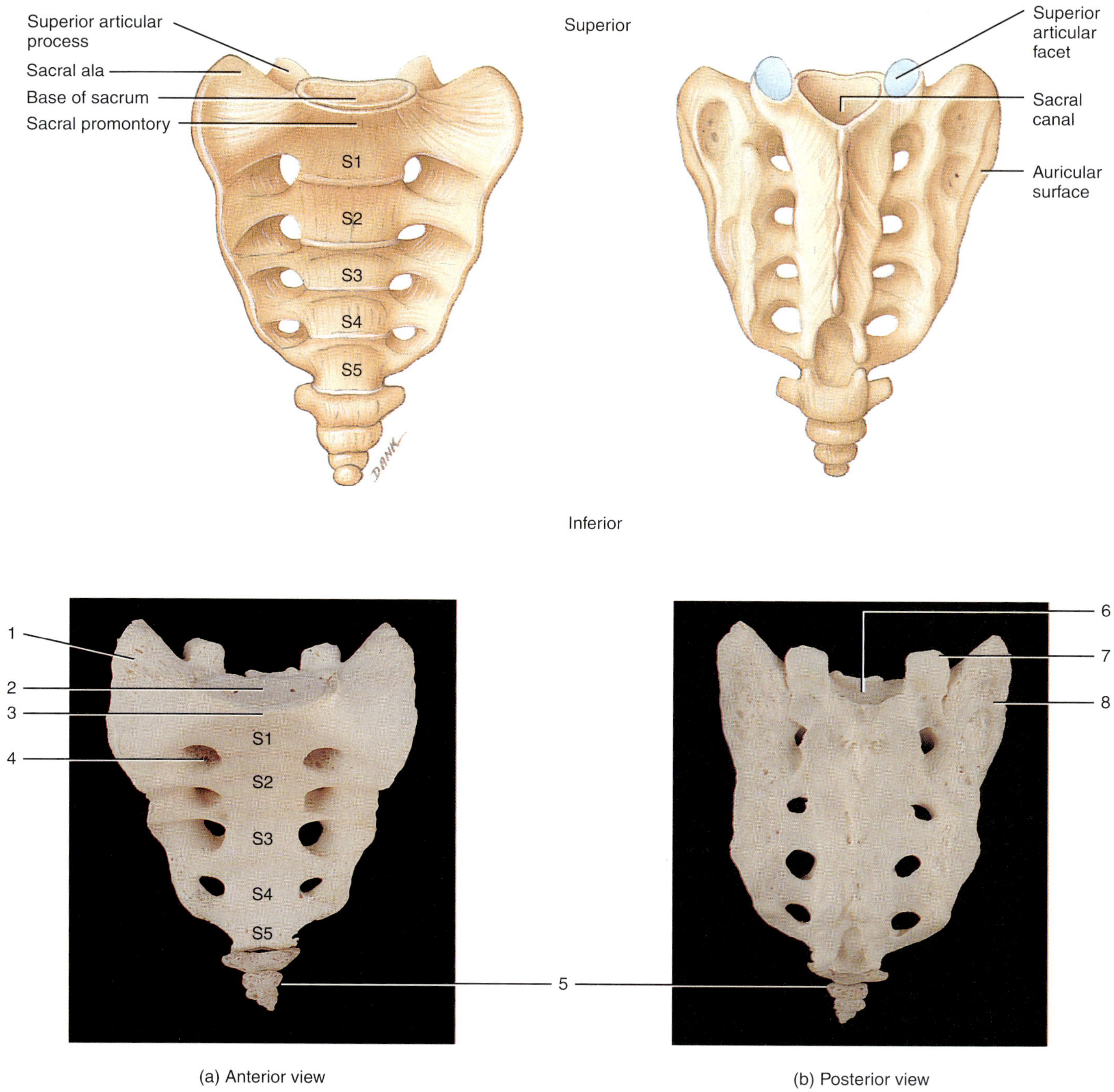

- auricular surface (for sacroiliac joint)
- base
- coccyx
- sacral ala
- sacral canal
- sacral foramen
- sacral promontory
- superior articular facet

1 ______________________

2 ______________________

3 ______________________

4 ______________________

5 ______________________

6 ______________________

7 ______________________

8 ______________________

FIGURE 7.21 **Sacrum and coccyx.**

4. Sacrum and Coccyx

The **sacrum** has a slightly curved, triangular shape and has two **superior articular processes** with facets that articulate with the fifth lumbar vertebra. The sacrum has **sacral foramina** that provide exits for spinal nerves. From the posterior view, the opening of the **sacral canal** is located just posterior to the body of the sacrum and is open all the way through the sacrum. (*Note:* On many plastic models, the sacral canal is closed.) The lateral surfaces of the sacrum, the **auricular surfaces,** are roughened to articulate with the iliac portion of the os coxa on each side, forming **sacroiliac joints.** The **sacral promontory** protrudes anteriorly and is an important landmark in females during labor and delivery. The vertebral column ends with the small **coccyx,** or tailbone. The tiny, fused vertebrae of the coccyx are attached to the sacrum with ligaments.

ACTIVITY 13 Sacrum and Coccyx

1 Locate the parts of the sacrum and coccyx in Figure 7.21.

2 Identify these structures on a model of the sacrum and coccyx.

3 Pronounce the terms as you point to them on the model.

5. Abnormal Spinal Curvatures

Three abnormal curves of the vertebral column are scoliosis, kyphosis, and lordosis. The vertebral column bends laterally in **scoliosis** (*scolio-* = crooked). **Kyphosis** is an exaggerated thoracic curve (kyphotic curvature) that results in a hunched back with rounded shoulders. **Lordosis** is an exaggerated lumbar curve (lordotic curvature) that appears as a sway-back with the abdomen protruding anteriorly.

ACTIVITY 14 Abnormal Curves of the Vertebral Column

Identify the three different types of abnormal curves in Figure 7.22(a), (b), and (c).

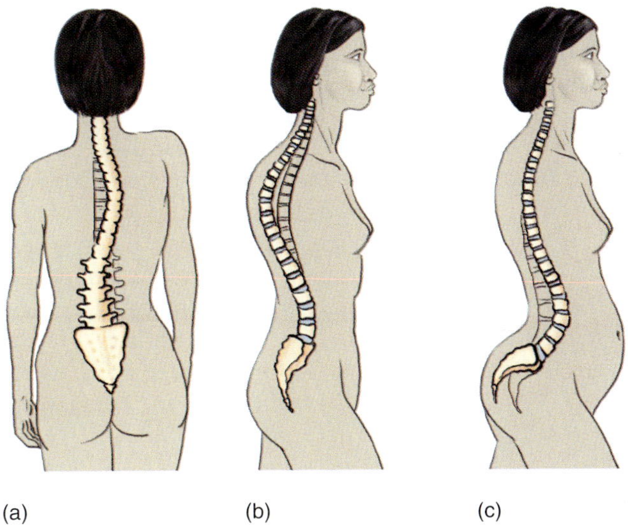

- kyphosis
- lordosis
- scoliosis

a ______________________

b ______________________

c ______________________

FIGURE 7.22 **Abnormal curves of the vertebral column.**

E. Thorax (Thoracic Cage)

The bony cage that encircles the chest is called the **thoracic cage,** or **thorax.** The thorax is composed of the sternum, ribs, costal cartilages, and bodies of the thoracic vertebrae.

The **sternum** is a narrow flat bone that is composed of three fused bones: the manubrium, the body of the sternum, and the xiphoid process. The **manubrium** (handle), the superior portion of the sternum, has a concave superior surface called the **suprasternal notch** or **jugular notch.** Between the **body** of the sternum and the manubrium is the **sternal angle,** an important clinical landmark indicating the second intercostal space. The manubrium and body articulate (*articul-* = pertaining to a joint) with the **costal cartilages** of the **ribs.** The **xiphoid process** (sword-like) is the inferior portion of the sternum that is shaped like a small sword.

There are 12 pairs of **ribs** in both males and females. The first seven pairs are called the **true ribs** or **vertebrosternal ribs** because their **costal (rib) cartilages** (hyaline) have a direct attachment to the sternum. The last five rib pairs (8–12) are called **false ribs.** Rib pairs 8–10 are

vertebrochondral ribs (*vertebro* = ribs; *chondral* = cartilage) because their costal cartilages do not have a direct attachment to the sternum, but attach to the costal cartilage of the seventh rib instead. Rib pairs 11 and 12 do not have any attachment to the sternum or cartilage and are called **floating ribs** or **vertebral ribs.** The space between the ribs is called the **intercostal space.**

The main parts of a rib are the head, neck, tubercle, and body. The **head** projects from the posterior part of the rib and articulates with **demifacets** of the bodies of thoracic vertebrae. The **neck** is the constricted part lateral to the head. The **tubercle** is a small, knoblike projection close to the neck that articulates with the facet of a transverse process. The **body** is the main part of the rib.

ACTIVITY 15 Thoracic Cage and Rib Articulations

1 Locate the parts of the thorax in Figure 7.23.
2 Identify these parts on an articulated thorax or skeleton.
3 Locate the parts of a rib in Figure 7.24(a) and its articulation with vertebrae on Figure 7.24(b) and (c).
4 Identify the four parts of a rib and its articulations on a skeleton.
5 Pronounce the name of each part as you point to it.
6 Palpate as many of these parts as you can on your body.

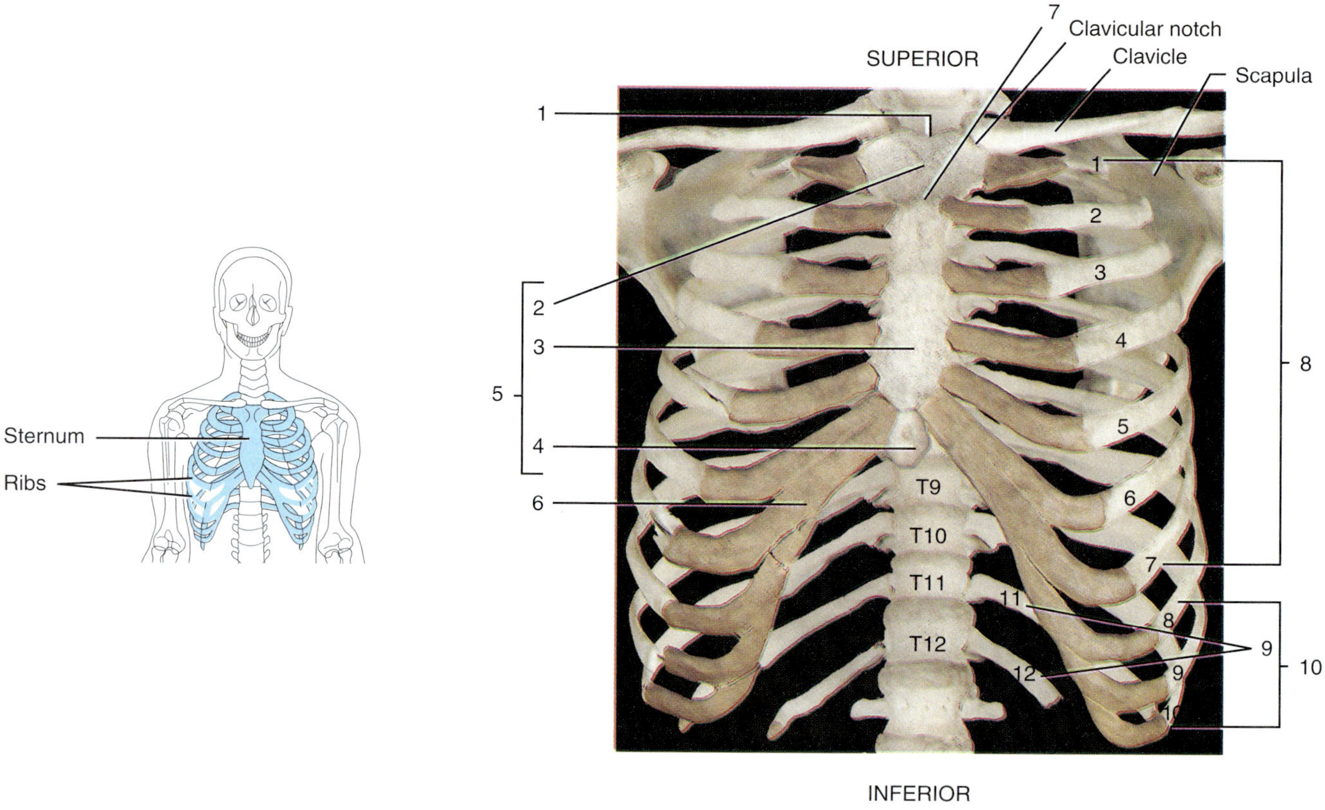

- body of sternum
- costal cartilage
- false ribs
- floating ribs
- manubrium
- sternal angle
- sternum
- suprasternal notch (jugular notch)
- true ribs
- xiphoid process

1 ____________ 6 ____________

2 ____________ 7 ____________

3 ____________ 8 ____________

4 ____________ 9 ____________

5 ____________ 10 ____________

FIGURE 7.23 Thoracic cage.

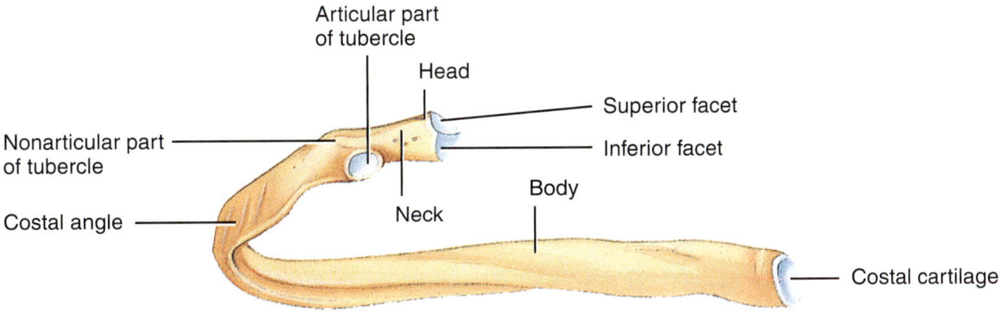

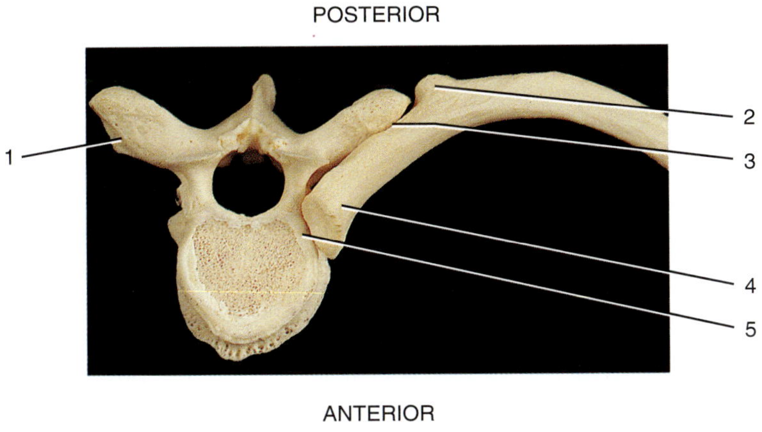

(a) Superior view

(a) Superior view
- articular part of tubercle
- demifacet of vertebra
- facet for articular part of tubercle
- head of rib
- tubercle (nonarticular part)

1 ______________________

2 ______________________

3 ______________________

4 ______________________

5 ______________________

(b) Right lateral view
- body of rib
- head of rib
- inferior demifacet of vertebra
- intervertebral foramen
- superior demifacet of vertebra
- tubercle (nonarticulating)

6 ______________________

7 ______________________

8 ______________________

9 ______________________

10 ______________________

11 ______________________

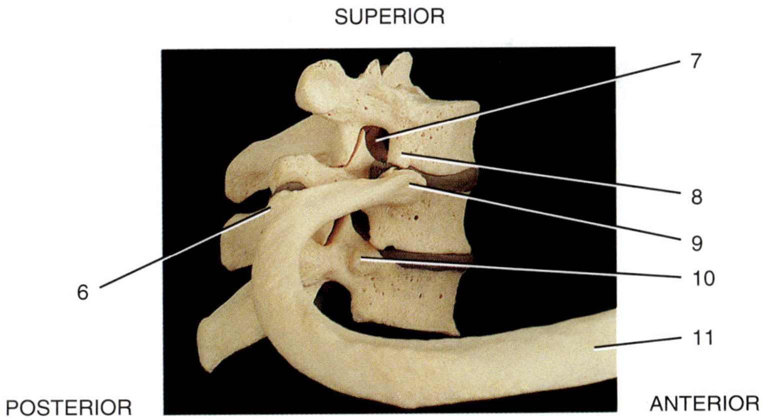

(b) Right lateral view

FIGURE 7.24 **Rib and its articulation with vertebrae.**

Name ______________________ Date ______________ Section ________________

EXERCISE 7

REVIEWING YOUR KNOWLEDGE

A. Bone Surface Markings

Name the depression, opening, process, or projection that describes the definition.

1. ______________________ Tubelike opening
2. ______________________ Rounded articular process
3. ______________________ Opening or hole through a bone (oval or round)
4. ______________________ Shallow depression
5. ______________________ Branchlike process
6. ______________________ Narrow slit or cleft in bone

B. Bones and Bone Surface Markings

Identify the cranial bones that have the following bone markings.

1. ______________________ middle nasal concha
2. ______________________ foramen magnum
3. ______________________ alveoli (2 bones)
4. ______________________ sella turcica
5. ______________________ external auditory meatus
6. ______________________ crista galli
7. ______________________ greater wing
8. ______________________ mastoid process
9. ______________________ occipital condyle
10. ______________________ optic foramen

C. Skull Bones and Bone Markings

Identify the bones and bone markings in Figure 7.25, anterior view of skull.

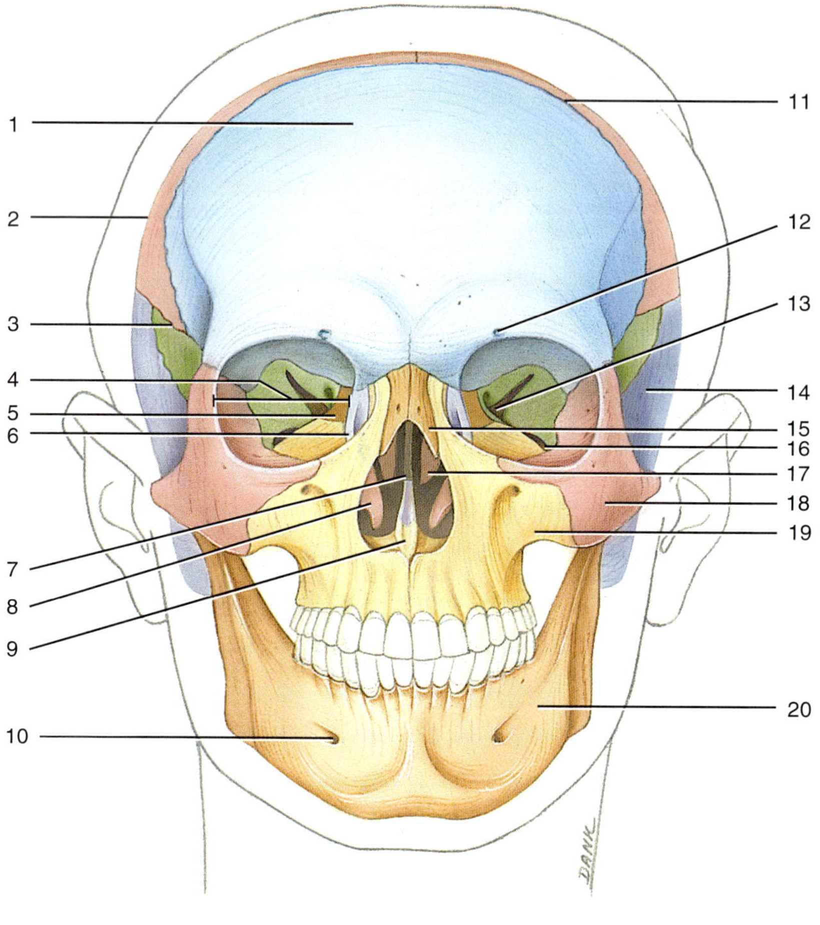

FIGURE 7.25 Anterior view of skull.

1. ______________________
2. ______________________
3. ______________________
4. ______________________
5. ______________________
6. ______________________
7. ______________________
8. ______________________
9. ______________________
10. ______________________
11. ______________________
12. ______________________
13. ______________________
14. ______________________
15. ______________________
16. ______________________
17. ______________________
18. ______________________
19. ______________________
20. ______________________

D. Skull Bones and Bone Markings, Lateral View

Identify the bones and bone markings in Figure 7.26, lateral view of skull.

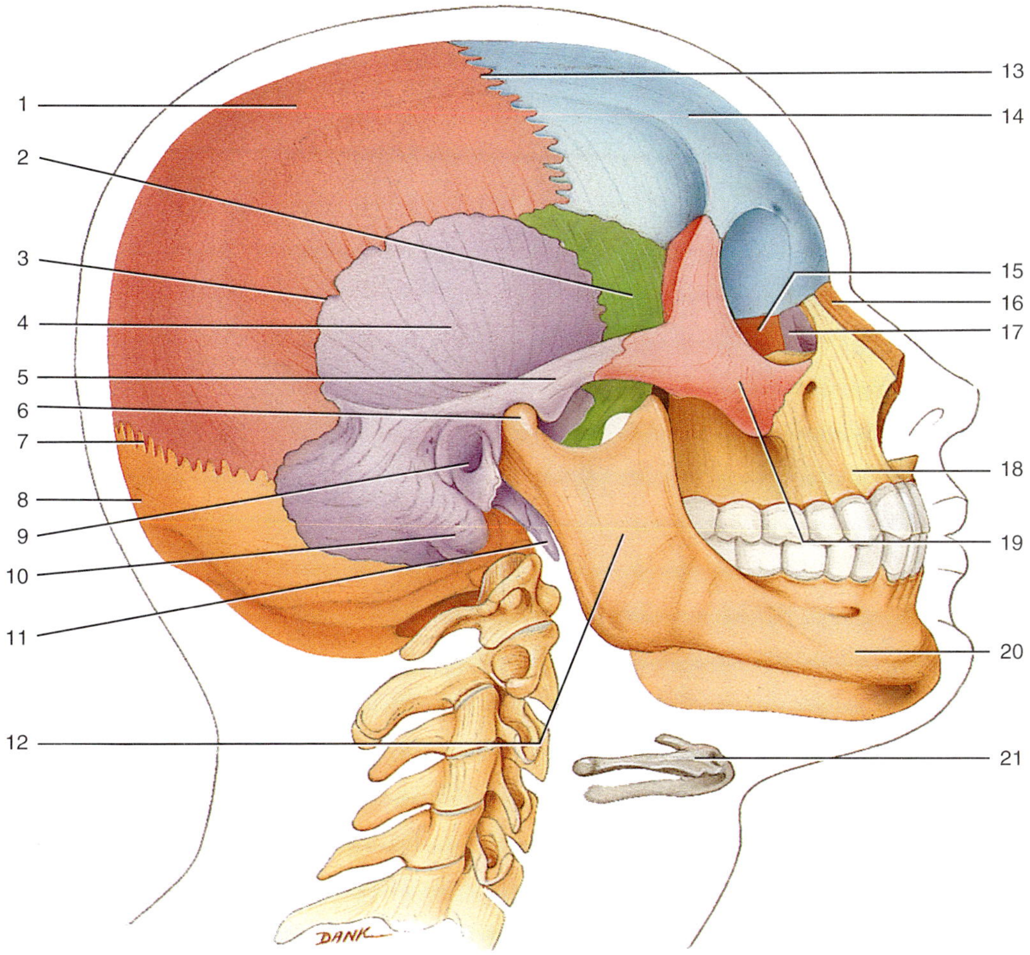

FIGURE 7.26 Right lateral view of skull.

1. ______________________
2. ______________________
3. ______________________
4. ______________________
5. ______________________
6. ______________________
7. ______________________
8. ______________________
9. ______________________
10. ______________________
11. ______________________
12. ______________________
13. ______________________
14. ______________________
15. ______________________
16. ______________________
17. ______________________
18. ______________________
19. ______________________
20. ______________________
21. ______________________

E. Skull Bones and Bone Markings, Inferior View of Skull

Identify the bones and bone markings in Figure 7.27, inferior view of skull.

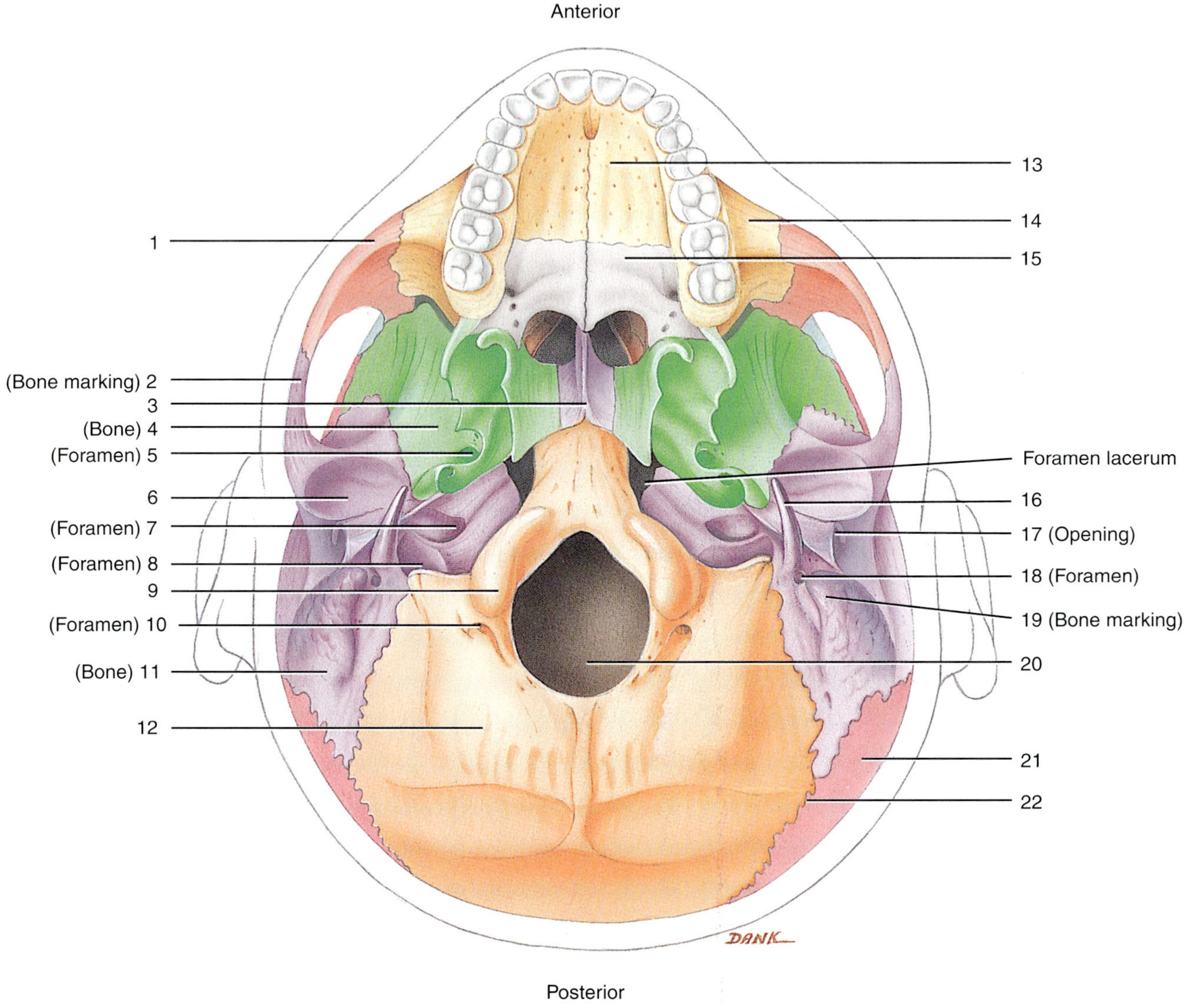

FIGURE 7.27 Inferior view of skull.

1. ______________
2. ______________
3. ______________
4. ______________
5. ______________
6. ______________
7. ______________
8. ______________
9. ______________
10. ______________
11. ______________
12. ______________
13. ______________
14. ______________
15. ______________
16. ______________
17. ______________
18. ______________
19. ______________
20. ______________
21. ______________
22. ______________

F. Skull Bones and Bone Markings, Superior View of Floor of Cranium

Identify the bones and bone markings in Figure 7.28, superior view of floor of cranium.

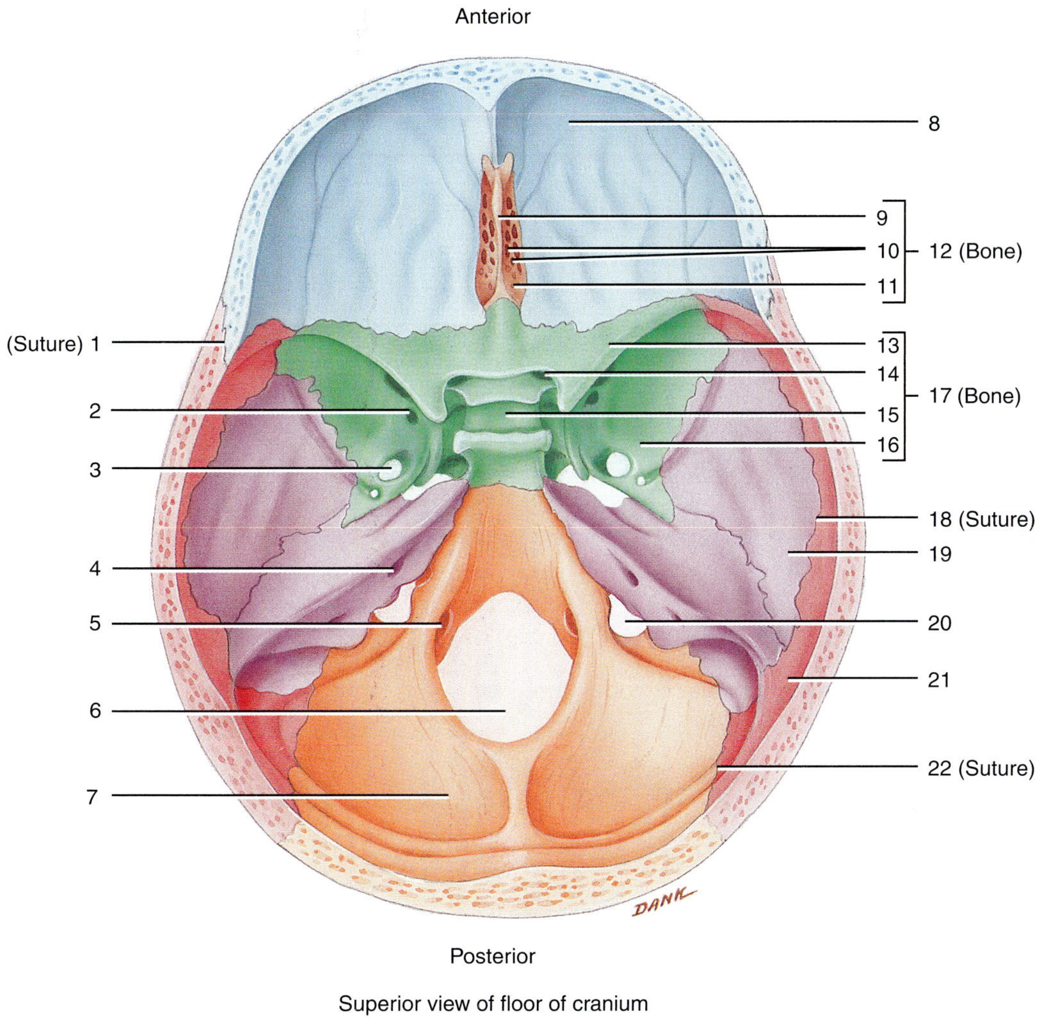

FIGURE 7.28 **Superior view of floor of cranium.**

1. ______________________
2. ______________________
3. ______________________
4. ______________________
5. ______________________
6. ______________________
7. ______________________
8. ______________________
9. ______________________
10. ______________________
11. ______________________
12. ______________________
13. ______________________
14. ______________________
15. ______________________
16. ______________________
17. ______________________
18. ______________________
19. ______________________
20. ______________________
21. ______________________
22. ______________________

G. Vertebral Column and Thorax

Match the skeletal term with the proper description.

____ 1. Softens jolts to the vertebral column

____ 2. Opening for spinal nerve exit

____ 3. Bony protection for thoracic organs

____ 4. First cervical vertebra

____ 5. Second cervical vertebra

____ 6. Articulates with rib posteriorly

____ 7. Tailbone

____ 8. Encloses and protects the spinal cord

____ 9. Lordotic curvatures

____ 10. Kyphotic curvatures

____ 11. Formed by the fusion of pedicles and lamina

____ 12. Passageway for vertebral arteries in cervical vertebrae

a. atlas
b. axis
c. cervical and lumbar curvatures
d. coccyx
e. intervertebral discs
f. intervertebral foramen
g. thoracic cage
h. thoracic and pelvic curvatures
i. thoracic vertebrae
j. transverse foramen
k. vertebral arch
l. vertebral column

H. Other Major Features of the Axial Skeleton

Identify the major skull feature or structure that is described.

1. ______________________ The suture that joins the occipital bone to the parietal bones.

2. ______________________ The facial bone that contains a paranasal sinus.

3. ______________________ The articulation between the mandible and skull.

4. ______________________ Neck and tongue muscles are attached to this bone.

5. ______________________ This structure allows the baby's cranium to compress during childbirth.

6. ______________________ A special feature present on the transverse process of cervical vertebrae.

7. ______________________ Special features present on thoracic vertebrae for rib articulations.

8. ______________________ A part of the rib that articulates with the body of the thoracic vertebrae.

9. ______________________ A part of the rib that articulates with the transverse process of the thoracic vertebrae.

10. ______________________ The odontoid process is a part of which bone?

11. ______________________ Name the superior bone of the nasal septum.

12. ______________________ Name the inferior bone of the nasal septum.

Name ______________________ Date ______________ Section ______________

EXERCISE 7

USING YOUR KNOWLEDGE

A. Identifying Bones and Bone Markings on Radiographs

Identify structures in Figure 7.29(a).

1. ______________________ (bone marking)
2. ______________________ (bone)
3. ______________________ (bone)
4. ______________________ (bone)
5. ______________________ (bone)

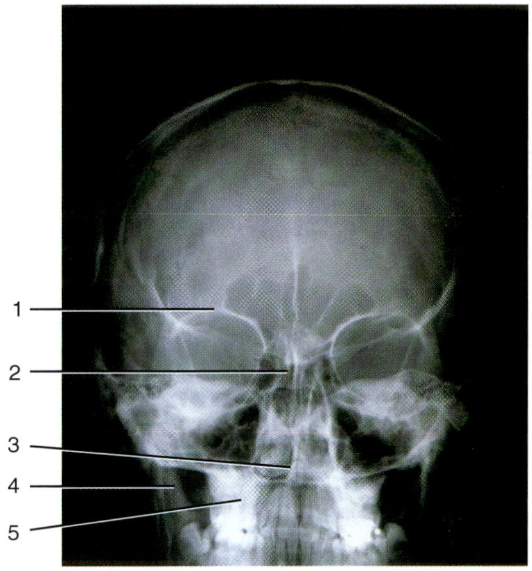

(a) Anterior view of skull

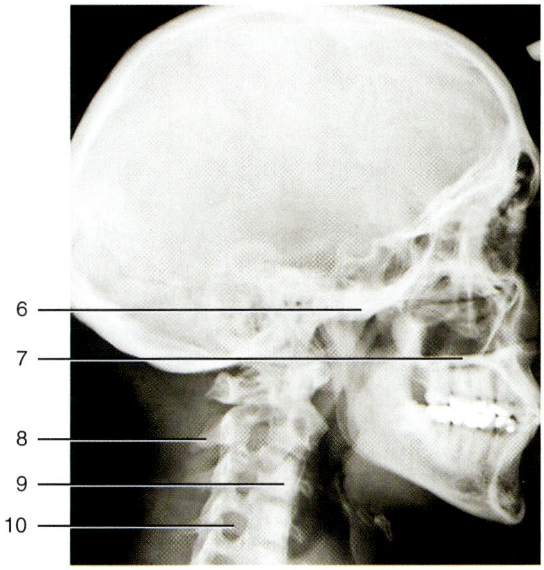

(b) Lateral view of skull and vertebral column.

Identify the structures in Figure 7.29(b).

6. ______________________ (bone marking)
7. ______________________ (bone marking)
8. ______________________ (bone marking)
9. ______________________ (bone marking)
10. ______________________ (space between bones)

FIGURE 7.29 Radiographs.

B. Identifying Bones and Bone Markings on CT Scans

Identify the structures in Figure 7.30(a), CT of lateral view of skull.

11. ______________________ (bone)

12. ______________________ (bone)

13. ______________________ (sinus)

14. ______________________ (bone marking in sphenoid)

15. ______________________ (opening)

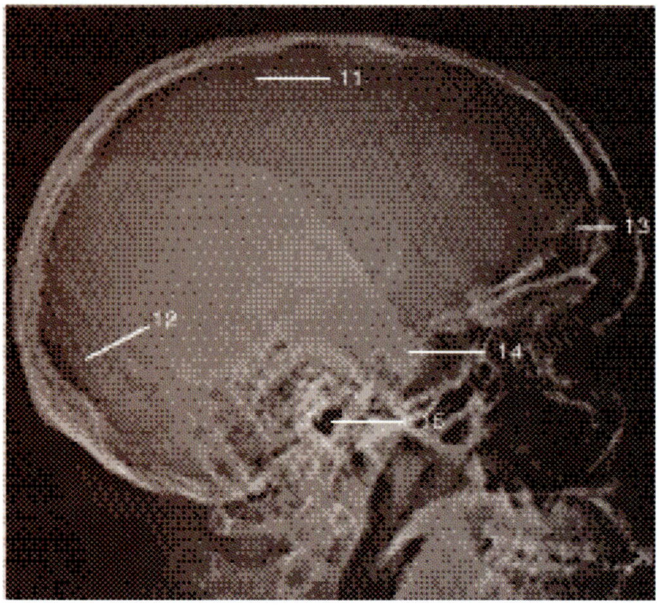

(a) Lateral view of skull.

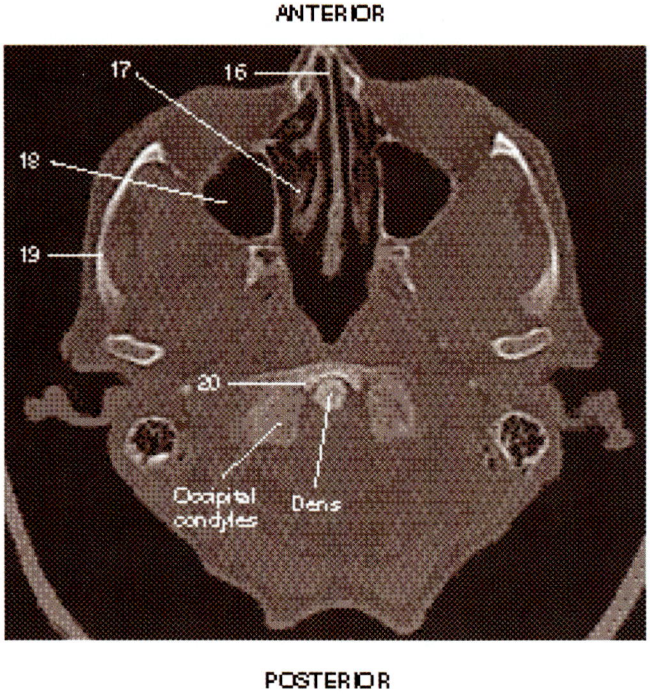

(b) Transverse section through skull at the level of the altas.

Identify the structures in Figure 7.30(b).

16. ______________________ (bone marking)

17. ______________________ (bone marking)

18. ______________________ (bone sinus)

19. ______________________ (bone marking)

20. ______________________ (bone)

FIGURE 7.30 CT scans.

EXERCISE 8

APPENDICULAR SKELETON

OUTLINE

OBJECTIVES

- Identify the principal bone markings of the pectoral (shoulder) girdle and the upper limb
- Describe the articulation of the pectoral girdle with the humerus
- Describe the articulation of the humerus with the forearm bones
- Identify the bone markings of the pelvic girdle and the lower limbs
- Describe the articulation of the bones of the pelvic girdle with the femur
- Describe the articulation of the femur with the leg bones

MATERIALS

- articulated skeleton
- disarticulated skeleton

The **appendicular skeleton** (*appendere* = to add something) has larger bones than the axial skeleton and bears more weight. The bones of this division are separated into four main areas: the **pectoral girdles** (*pectus* = breast; *girdle* = any curved structure), the **upper limbs** or **extremities** (*extremetas* = arm or leg), the **pelvic girdle** (*pelvis* = basin), and the **lower limbs** or **extremities**. The bone markings include sites of muscle attachment and articulations with other bones to form a joint. Bone surface markings that pertain to the appendicular skeleton are given in Table 8.1.

A. Pectoral Girdle

There are two pectoral girdles and each attaches an upper limb to the axial skeleton. Each **pectoral** (or shoulder) **girdle** is composed of a **scapula** (shoulder blade) and a **clavicle** (*clavicle* = key).

1. Bones and Selected Bone Markings of the Pectoral Girdle

Clavicle (Collar Bone)

- **sternal extremity** – blunt, medial end
- **acromial extremity** (*acrom-* = topmost) – broader, flat, roughened, lateral end

Scapula (Shoulder Blade)

- **spine** – sharp ridge located on posterior side
- **acromion** – flattened process at lateral end of spine
- **glenoid cavity** (*glene* = joint socket) or **fossa** – depression inferior to acromion
- **coracoid process** (*coracoid* = crow's beak) – superior and medial to glenoid cavity
- **supraspinous fossa** (*supra-* = above; *spinous* = spine) – depression superior to spine
- **infraspinous fossa** (*infra-* = below) – depression inferior to spine
- **subscapular fossa** (*sub-* = under) – depression on anterior surface of scapula
- **lateral** or **axillary border** – thicker edge near axilla
- **medial** or **vertebral border** – thinner edge near vertebral column

The acromial end of the clavicle articulates with the acromion (acromial process) of the scapula laterally, forming the pectoral girdle. The sternal end of the clavicle articulates with the manubrium of the sternum medially, attaching the pectoral girdle to the axial skeleton. The scapula does not articulate directly with the axial skeleton, but is attached to it with muscles.

ACTIVITY 1 Bones of the Pectoral Girdle

1 Identify the parts of the clavicle and scapula in Figure 8.1.

2 Locate these parts on disarticulated bones.

3 Pronounce the terms as you point to them.

4 Palpate these parts on your own body: clavicle, acromion (process), spine of scapula, and muscles located in the supraspinous and infraspinous fossae.

TABLE 8.1 Selected Bone Surface Markings of the Appendicular Skeleton

MARKING	DESCRIPTION	PURPOSE
Processes		
1. Crest	Prominent ridge	muscle attachment
2. Condyle	Smooth, rounded articular process	articulation
3. Epicondyle	Projection above a condyle	muscle attachment
4. Foramen	Opening or hole	opening for blood vessels and nerves
5. Fossa	Shallow depression	muscle attachment or articulation
6. Head	Rounded articular projection supported on the neck of a bone.	articulation
7. Line	Long, narrow ridge (less prominent than a crest)	muscle attachment
8. Trochanter	Very large projection	muscle attachment
9. Tubercle	Small, rounded projection	muscle attachment
10. Tuberosity	Large, roughened projection	muscle attachment

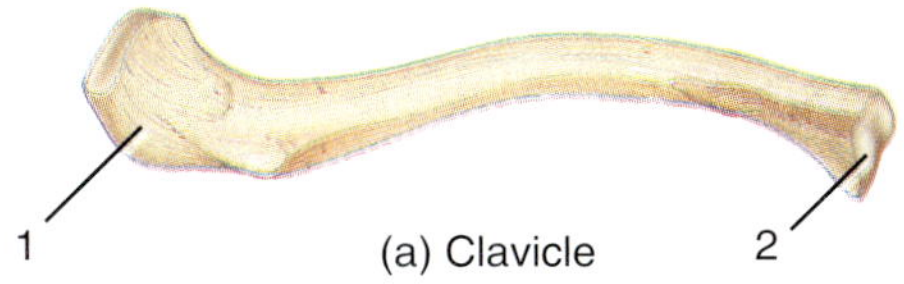

(a) Clavicle

(a) Clavicle
- acromial end (a-CROHM-ee-al)
- sternal end

1 ______________________________

2 ______________________________

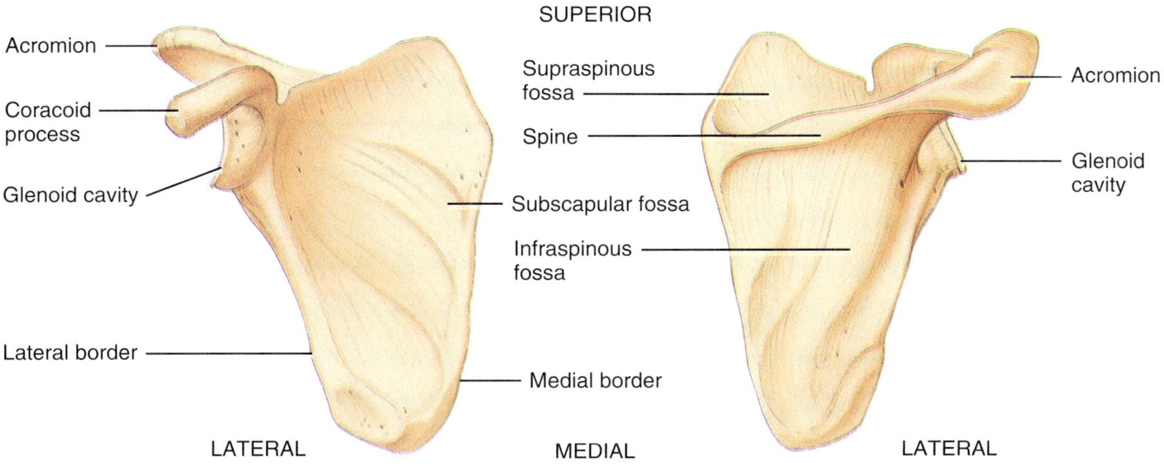

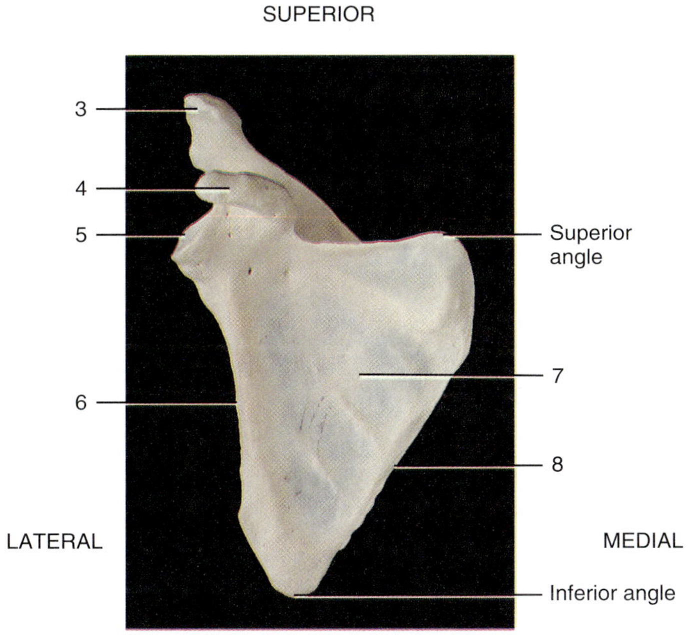

(b) Scapula, anterior view

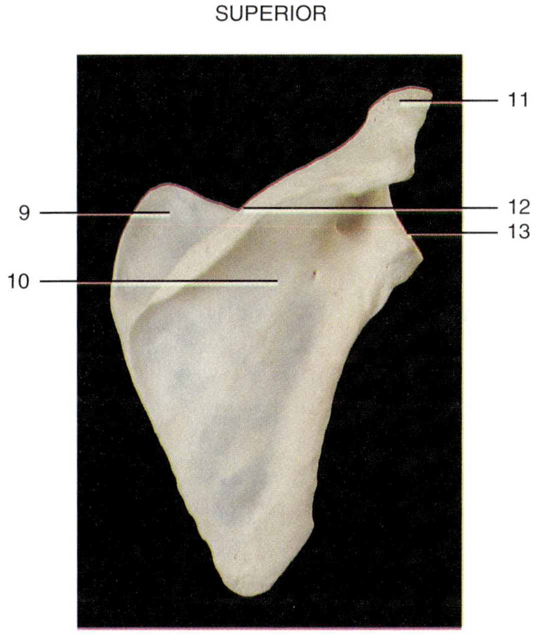

(c) Scapula, posterior view

(b) Scapula, anterior view
- acromion or acromial process (a-CROW-mee-yon)
- axillary or lateral border (AX-il-lary)
- coracoid process (COR-a-coid)
- glenoid cavity or fossa (GLEN-oid)
- subscapular fossa (sub-SCAP-u-lar)
- vertebral or medial border (ver-TEE-bral)

(c) Scapula, posterior view
- acromion or acromion process
- glenoid cavity
- infraspinous fossa (in-fra-SPINE-us FOS-sa)
- spine of scapula
- supraspinous fossa (su-pra-SPINE-ous)

3 ____________________ 6 ____________________

4 ____________________ 7 ____________________

5 ____________________ 8 ____________________

9 ____________________ 12 ____________________

10 ____________________ 13 ____________________

11 ____________________

FIGURE 8.1 **The right pectoral girdle.**

B. Upper Limb (Extremity)

The upper limb consists of the **humerus, ulna, radius, carpals, metacarpals,** and **phalanges**. Of the 30 bones in each upper limb, 1 is in the arm, 2 in the forearm, and the other 27 are in the hand.

1. Bones and Selected Bone Markings of the Arm and Forearm

Humerus (Arm Bone)

- **head** – rounded, proximal end
- **anatomical neck** – constriction immediately distal to head
- **greater tubercle** (*tuber* = swelling) – lateral projection distal to anatomical neck
- **lesser tubercle** – smaller, anterior projection distal to anatomical neck
- **surgical neck** – constriction distal to the tubercles
- **deltoid tuberosity** – raised area between the proximal and distal ends of humerus
- **trochlea** (*trochlea* = pulley) – spool-shaped medial condyle on distal end
- **capitulum** (*caput* = head) – rounded, knob-like condyle lateral to trochlea
- **medial epicondyle** (*epi-* = upon) – rough projection above trochlea
- **lateral epicondyle** – rough projection above capitulum; smaller than medial epicondyle
- **coronoid fossa** (*corona* = crown) – shallow anterior depression on distal end
- **olecranon fossa** (*olekranon* = tip of the elbow) – largest depression on posterior, distal end

Ulna (Medial bone of forearm)

- **olecranon** – large, curved lip-like projection on posterior side of proximal end
- **coronoid process** – smaller, curved lip-like projection on anterior side of proximal end; distal to olecranon
- **trochlear notch** – deep, curved area between olecranon and coronoid process
- **styloid process** (*stylos* = pole; *-oid* = like) – slender, pointed projection on distal end

Radius (Lateral bone of forearm)

- **head** – flat, disc-shaped proximal end
- **styloid process** – slender, pointed projection; distal end

The shoulder joint that connects the upper limb to the pectoral girdle is formed by the head of the humerus (*humeri* = shoulder), articulating with the glenoid cavity of the scapula. The olecranon and coronoid process of the ulna fit into the olecranon and coronoid fossae of the humerus. The trochlea of the humerus articulates with the trochlear notch of the ulna. The head of the radius articulates with the capitulum of the humerus at the elbow joint and with the radial notch of the ulna at the proximal radioulnar joint.

ACTIVITY 2 The Upper Limb Bones and Bone Markings

1 Identify the parts of the humerus on Figure 8.2a and Figure 8.2b, and the ulna and radius on Figure 8.3a and Figure 8.3b.

2 Locate these bones and their bone markings on disarticulated bones.

3 Pronounce the terms as you point to them.

4 Palpate the following bone parts on your own body: medial and lateral epicondyle of the humerus and olecranon of the ulna.

(a) Anterior view
- anatomical neck
- capitulum (ca-PIT-u-lum)
- coronoid fossa (COR-a-noid)
- deltoid tuberosity (DEL-toid tu-ber-OS-ity)
- greater tubercle (TU-ber-cul)
- head
- intertubercular groove (in-ter-tu-BER-cue-lar)
- lateral epicondyle (epi-CON-dile)
- lesser tubercle
- medial epicondyle
- trochlea (TRO-clee-a)

1 ______________________

2 ______________________

3 ______________________

4 ______________________

5 ______________________

6 ______________________

7 ______________________

8 ______________________

9 ______________________

10 ______________________

11 ______________________

(b) Posterior view
- lateral epicondyle
- medial epicondyle
- olecranon fossa (o-LEH-cra-non)

12 ______________________

13 ______________________

14 ______________________

FIGURE 8.2 Right humerus.

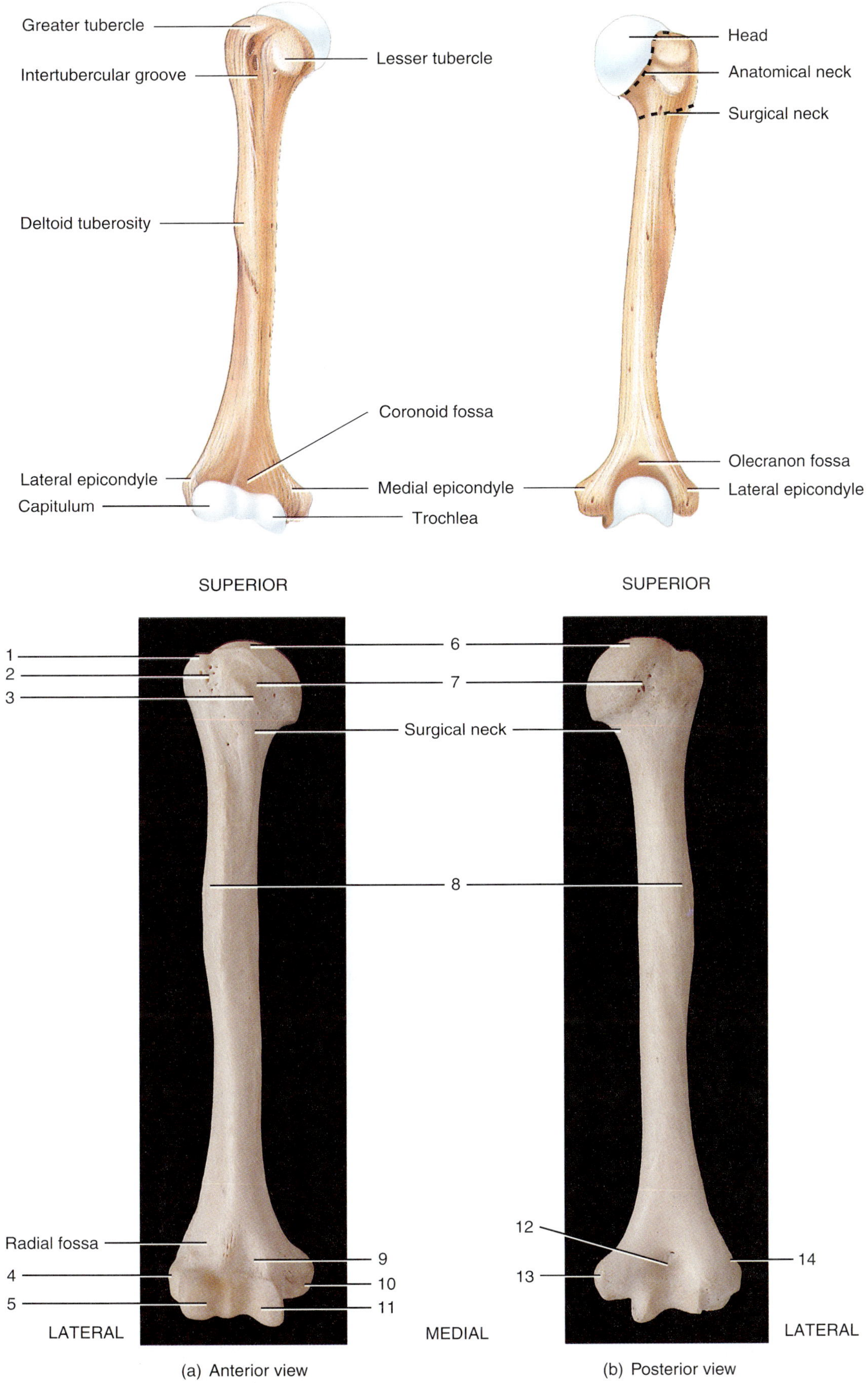

FIGURE 8.2 **Right humerus,** ***continued.***

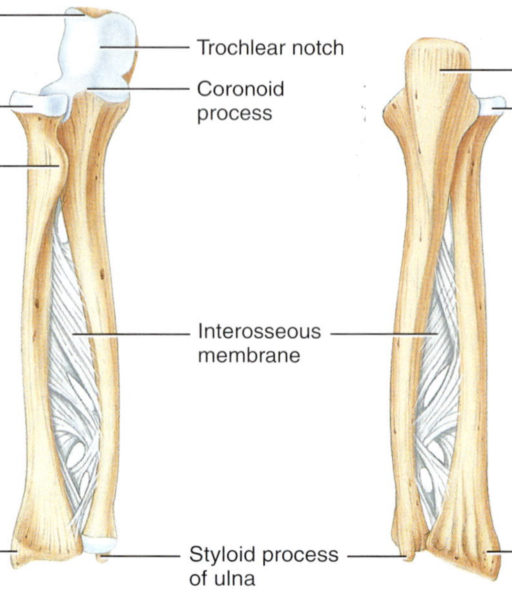

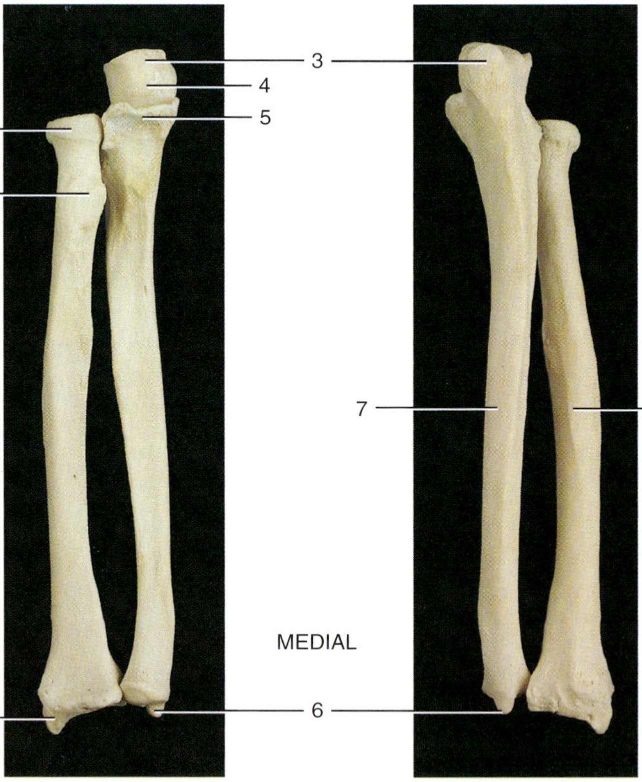

(a) Anterior view (b) Posterior view

(a) Anterior view
- coronoid process
- head of radius
- olecranon (process)
- styloid process of radius (STY-loid)
- styloid process of ulna
- trochlear notch (semilunar)

(b) Posterior view
- radius
- ulna

1 ______________________ 4 ______________________

2 ______________________ 5 ______________________ 7 ______________________

3 ______________________ 6 ______________________ 8 ______________________

FIGURE 8.3 Right ulna and radius.

2. Bones of the Hand: Carpals, Metacarpals, and Phalanges

Carpus (Wrists)

The carpus is composed of eight short bones of the wrist, the **carpal** bones, that are lined up to form a proximal and a distal row of bones. Two of the carpal bones articulate with the radius, but there is no articulation of the carpal bones with the ulna.

Metacarpus (Palm of Hand)

The metacarpus is composed of five **metacarpal** bones that make up the palm of the hand. They are numbered as Roman numerals I–V from the metacarpal of the thumb (lateral side) to the little finger side. The metacarpals articulate with the carpals proximally and with the phalanges distally.

Phalanges (Fingers)

The phalanges (phalanx, singular) make up the fingers or digits. They are also numbered I–V from the thumb to little finger. The thumb has two phalanges, proximal and distal. Digits II through V each have **proximal, middle,** and **distal phalanges** (*phalanges* = line of soldiers).

ACTIVITY 3 Bones of the Hand

1. Identify the parts of the hand on Figure 8.4.
2. Locate the bones of the hand on an articulated hand or skeleton.
3. Pronounce the terms as you point to them.

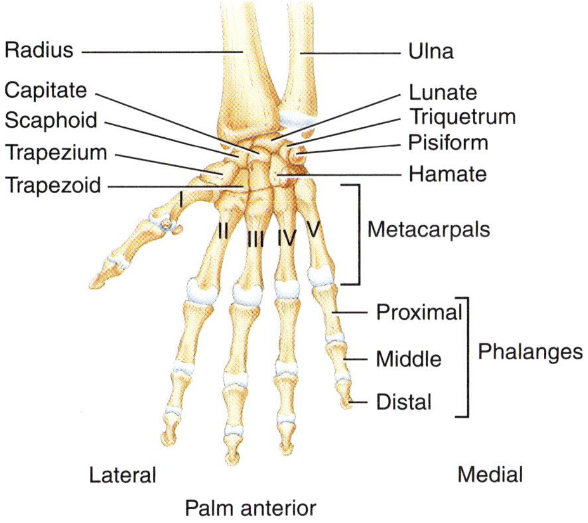

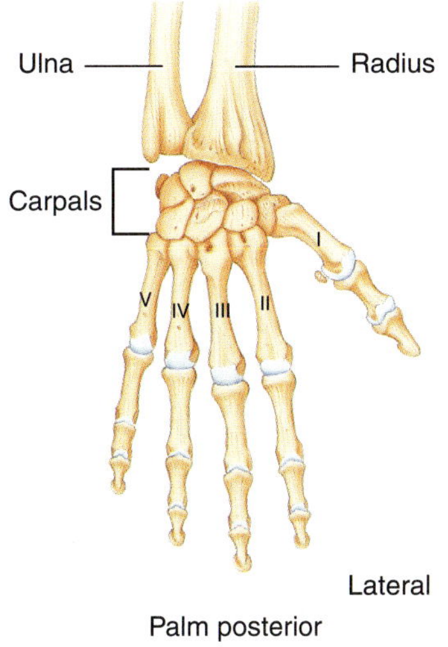

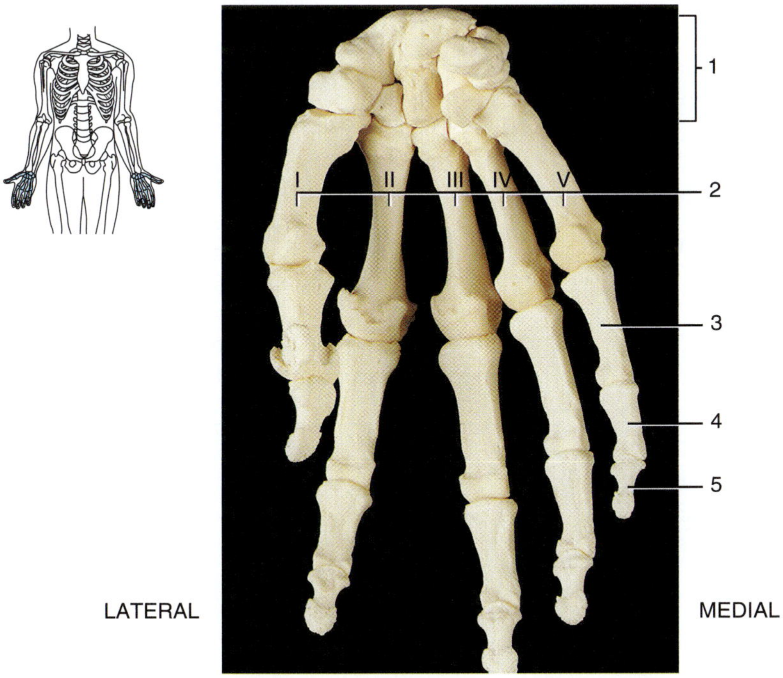

- carpals (CAR-puls)
- distal phalanx (FAY-lanx)
- metacarpals (meta-CAR-pul)
- middle phalanx
- proximal phalanx

1 ______________________

2 ______________________

3 ______________________

4 ______________________

5 ______________________

FIGURE 8.4 Right hand and wrist.

C. Pelvic Girdle

The **pelvic girdle** (*pelvis* = basin) is composed of two hip or coxal bones called the **os coxae** (*os-* = bone; *cox-* = hip) that attach the lower limb to the axial skeleton. Each **os coxae** is formed by the fusion of three separate bones: the **ilium** (*ilia* = flank), **ischium** (*ishion* = hip joint), and **pubis** (*pub-* = grown up or adult) bones. These three bones are identifiable as separate bones in children.

1. Bones and Selected Bone Markings of the Pelvic Girdle

Os coxa

ilium – largest and most superior of the 3 components of os coxa

- **iliac crest** – superior border of ilium
- **anterior superior iliac spine** – anterior end of iliac crest
- **greater sciatic notch** – large notch on posterior side
- **iliac fossa** – depression on anterior surface

ischium – inferior, posterior portion of os coxa

- **ischial tuberosity** – large, roughened projection on posterior and inferior edge
- **ischial spine** – posterior projection between greater and lesser sciatic notches
- **lesser sciatic notch** – smaller indentation between ischial spine and ischial tuberosity

pubis – anterior, inferior portion of os coxa

- **pubic symphysis** (*symphysis* = growing together) – joint where the 2 pubic bones join anteriorly

bone markings formed by ilium, ischium and pubis

- **acetabulum** (*acetabulum* = little saucer) – deep indentation or cup for head of the femur
- **obturator foramen** – largest foramen in the skeleton

Pelvis

- **pelvic brim** – divides the false pelvis from the true pelvis; begins at the sacral promontory and extends laterally and inferiorly to end at the pubic symphysis
- **false pelvis** – portion of pelvis superior to pelvic brim; wide area extending to top of iliac crest
- **true pelvis** – portion of pelvis inferior to pelvic brim; surrounds the pelvic cavity
- **pelvic inlet** – superior opening of true pelvis; bordered by pelvic brim
- **pelvic outlet** – inferior opening of true pelvis; bordered by the coccyx, ischial spine, and ischial tuberosities

The **hip** or **coxal joint** is formed by the acetabulum articulating with the head of the femur to form a ball and socket joint. There is a strong ligament that connects these two structures deep inside the joint itself. When articulated os coxae are united posteriorly with the sacrum at the **sacroiliac joints** (*sacro-* = sacrum; *iliac* = ilium), they form the bony **pelvis** and the connection of the lower extremity with the axial skeleton.

There are definite anatomical differences between the male and female pelves (plural). The bones of the male are typically heavier and rougher, with larger bone markings than the, female. The **male pelvis** is more vertical and narrower, has a pelvic inlet that is heart-shaped, and has a 90° or less pubic arch angle. The **female pelvis** generally has more space in the true pelvis for childbirth, and her pelvis is tilted backward and flared. The pelvic inlet is round or oval, and the angle of the pubic arch is generally greater than 100°.

ACTIVITY 4 The Os Coxae and Pelvis

1. Identify the bone markings of the os coxae in Figure 8.5.
2. Locate the markings on a disarticulated os coxa and on an articulated pelvis.
3. Pronounce the terms as you point to them.
4. Palpate the iliac crest, the anterior superior iliac spine, and the pubic symphysis on your own body.
5. Identify the bone markings of the pelvis in Figure 8.6.
6. Locate these markings on an articulated pelvis or skeleton.
7. Identify the differences between male and female pelves on models or articulated skeletons.

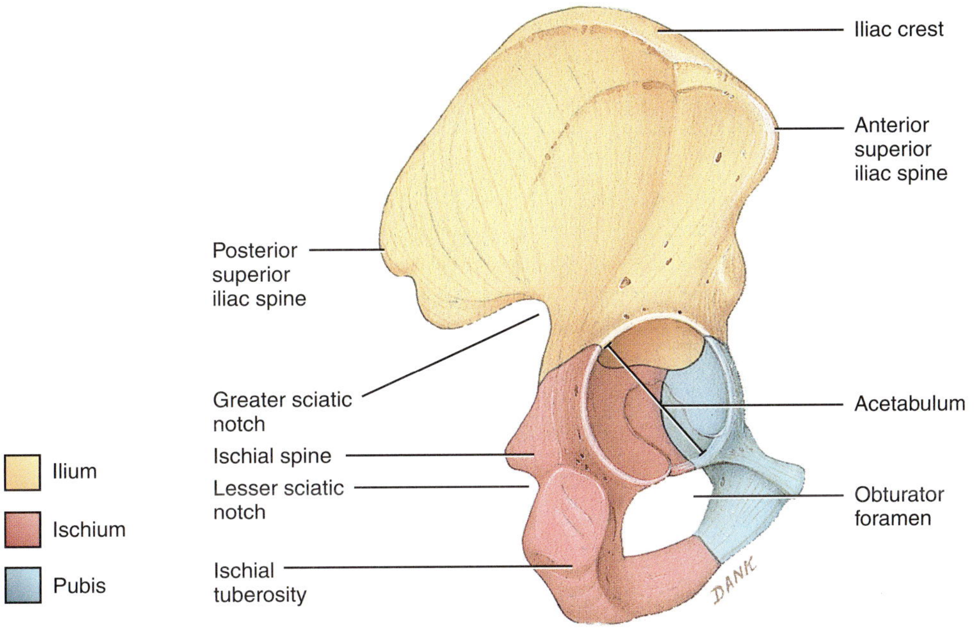

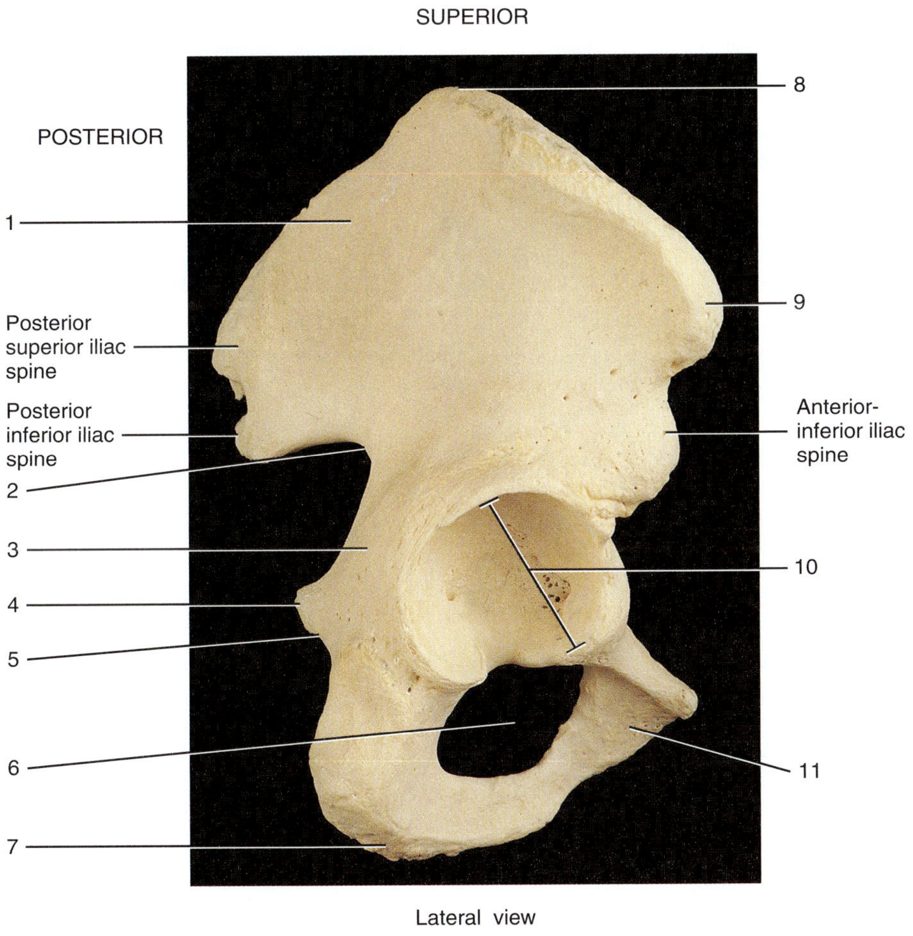

- acetabulum (asa-TAB-u-lum)
- anterior superior iliac spine
- greater sciatic notch (sigh-A-tic)
- iliac crest
- ilium (IL-lee-um)
- ischial spine (ISH-ee-ul)
- ischial tuberosity (tu-ber-OS-ity)
- ischium (ISH-ee-um)
- lesser sciatic notch
- obturator foramen (OB-tur-a-tur for-AY-men)
- pubis (PYU-bis)

1 ______________________

2 ______________________

3 ______________________

4 ______________________

5 ______________________

6 ______________________

7 ______________________

8 ______________________

9 ______________________

10 ______________________

11 ______________________

FIGURE 8.5 Right os coxa.

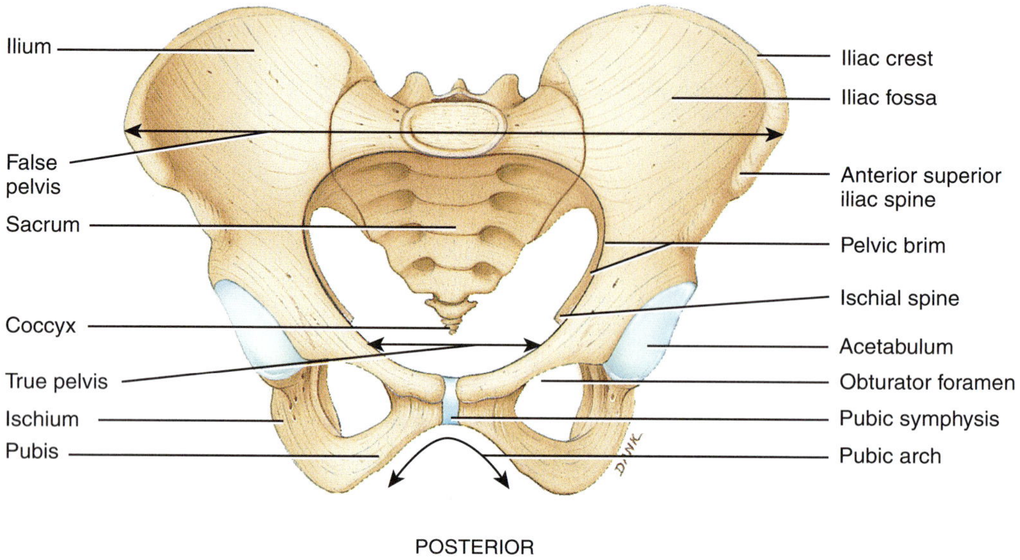

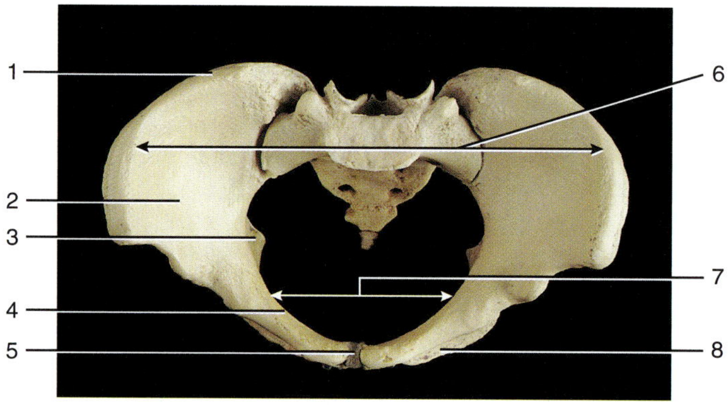

(a) Superior view of female pelvis

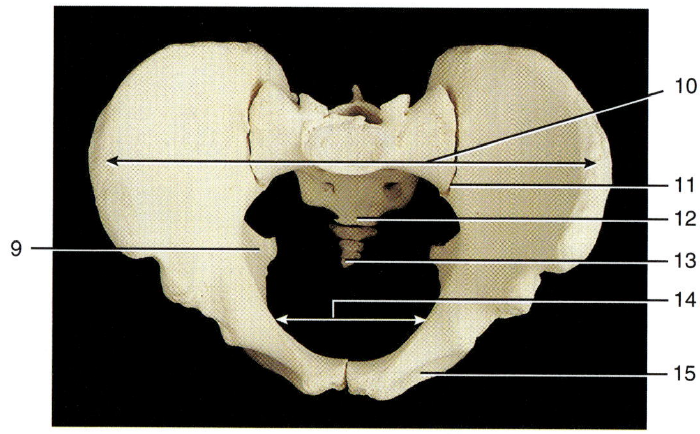

(b) Superior view of male pelvis

(a) Female pelvis

- false pelvis
- iliac crest
- ilium
- ischial spine
- pelvic brim
- pubic symphysis (PYU-bic SYM-fah-sis)
- pubis (PYU-bis)
- true pelvis

(b) Male pelvis

- coccyx (COCK-six)
- false pelvis
- ischial spine
- pubis
- sacroiliac joint (say-crow-ILL-ee-ac)
- sacrum (SAY-crum)
- true pelvis

1 ____________________ 5 ____________________

2 ____________________ 6 ____________________

3 ____________________ 7 ____________________

4 ____________________ 8 ____________________

9 ____________________ 13 ____________________

10 ____________________ 14 ____________________

11 ____________________ 15 ____________________

12 ____________________

FIGURE 8.6 **Pelvis.**

D. Lower Limb (Extremity)

The lower limb includes bones of the **femur, patella, tibia, fibula, tarsals, metatarsals,** and the **phalanges.** Of the 30 bones in each lower limb, 4 are in the thigh and leg, and the other 26 are in the foot.

1. Bones and Selected Bone Markings of the Thigh and Leg

Femur (Thigh Bone)

The femur is the largest and strongest bone in the human skeleton. This bone is bowed anteriorly in a slight curve. Its head articulates with the acetabulum, and the distal end articulates with the tibia and patella.

- **head** – large, rounded knob-like proximal end
- **neck** – narrower, constriction distal to head
- **greater trochanter** (*trochanter* = runner) – large and roughened superior projection; lateral to neck
- **lesser trochanter** – smaller, posterior-medial prominence distal to greater trochanter
- **medial condyle** – rounded, medial process on posterior side of distal end
- **lateral condyle** – similar to medial condyle on lateral side
- **intercondylar fossa** – deep fossa between medial and lateral condyles
- **medial epicondyle** – bump-like projection superior to medial condyle
- **lateral epicondyle** – bump-like projection superior to lateral condyle; a little smaller
- **gluteal tuberosity** – posterior surface of body of femur; roughened projection inferior to lesser trochanter
- **linea aspera** – vertical ridge on posterior surface

Patella (Kneecap)

This small, triangular bone has an anterior surface that is smoother than the posterior surface. Shallow, irregular-shaped articular facets are on the posterior surface that articulate with the condyles of the femur.

Tibia (Leg Bone)

The tibia is the weight-bearing bone of the two leg bones and is medially located. Laterally, the tibia forms a joint with the fibula.

- **medial condyles** – flattened, expanded medial projections on proximal end
- **lateral condyles** – similar to medial condyle on lateral side
- **tibial tuberosity** – large, roughened projection on anterior surface, inferior to condyles
- **anterior border (crest)** – slender ridge on anterior surface
- **medial malleolus** – medial process on distal end, forms medial bump of ankle

Fibula (Leg Bone)

The slender fibula is the lateral leg bone that is important for muscle attachment, but not for bearing weight. The **head** of the fibula is proximal and articulates with the tibia, but not the femur. The **lateral malleolus** is distal and articulates with the talus laterally.

- **head** – proximal end
- **lateral malleolus** – distal end, forms lateral bump of ankle

ACTIVITY 5 Bones and Bone Markings of the Thigh and Leg

1 Identify the bones and bone markings of the femur on Figure 8.7a and Figure 8.7b, and the patella, tibia, and fibula on Figures 8.8a and 8.8b.

2 Locate the bones and bone markings on disarticulated bones as well as on an articulated skeleton.

3 Pronounce the terms as you point to them.

4 Palpate these bone markings on your own body: greater trochanter, medial and lateral epicondyles, patella, head of the fibula, tibial tuberosity, anterior crest (shin) of the tibia and medial malleolus.

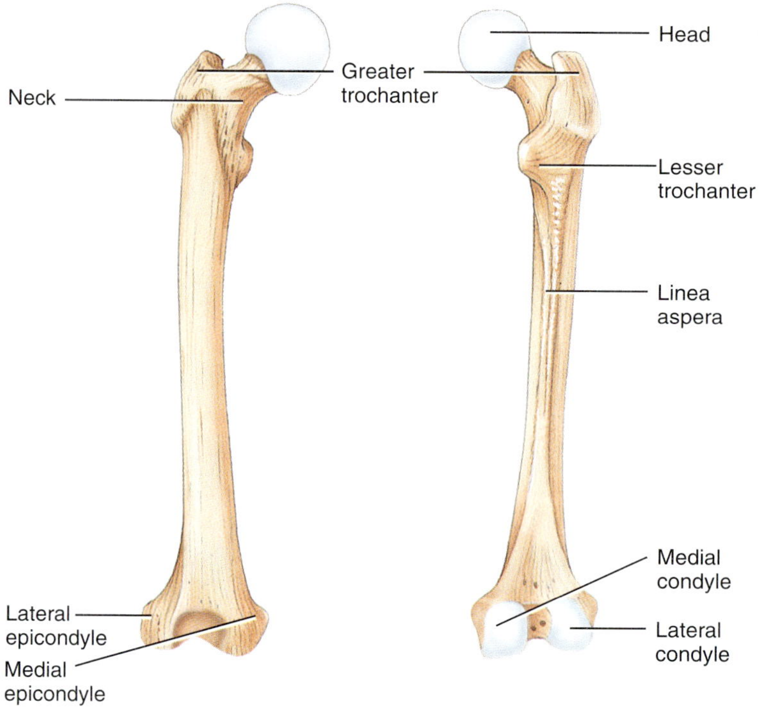

- greater trochanter (tro-CAN-ter)
- head of femur
- lateral condyle (CON-dile)
- lateral epicondyle (epi-CON-dile)
- lesser trochanter
- linea aspera (LIN-ee-uh ASP-er-uh)
- medial condyle
- medial epicondyle
- neck

(a) Anterior view

1 ______________________________

2 ______________________________

3 ______________________________

4 ______________________________

5 ______________________________

6 ______________________________

(b) Posterior view

7 ______________________________

8 ______________________________

9 ______________________________

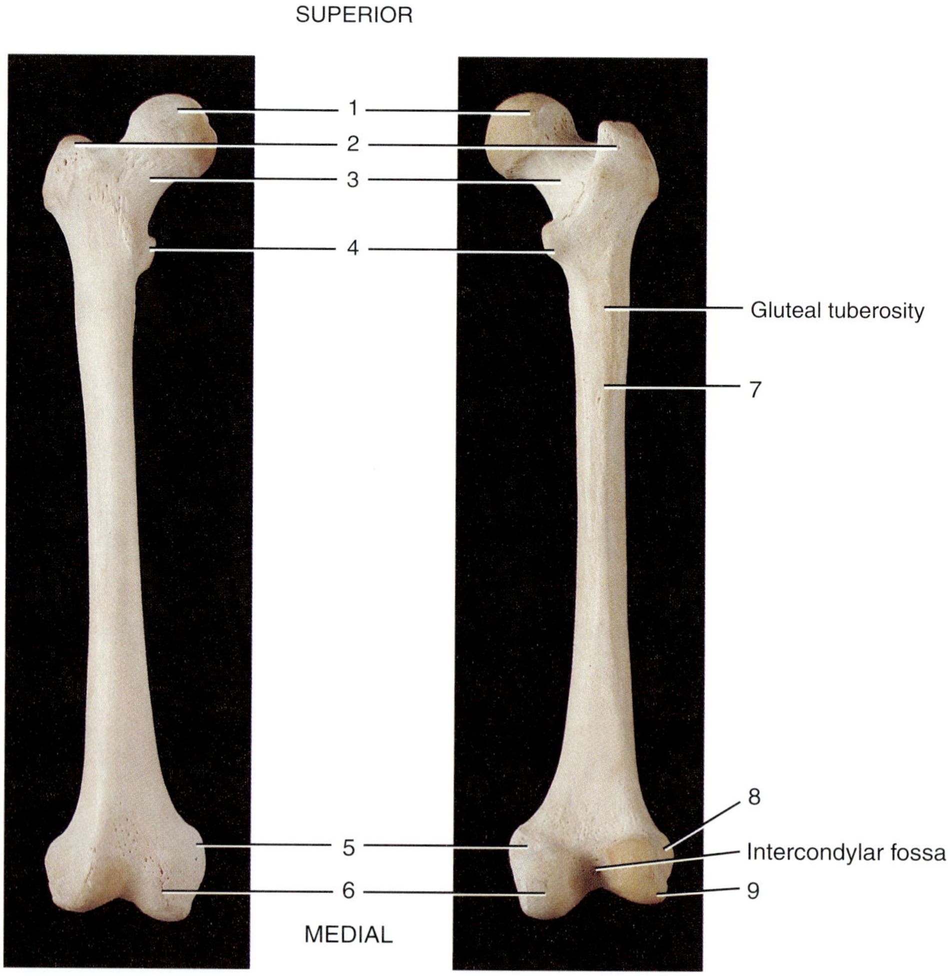

(a) Anterior view (b) Posterior view

FIGURE 8.7 **Right femur.**

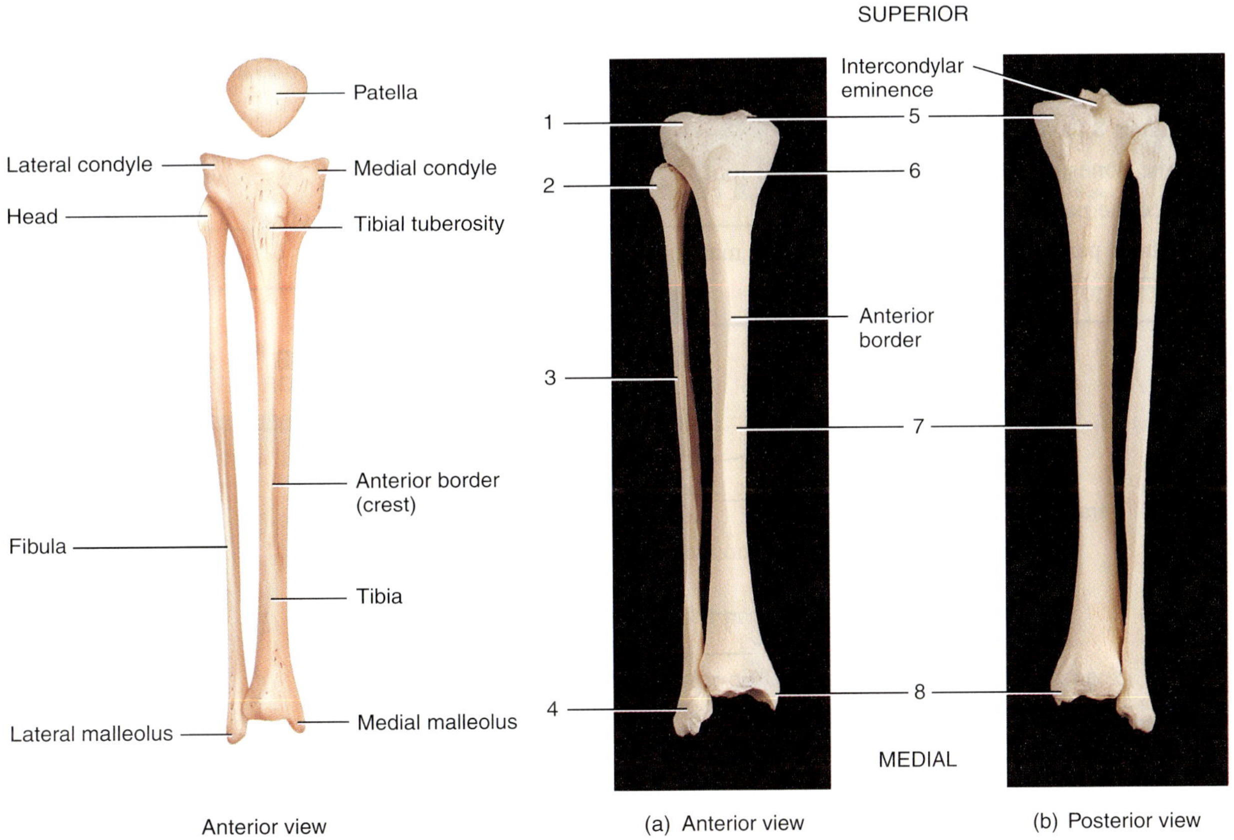

- fibula (FIB-u-la)
- head of fibula
- lateral condyle
- lateral malleolus (mal-LAY-e-lus)
- medial condyle
- medial malleolus
- tibia
- tibial tuberosity

1 ______________________

2 ______________________

3 ______________________

4 ______________________

5 ______________________

6 ______________________

7 ______________________

8 ______________________

FIGURE 8.8 **Right tibia, fibula, and patella.**

2. Bones of the Foot: Tarsals, Metatarsals, and Phalanges

Tarsus (Ankles)

The tarsus is composed of seven tarsal bones of the foot, with two of them being larger than the rest. The largest tarsal bone is the **calcaneus** (*calcaneum* = heel), also known as the heel bone. The other large tarsal bone is the **talus** (*talus* = ankle) that articulates with the tibia.

Metatarsus (Anterior portion of the Instep)

The metatarsus is composed of five metatarsal bones (*meta-* = after or next) that coincide with the metacarpals in the hand. They are numbered the same way, I to V from the great toe to the little toe.

Phalanges (Toes)

The phalanges (toes or digits) are similar to the phalanges in the hand. They are numbered I to V from the great toe to the little toe. The great toe is made of two phalanges (**proximal** and **distal**) and digits II–V have three bones each, **proximal, middle** and **distal phalanges.**

B. Identify the Bones and Bone Markings on Surface Anatomy Photographs

Figure 8.13a Surface anatomy of the upper limb.

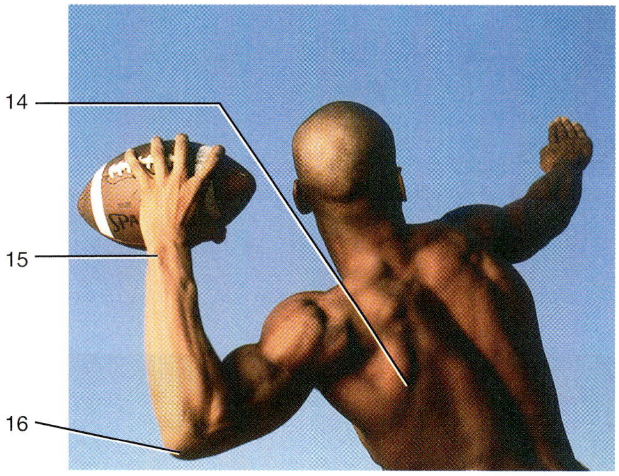

14. ________________ (bone marking)

15. ________________ (bone marking)

16. ________________ (bone marking)

FIGURE 8.13a Surface anatomy of the upper limb and pectoral girdle.

Figure 8.13b Surface anatomy of the hip and lower limb.

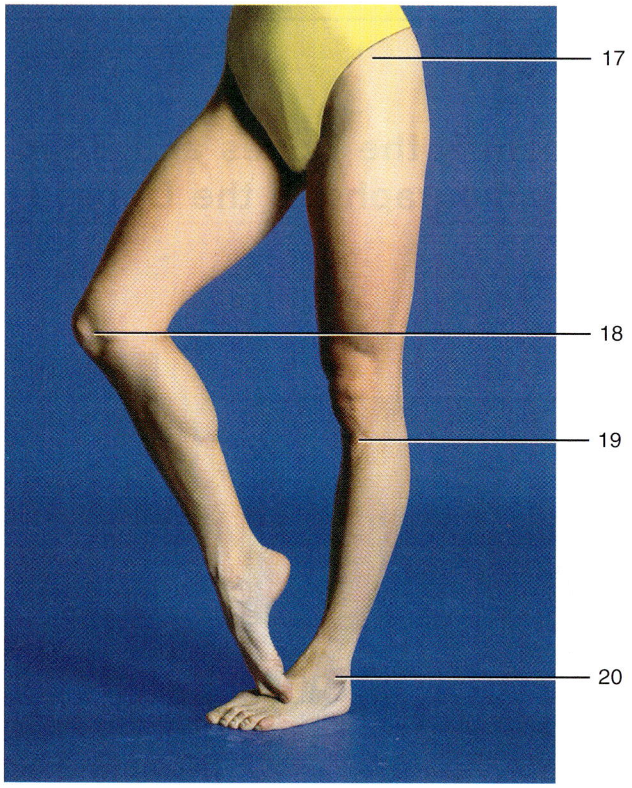

17. ________________ (bone marking)

18. ________________ (bone)

19. ________________ (bone marking)

20. ________________ (bone marking)

FIGURE 8.13b Surface anatomy of the hip.

EXERCISE 12

SKELETAL MUSCLES AND THEIR ACTIONS

OUTLINE

OBJECTIVES

After completing this exercise, you should be able to:

- Describe how skeletal muscles are named
- Identify major skeletal muscles
- Describe the function of major skeletal muscles

MATERIALS

- Muscle models, anatomical charts, and/or cadaver photographs
- Articulated skeleton (to simulate skeletal muscle actions)
- Colored pencils (optional)

A. Criteria for Naming Skeletal Muscles

Learning the criteria used to name skeletal muscles will assist you in identifying and learning the function of these muscles. Skeletal muscles are named for their orientation relative to the midline of the body, size, shape, action, number of origins, location, or origin and insertion. The muscle attachment points, the origin and insertion, are usually skin or bone. The **origin** is the nonmoving point of attachment when a muscle contracts and the **insertion** point moves toward the origin. Table 12.1 identifies criteria for naming skeletal muscles.

ACTIVITY 1 Criteria for Naming Skeletal Muscles

Each word in a skeletal muscle name gives information about the muscle. Give the criteria used for each word below.

Name	Criteria
1 orbicularis oculi	orbicularis—direction of fibers (circular) oculi—location (eye)
2 biceps brachii	____________________
3 rectus femoris	____________________
4 gluteus maximus	____________________
5 deltoid	____________________
6 sternocleidomastoid	____________________

TABLE 12.1 Criteria for Naming Skeletal Muscles

NAME	DEFINITION	NAME	DEFINITION
Orientation of Muscle Relative to Body Midline		**Muscle Action**	
Rectus	Muscle parallel to body midline	Flexor	Decreases joint angle
Transverse	Muscle perpendicular to body midline	Extensor	Increases joint angle
Oblique	Muscle diagonal to body midline	Abductor	Moves bone away from midline
		Adductor	Moves bone close to midline
		Levator	Elevates
Muscle Size		Depressor	Depresses
Maximus	Largest	Supinator	Turns palm superiorly or anteriorly
Medius	Middle	Pronator	Turns palm inferiorly or posteriorly
Minimus	Smallest	Sphincter	Decreases size of opening
Magnus	Large	Tensor	Makes a body part rigid
Brevis	Shortest	Rotator	Moves bone around longitudinal axis
Latissimus	Wide		
Major	Larger	**Number of Origins**	
Minor	Smaller	Biceps	Two origins
Vastus	Great	Triceps	Three origins
		Quadriceps	Four origins
Muscle Shape			
Deltoid	Triangular		
Trapezius	Trapezoid	**Location**	*(example given)*
Serratus	Saw-toothed	Frontalis	Located on the frontal bone
Rhomboid	Diamond-shaped		
Orbicularis	Circular		
Pectinate	Comblike		
Piriformis	Pear-shaped	**Origin and Insertion**	*(example given)*
Platysma	Flat	Sternohyoid	Originates on the sternum; inserts on the hyoid bone
Quadratus	Square		
Gracilis	Slender		

B. Skeletal Muscle Identification

Word derivatives and the muscle location are provided to help you identify the muscle. Within a location, some muscles are grouped according to whether they are **superficial** or **deep.**

A core group of muscles was selected for Activity 2 to which your instructor may add additional muscles. These muscles can be written in the spaces provided in the tables.

ACTIVITY 2 Skeletal Muscle Identification

1 Label Figures 12.1 to 12.8.

2 Use the name, word derivative, and the location in Tables 12.2–12.9 to point to the muscles on models, charts, and/or cadaver photographs. Pronounce the names as you point to them. Use Figures 12.1–12.9 when necessary.

3 Optional: Color black and white muscles in contrasting colors. Color in the same direction as the muscle fibers.

1. Muscles of the Head

Muscles located in the head include those involved in facial expression, mastication, blinking, and eye movement. The muscles that move the eye will be studied in the exercise on "Special Senses."

TABLE 12.2 Muscles of the Head

MUSCLE	LOCATION
Epicranius muscle (*epi-* = upon; *cranius* = cranium)	Combination of frontalis and occipitalis muscle connected by an aponeurosis (a flat, broad tendon)
Frontalis (*frontalis* = in front)	Lies over frontal bone
Occipitalis (*occipito* = base of skull)	Lies over occipital bone
Temporalis (*tempora* = temples)	Lies over temporal bone
Orbicularis oculi (*orbicularis* = little circle; *oculi* = eye)	Encircles the eye; circular muscle
Zygomaticus major and minor (*zygoma* = bar)	Between zygomatic bone and corner of mouth
Orbicularis oris (*oris* = mouth)	Encircles the mouth; circular muscle
Masseter (*maseter* = chewer)	Between zygomatic arch and posterior portion of mandible
Deep Muscles	
Buccinator (*bucca* = cheek)	Deep to masseter. Fibers run transversely and form fleshy part of cheek
Lateral pterygoid (*pterygoid* = like a wing)	Deep to masseter. Transverse muscle fibers between pterygoid process of sphenoid and mandible, external to medial pterygoid
Medial pterygoid	Deep to masseter. Verticle muscle fibers between pterygoid process of sphenoid and mandible
Additional Muscles	

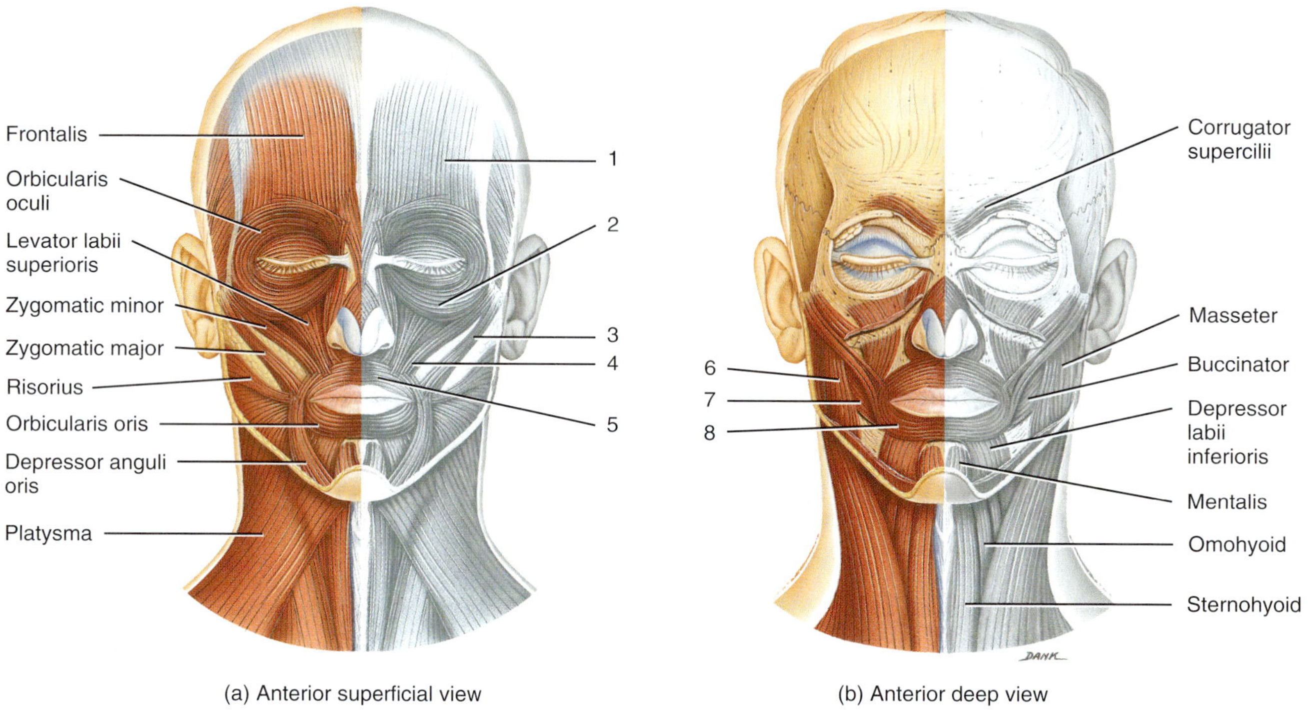

- frontalis (fron-TA-lis)
- orbicularis oculi (or-bi-kyoo-LAR-is OK-yoo-lie)
- orbicularis oris (OR-is)
- zygomaticus major (zy-go-MA-ti-kus)
- zygomaticus minor

1 ____________________

2 ____________________

3 ____________________

4 ____________________

5 ____________________

- buccinator (BUK-sih-nay-tor)
- masseter (MAS-se-ter)
- orbicularis oris

6 ____________________

7 ____________________

8 ____________________

FIGURE 12.1 **Selected muscles of the head.**

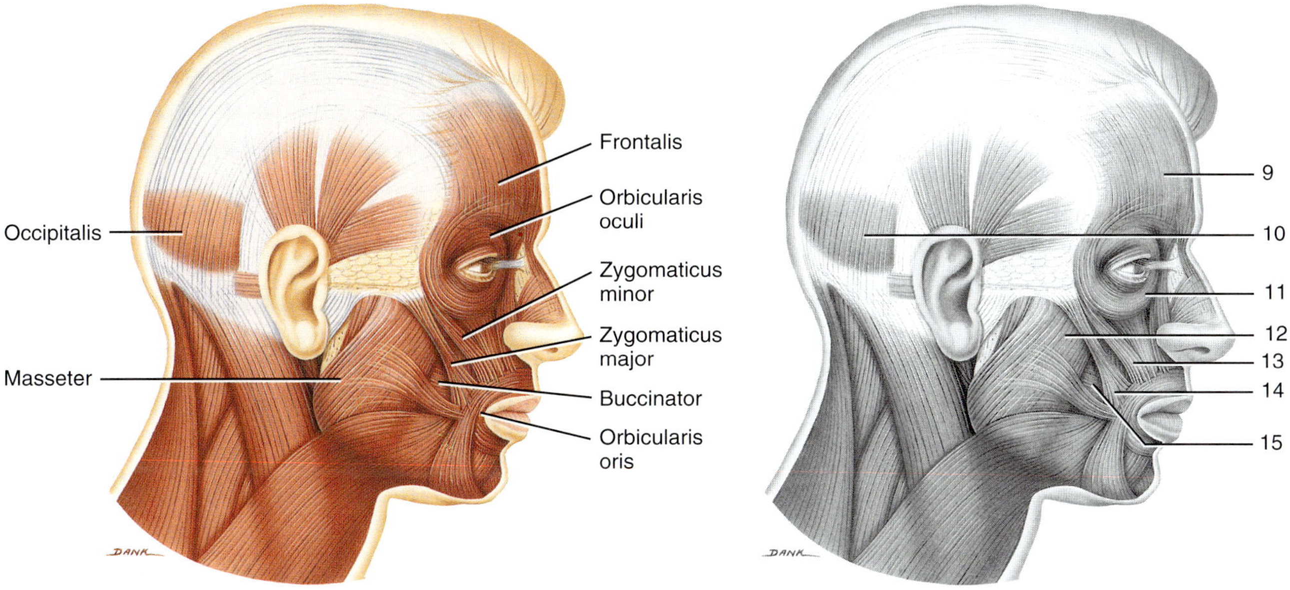

(c) Lateral superficial view

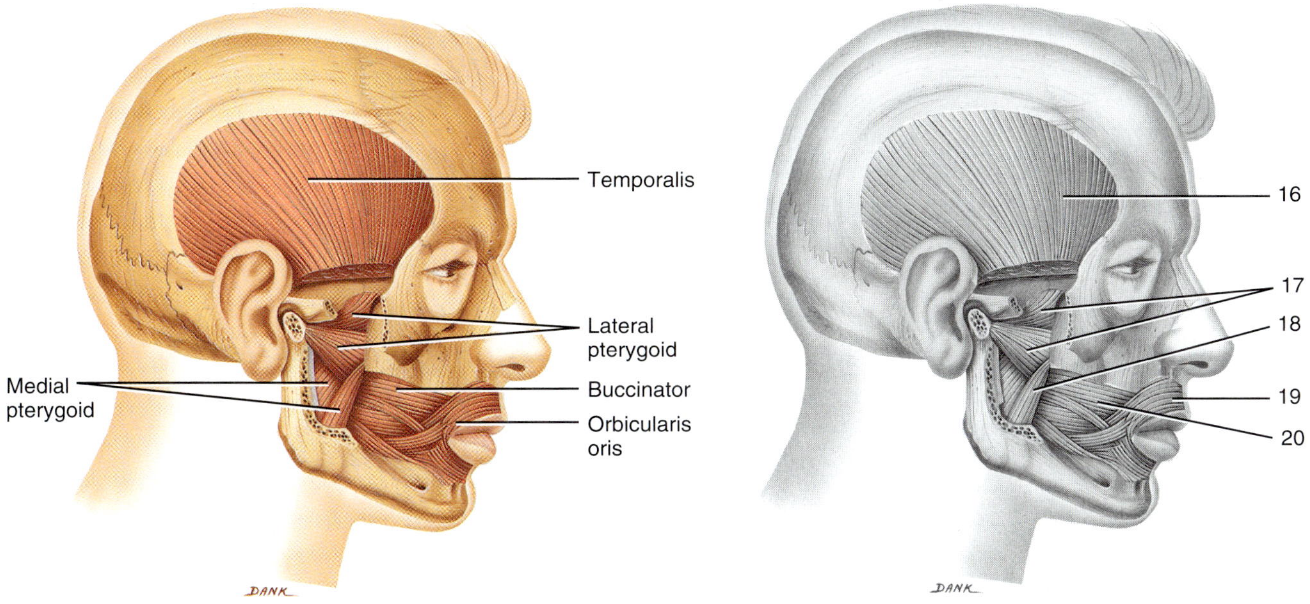

(d) Lateral deep view

- buccinator
- frontalis
- masseter
- occipitalis (ok-si-pi-TA-lis)
- orbicularis oculi
- zygomaticus major
- zygomaticus minor

9 ____________________

10 ____________________

11 ____________________

12 ____________________

13 ____________________

14 ____________________

15 ____________________

- buccinator
- lateral pterygoid (TER-ih-goid)
- medial pterygoid
- orbicularis oris
- temporalis (tem-por-A-lis)

16 ____________________

17 ____________________

18 ____________________

19 ____________________

20 ____________________

FIGURE 12.1 **Selected muscles of the head, *continued.***

2. Muscles of the Neck

Muscles of the neck include those that are attached to the hyoid bone and play a role in swallowing, and those that move the head and neck. The sternocleidomastoid muscle, a muscle that runs diagonally from the sternum and clavicle to the mastoid process of the temporal bone, divides each side of the neck into an anterior and posterior triangle. The anterior triangle includes the carotid artery and the internal jugular vein while the posterior triangle includes the external jugular vein and part of the subclavian artery.

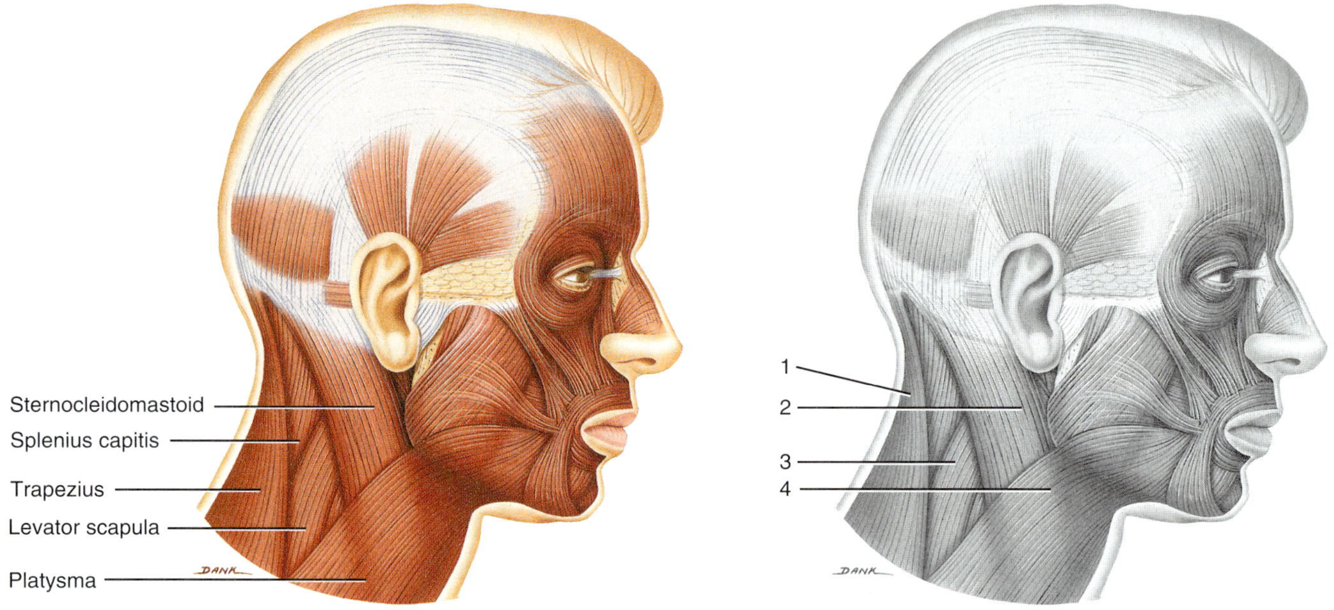

(a) Lateral superficial view

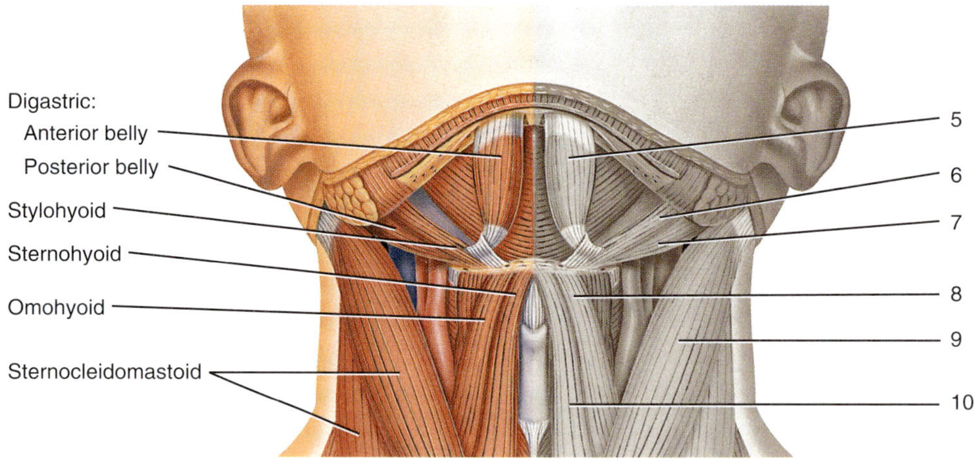

(b) Anterior view with platysma removed

- levator scapulae (le-VAY-tor SKA-pyoo-lee)
- platysma (pla-TIZ-ma)
- sternocleidomastoid (ster-no-kli-do-MAS-toid)
- trapezius (tra-PEE-zee-us)

1 ____________________

2 ____________________

3 ____________________

4 ____________________

- digastric, anterior belly
- digastric, posterior belly
- omohyoid
- sternocleidomastoid
- sternohyoid
- stylohyoid

5 ____________________

6 ____________________

7 ____________________

8 ____________________

9 ____________________

10 ____________________

FIGURE 12.2 **Selected muscles of the chin and neck.**

TABLE 12.3 Muscles of the Neck

MUSCLE	LOCATION
Platysma (*platy* = flat, broad)	Covers lower mandible and entire anterior neck; ends on chest; wide, flat muscle
Sternocleidomastoid or **SCM** (*sterno-* = breastbone; *cleido* = clavicle; *mastoid* = mastoid process)	On anterior and lateral neck; fibers run diagonally across the neck between mastoid process, sternum, and clavicle; strap-like muscle
Digastric (*di* = two; *gastric* = belly)	
Anterior belly	Straplike muscle of chin that is parallel to midline of chin and extends from posterior belly
Posterior belly	Runs along posterior border of chin
Stylohyoid	Chin muscle, medial to posterior belly of digastric
Mylohyoid	Deep muscle of chin extending from right side of mandible to left side
Sternohyoid	Runs along midline of anterior neck
Omohyoid	Lateral to sternohyoid
Scalenes (*scalenos* = uneven; located deep to SCM; anterior, middle, and posterior scalenes)	Three muscles in lateral neck deep to the sternocleidomastoid
Levator scapulae (*levare* = to raise)	Posterior to sternocleidomastoid; runs diagonally from posterior head to scapula
Trapezius (superior portion)	Superficial muscle; upper back and posterior neck
Splenius capitis (*splenion* = bandage; *caput* = head)	Posterior neck deep to trapezius
Additional Muscles	

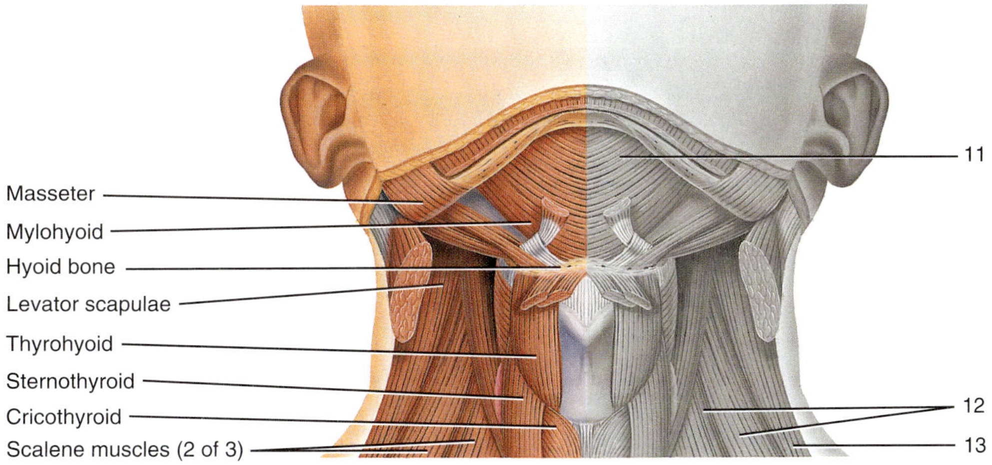

(c) Anterior deep view

- levator scapulae
- mylohyoid
- scalenes (SKAY-leens)

11 ____________________

12 ____________________

13 ____________________

FIGURE 12.2 Selected muscles of the chin and neck, *continued.*

3. Muscles of the Anterior Trunk

Muscles of the anterior trunk have a variety of functions. The anterior trunk contains muscles that move the arm, raise and lower the thoracic cage, flex the trunk, and compress abdominal content.

TABLE 12.4 Muscles of the Anterior Trunk

MUSCLE	LOCATION
Superficial Muscles	
Pectoralis major (*pectus* = chest)	Large muscles on superior, anterior chest between sternum and arm
Serratus anterior (*serratus* = saw-toothed)	Serrated-looking muscles on the lateral trunk inferior to arms and ribs
External oblique	Lateral and anterior sheet-like abdominal muscles whose fibers run obliquely toward midline (linea alba)
Rectus abdominis (*rectus* = parallel fibers)	Midline abdominal muscles located between sternum and inguinal ligament.
Deep Muscles	
Pectoralis minor	Deep to pectoralis major attaching to 3rd–5th ribs
External intercostal (*inter-* = between; *costal* = ribs)	Oblique muscles located between ribs lateral to internal intercostals
Internal intercostal	Oblique muscles located between ribs near sternum and medial to external obliques
Internal oblique	Abdominal muscles deep to external oblique whose fibers run obliquely toward linea alba
Transversus abdominis	Abdominal muscles deep to internal oblique whose fibers run transversely
Diaphragm	Dome-shaped muscle inside the ventral body cavity separating it into the thoracic and abdominal cavities; contains openings for the esophagus, aorta, and vena cava
Additional Muscles	

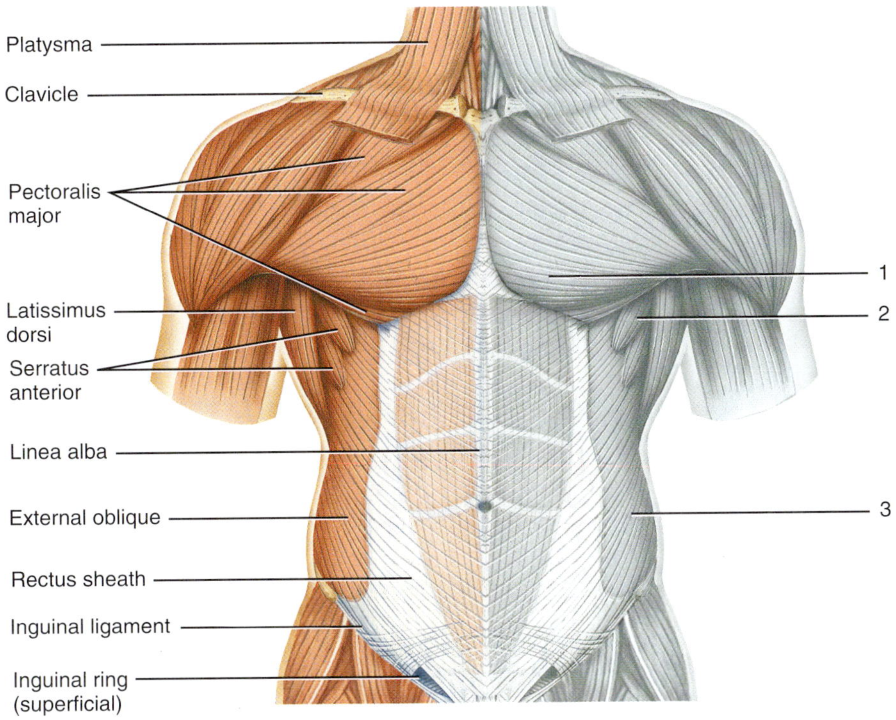

(a) Anterior superficial view

- external oblique
- pectoralis major (pek-tor-A-lis)
- serratus anterior (ser-RAY-tus)

1 ______________________

2 ______________________

3 ______________________

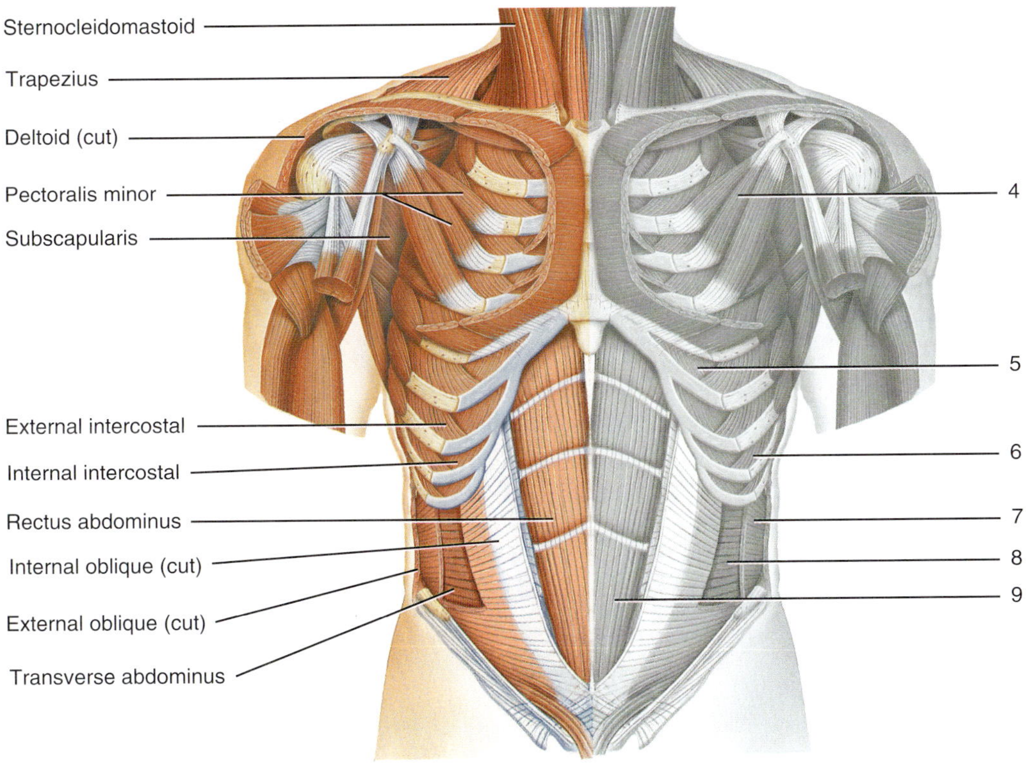

(b) Anterior deep view

- external intercostal
- internal intercostal
- internal oblique
- pectoralis minor
- rectus abdominis (REK-tus ab-DOM-in-is)
- transversus abdominis

4 ______________________

5 ______________________

6 ______________________

7 ______________________

8 ______________________

9 ______________________

FIGURE 12.3 Muscles of the anterior trunk.

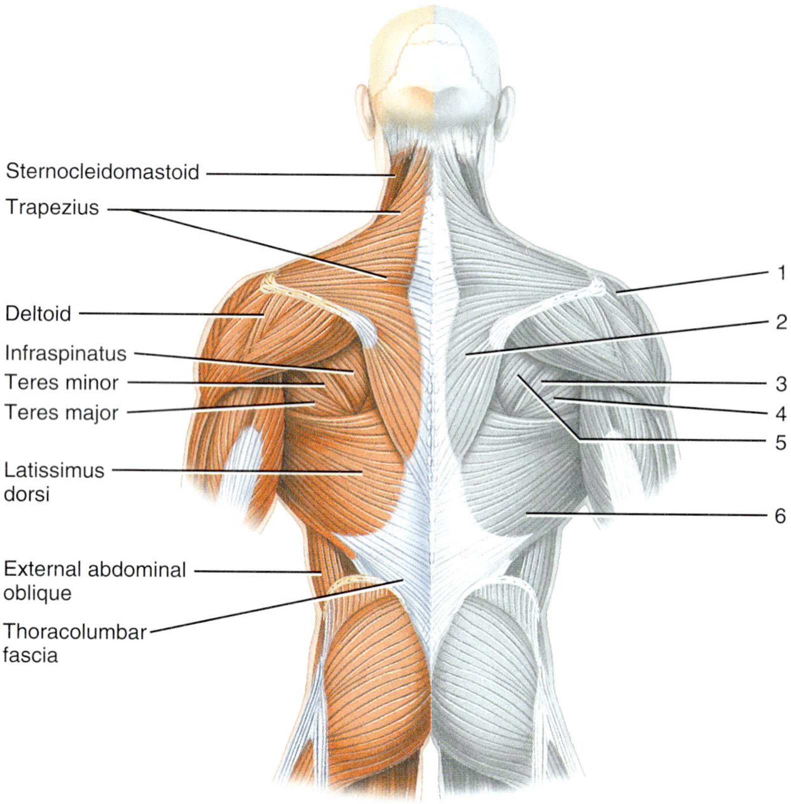

(a) Posterior superficial view

- deltoid
- infraspinatus (in-fra-spi-NAY-tus)
- latissimus dorsi (la-TIS-i-mus DOR-sigh)
- teres major (TEH-rez)
- teres minor
- trapezius (tra-PEE-zee-us)

1 ______________________________

2 ______________________________

3 ______________________________

4 ______________________________

5 ______________________________

6 ______________________________

- infraspinatus
- rhomboid major (ROM-boid)
- rhomboid minor
- supraspinatus (soo-pra-spi-NAY-tus)
- teres major (TE-rez)
- teres minor

7 ______________________________

8 ______________________________

9 ______________________________

10 ______________________________

11 ______________________________

12 ______________________________

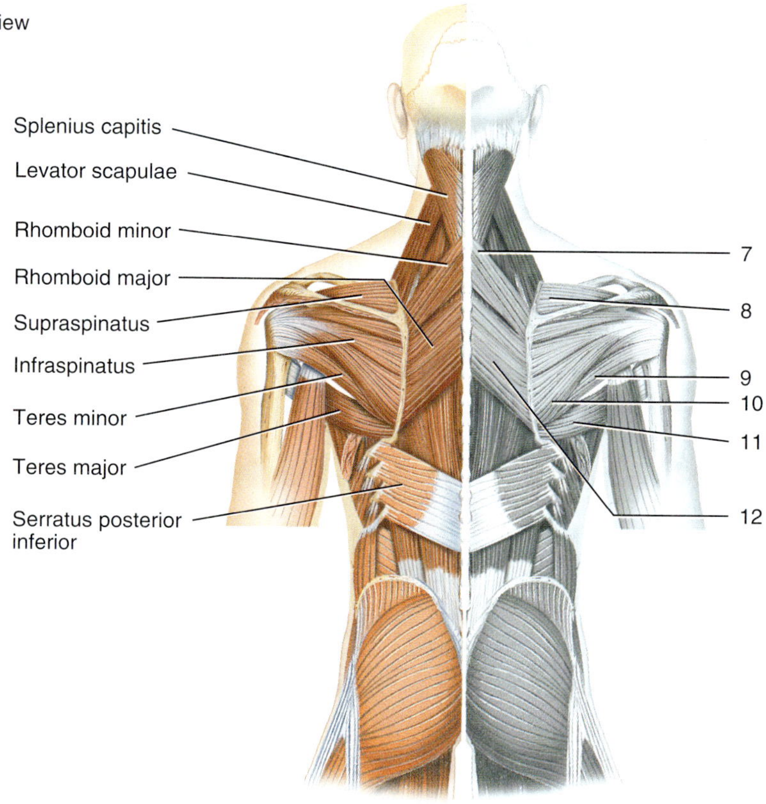

(b) Posterior deep view

FIGURE 12.4 Muscles of the posterior trunk.

4. Muscles of the Posterior Trunk

The posterior trunk contains muscles that move the neck, arm, scapula, and vertebral column.

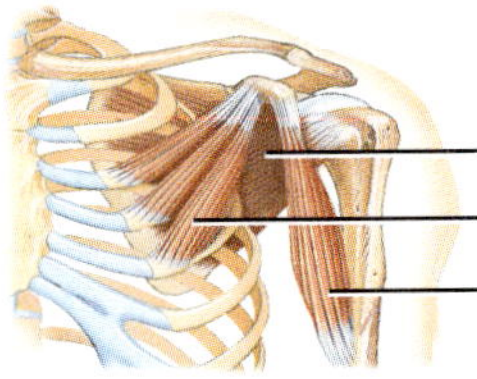

(c) Anterior view of scapula

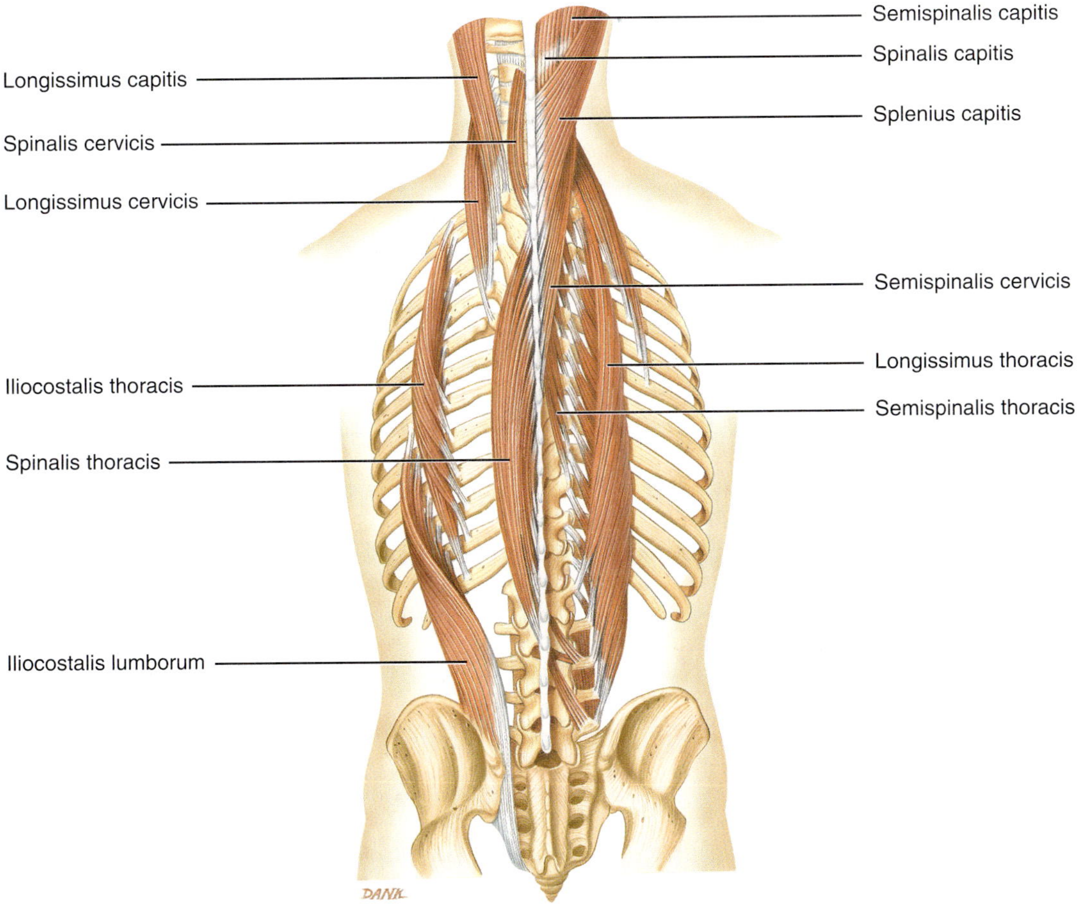

(d) Deep erector spinal muscles of the back

FIGURE 12.4 **Muscles of the posterior trunk, *continued.***

TABLE 12.5 Muscles of the Posterior Trunk

MUSCLE	LOCATION
Superficial Muscles	
Deltoid (delta; triangle)	Large, rounded, triangular, shoulder muscle
Trapezius (*trapezoides* = trapezoid shape)	Diamond-shaped muscle of posterior neck and upper back that extends from the skull to spine of scapula to vertebral column
Infraspinatus (*infra-* = below: *spinatus* = spine of scapula)	Located in infraspinous fossa (inferior to spine of scapula); partially covered by deltoid
Teres minor (*teres* = long and round)	Inferior to infraspinatus; partially covered by deltoid
Teres major	Inferior to teres minor and partially covered by deltoid
Latissimus dorsi (*latissimus* = widest; *dorsum* = back)	Main large, flat muscle of middle and lower back that runs laterally and attaches to superior portion of humerus
Deep Muscles	
Supraspinatus (*supra-* = above)	Located in supraspinous fossa (superior to spine of scapula) and totally covered by deltoid
Subscapularis	On ventral side of the scapula in the subscapular fossa
Rhomboid major and minor (*rhomboides* = diamond-shaped)	Deep to trapezius in upper back; between the vertebrae and scapula; rhomboideus minor is superior to the rhomboideus major
Erector spinae (*erector* = erect posture; *spinae* = spinal column; consists of iliocostalis, longissimus, and spinalis groups)	Group of muscles next to the vertebral column deep to the trapezius, latissimus dorsi, and scapula
Additional Muscles	

5. Muscles of the Arm

Muscles located in the arm have insertions that cross the elbow joint. When these muscles contract, they flex or extend the forearm. The structure of the elbow does not permit any other movements at this joint.

TABLE 12.6 Muscles of the Arm

MUSCLE	LOCATION
Anterior Surface	
Biceps brachii (*biceps* = 2 heads; *brachii* = arm)	Largest muscle in anterior compartment of arm; two heads
Brachialis	Posterior to biceps brachii and anterior to humerus
Posterior Surface	
Triceps brachii (*triceps* = 3 heads)	Large muscle with three heads
Long head	Originates on scapula, inferior to glenoid cavity
Medial head	Originates on humerus, runs medially
Lateral head	Originates on humerus, runs laterally
Additional Muscles	

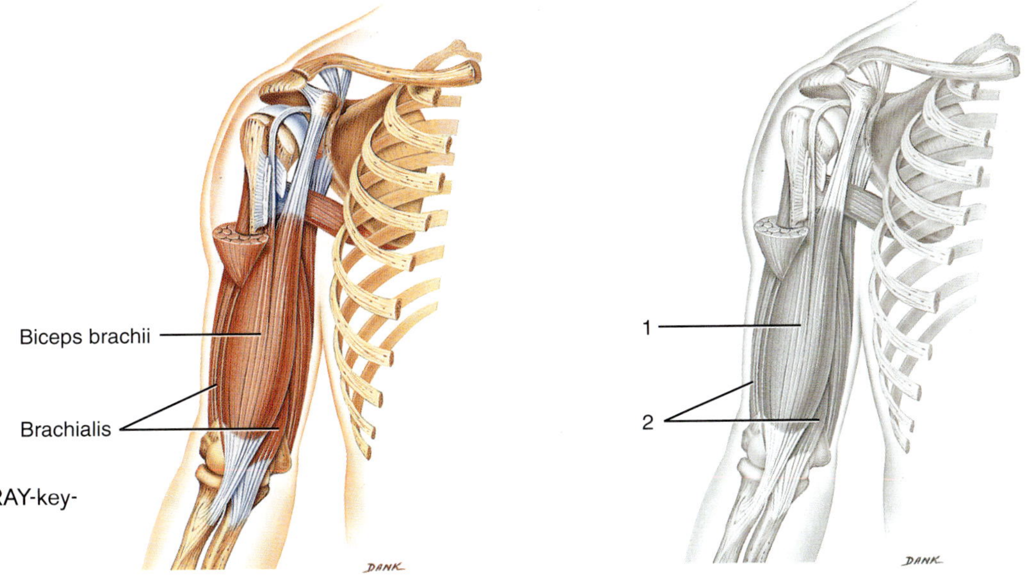

- biceps brachii (BI-ceps BRAY-key-eye)
- brachialis (bray-key-AL-is)

1 ______________________

2 ______________________

(a) Anterior view

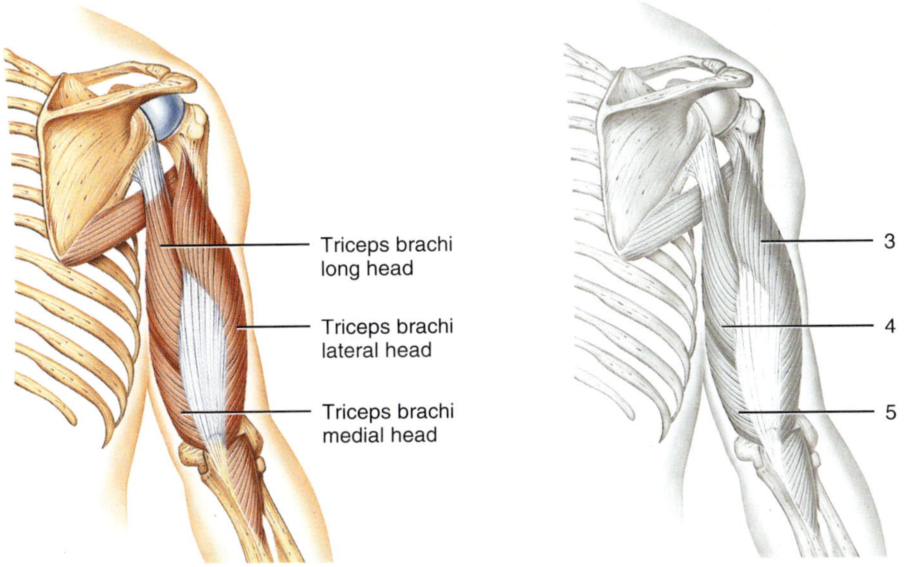

- triceps, long head
- triceps, medial head
- triceps brachii, lateral head

3 ______________________

4 ______________________

5 ______________________

(b) Posterior view

FIGURE 12.5 Muscles of the arm.

6. Muscles of the Forearm, Wrist, and Hands

Muscles located in the forearm flex, extend, abduct, or adduct the wrist and digits. The flexors are found on the anterior surface of the arm and originate on the medial condyle of the humerus, whereas the extensors are found on the posterior surface of the arm and originate on the lateral epicondyle.

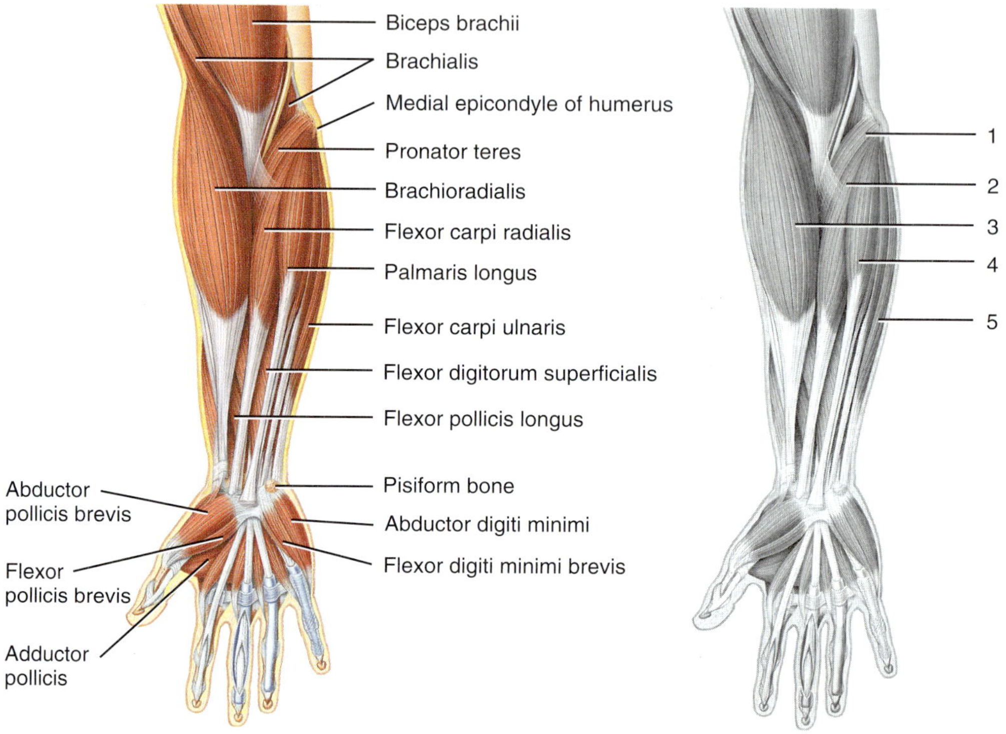

(a) Anterior superficial view

(a)
- brachioradialis (BRAY-kee-oh-ray-dee-AL-is)
- flexor carpi radialis (KAR-pee)
- flexor carpi ulnaris
- palmaris longis (pall-MARE-is)
- pronator teres (PRO-nay-tor)

1 ____________________

2 ____________________

3 ____________________

4 ____________________

5 ____________________

(b)
- flexor digitorum profundus
- flexor pollicus longus (POL-ih-kis)
- supinator

6 ____________________

7 ____________________

8 ____________________

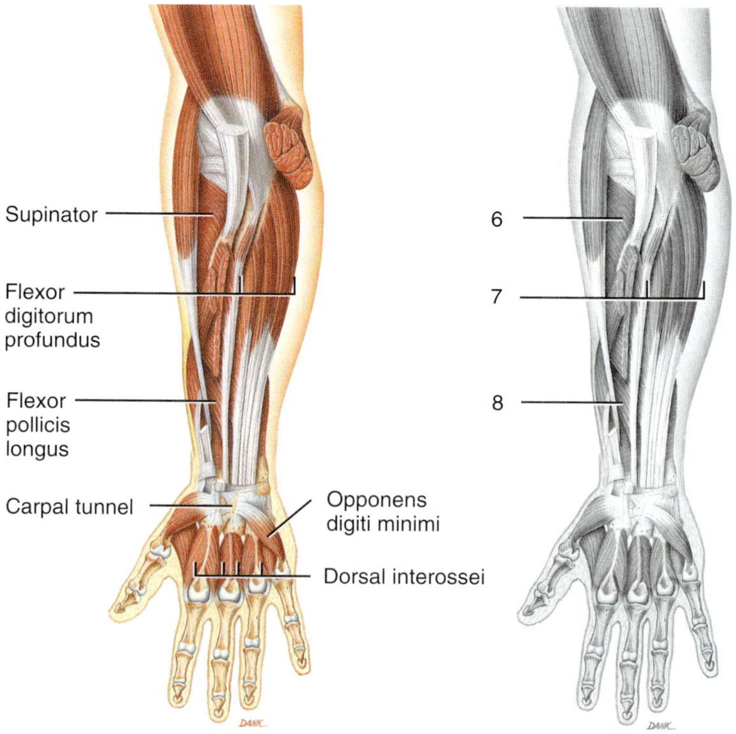

(b) Anterior deep view

FIGURE 12.6 Muscles of the forearm, wrist, and hands.

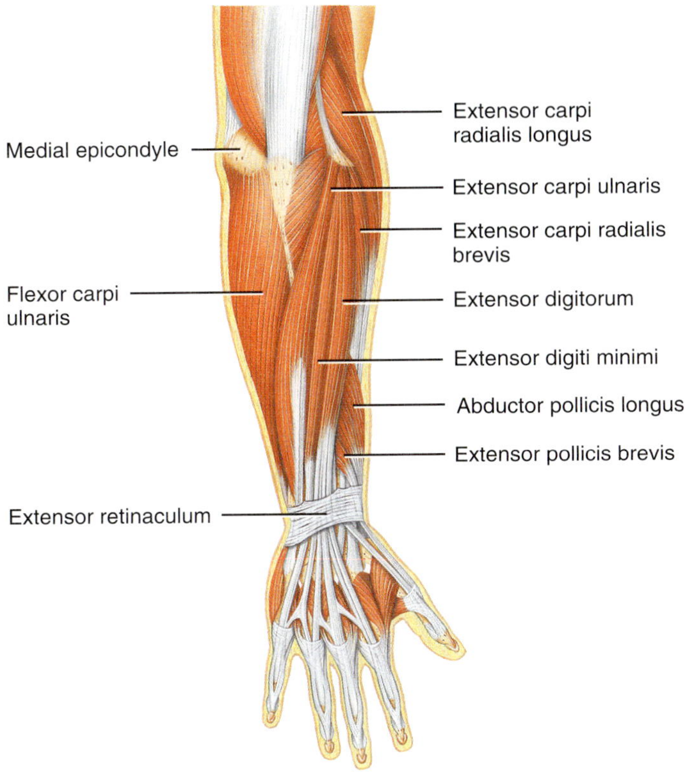

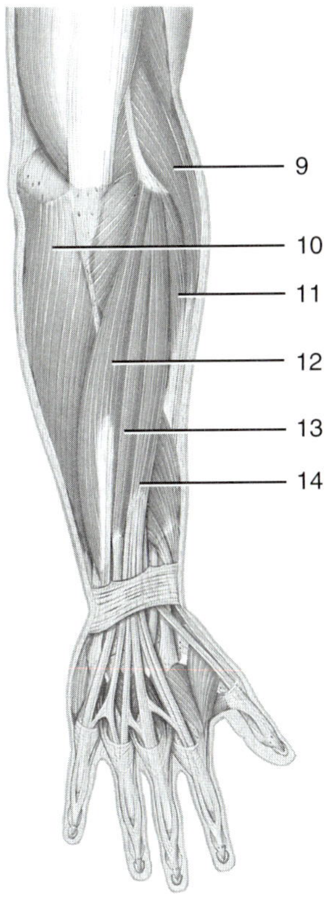

(c) Posterior superficial view

- extensor carpi radialis brevis
- extensor carpi radialis longus
- extensor carpi ulnaris
- extensor digitorum
- extensor digiti minimi
- flexor carpi ulnaris

9 ______________________

10 ______________________

11 ______________________

12 ______________________

13 ______________________

14 ______________________

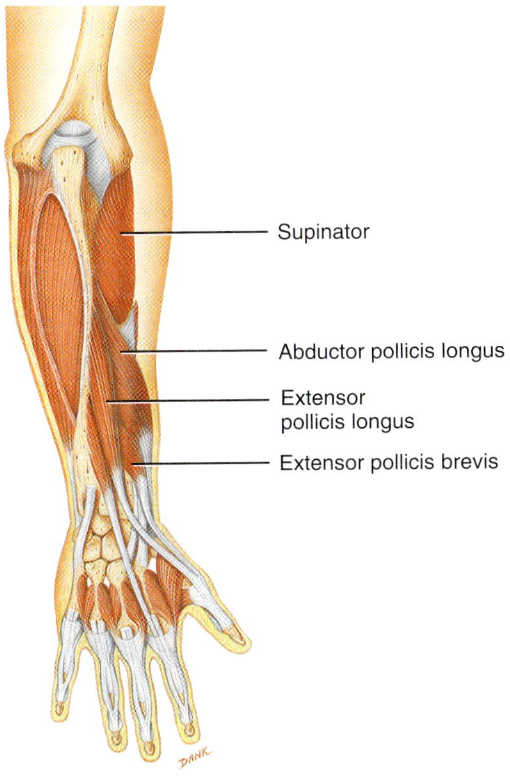

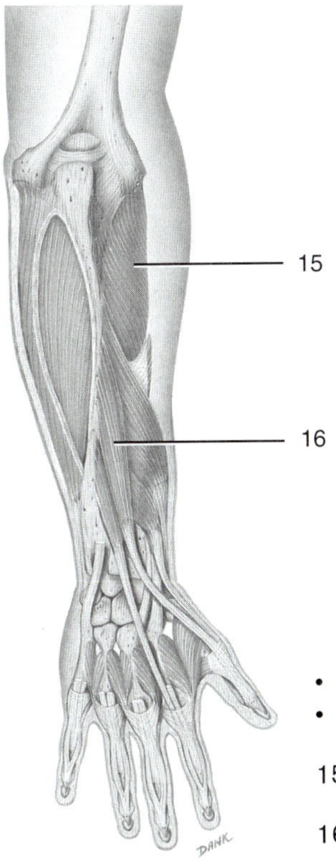

- extensor pollicis longus
- supinator (SOUP-ih-nay-tor)

15 ______________________

16 ______________________

FIGURE 12.6 **Muscles of the forearm, wrist, and hands, *continued.***

TABLE 12.7 Muscles of the Forearm, Wrist, and Hands

MUSCLE	LOCATION
Anterior Surface–Superficial Muscles (lateral to medial)	
Brachioradialis (*brachi-* = arm; *radialis* = radius)	Anterior forearm; large, superfical lateral muscle
Pronator teres (*pronare* = to bend forward; *teres* = long, cylindrical)	Fibers cross obliquely from medial epicondyle across antecubital fossa area near median nerve
Flexor carpi radialis (*carpi-* = wrist)	Medial and inferior to pronator teres; medial to brachioradialis in forearm
Palmaris longus (*palma* = palm)	Medial to flexor carpi radialis
Flexor carpi ulnaris	Small part of muscle is seen anteriorly; most medial muscle of posterior forearm
Anterior Surface–Deep Muscles	
Supinator (*supinate* = supine; palm upward)	Anterior portion is deep to brachioradialis
Flexor digitorum superficialis	Deep to tendons of the medial anterior forearm muscles in the distal part of forearm
Flexor pollicis longus (*pollex* = thumb)	Inferior and lateral to flexor digitorum superficialis
Posterior Surface–Superficial Muscles (medial to lateral)	
Extensor carpi ulnaris	Lateral to flexor carpi ulnaris; originates on lateral epicondyle of humerus
Extensor digitorum (*digitorum* = digits)	Lateral to extensor carpi ulnaris; originates on lateral epicondyle of humerus
Extensor carpi radialis longus and **brevis**	Lateral to extensor digitorum longus; crosses elbow joint
Posterior Surface–Deep Muscles	
Supinator	Posterior portion is deep to lateral muscles of posterior forearm
Extensor pollicis longus	Deep to lateral extensor muscles on posterior forearm
Additional Muscles	

7. Muscles of the Thigh

Muscles of the thigh flex, extend, abduct, adduct, circumduct and rotate the thigh. The **femoral triangle** is an important landmark formed by the inguinal ligament (superior border), the medial edge of the sartorius muscle (lateral border), and the medial edge of the adductor longus muscle. Within this triangle is located the femoral nerve, artery, and vein. This area is cut into during cardiac catheterization.

The **piriformis,** a deep muscle of the posterior thigh, serves as an important landmark for the sciatic nerve. The sciatic nerve is deep to the piriformis. The piriformis is palpated and avoided when giving injections in the gluteal area. Also, sitting on your piriformis for prolonged periods may cause numbness in the legs due to the pressure on the sciatic nerve.

TABLE 12.8 Muscles of the Thigh

MUSCLE	LOCATION
Anterior Surface (lateral to medial)	
Tensor fasciae latae (*tensor* = to stretch; *fascia* = band; *latus* = wide)	Small lateral hip muscle with fascia lata (deep fascia) that extends down the thigh
Quadriceps femoris (*quad* = four; *cep-* or *caput* = head or origins)	Four muscles on femur
Rectus femoris	Located along midline of thigh
Vastus lateralis	Lateral to rectus femoris
Vastus medialis	Medial to rectus femoris
Vastus intermedius	Intermediate to vastus lateralis and vastus medialis and deep to rectus femoris
Sartorius (*sartor* = tailor)	Diagonal muscle; extends from tensor fascia latae to beyond medial knee
Iliopsoas combination of **Psoas major** **Iliacus** (*psoas* = loin; *iliacus* = ilium)	A small portion of these muscles are observed in anterior/medial compartment of thigh inferior to inguinal ligament
Pectineus (*pecten* = comb)	Medial to iliopsoas
Adductor longus	Medial to pectineus
Adductor magnus	Observed medial and inferior to adductor longus; a larger portion of this muscle is deep to the adductor longus
Gracilis (*gracile* = long and slender)	Medial to adductor magnus; straight muscle on inside of thigh
Adductor brevis	Deep to adductor longus; totally covered by superficial muscles
Posterior Surface	
Gluteus maximus (*gluteus* = buttocks)	Largest buttocks muscle
Gluteus medius and **minimus**	Gluteus medius is observed superior to gluteus maximus, but is partially covered; gluteus minimus not seen superficially and is covered by gluteus medius
Piriformus (*pirum* = pear; *forma* = shape)	Deep muscle inferior to gluteus minimus; important landmark for sciatic nerve; sciatic nerve passes deep to the piriformis
Hamstrings	Three muscles on posterior thigh
Biceps femoris	Most lateral hamstring
Semitendinosus (*semi-* = one half medial hamstrings; *tendinosus* = long tendon)	1 of 2 medial hamstrings; between biceps femoris and semitendinosus
Semimembranosus (*membranosus* = partly membrane)	Most medial of the 3 hamstrings (remember, m for medial)
Additional Muscles	

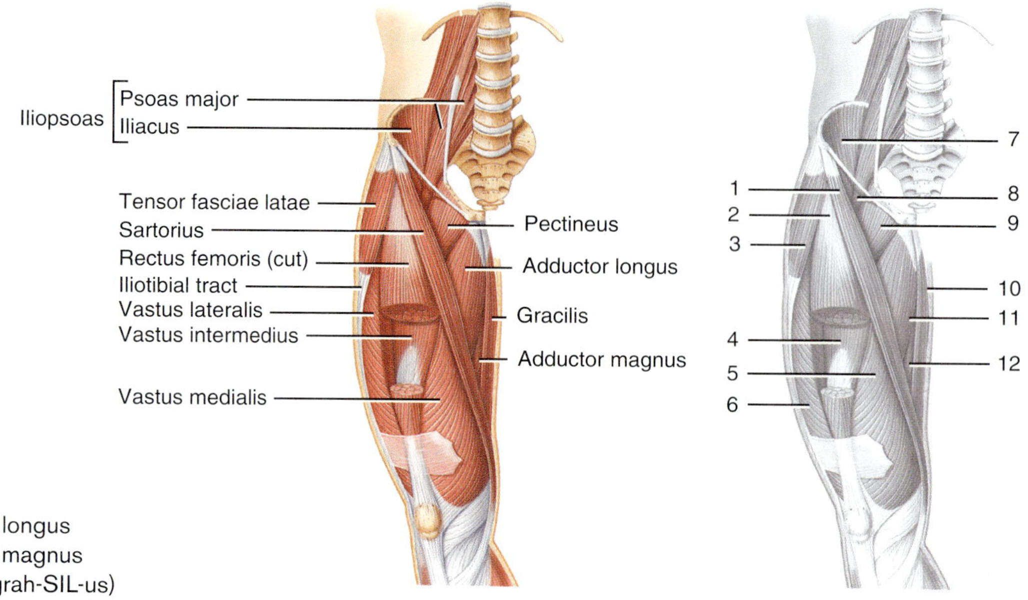

(a) Anterior superficial view

- adductor longus
- adductor magnus
- gracilis (grah-SIL-us)
- iliacus (il-ee-AK-us)
- pectineus (pek-TIN-ee-us)
- psoas major (SO-us)
- rectus femoris (FEM-or-is)
- sartorius (sar-TOR-ee-us)
- tensor fasciae latae (FA-schee LA-tee)
- vastus intermedius
- vastus lateralis
- vastus medialis

1 ____________ 5 ____________ 9 ____________

2 ____________ 6 ____________ 10 ____________

3 ____________ 7 ____________ 11 ____________

4 ____________ 8 ____________ 12 ____________

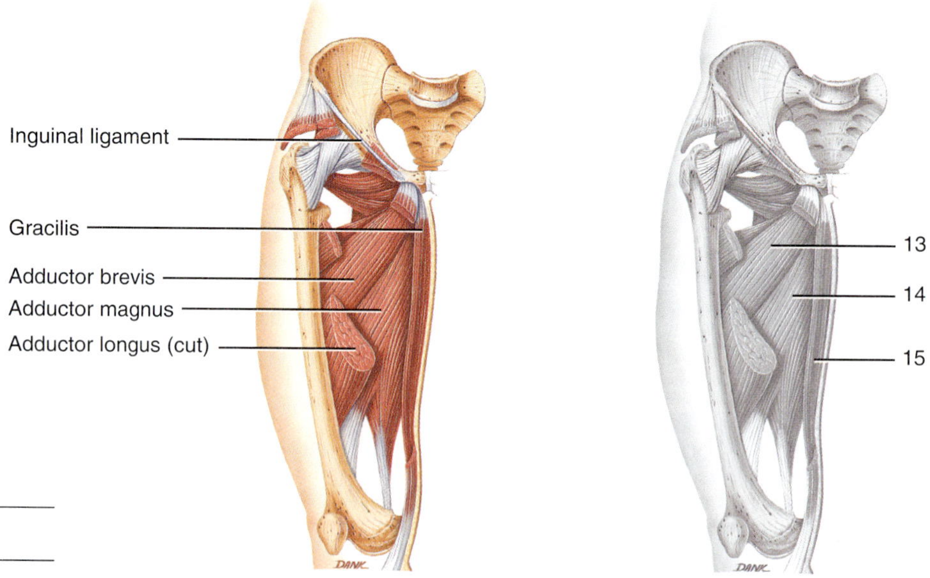

(b) Anterior deep view

- adductor brevis
- adductor magnus
- gracilis

13 ____________

14 ____________

15 ____________

FIGURE 12.7 Muscles of the thigh.

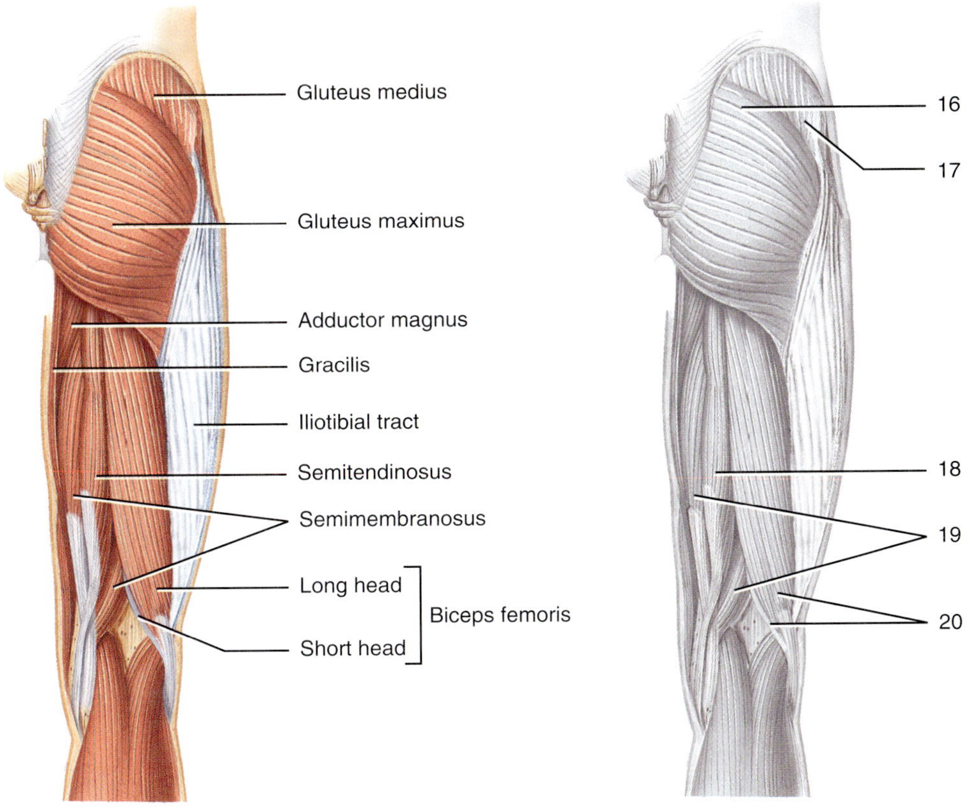

(c) Posterior superficial view

- biceps femoris
- gluteus maximus
- gluteus medius
- semimembranosus
- semitendinosus

16 ______________

17 ______________

18 ______________

19 ______________

20 ______________

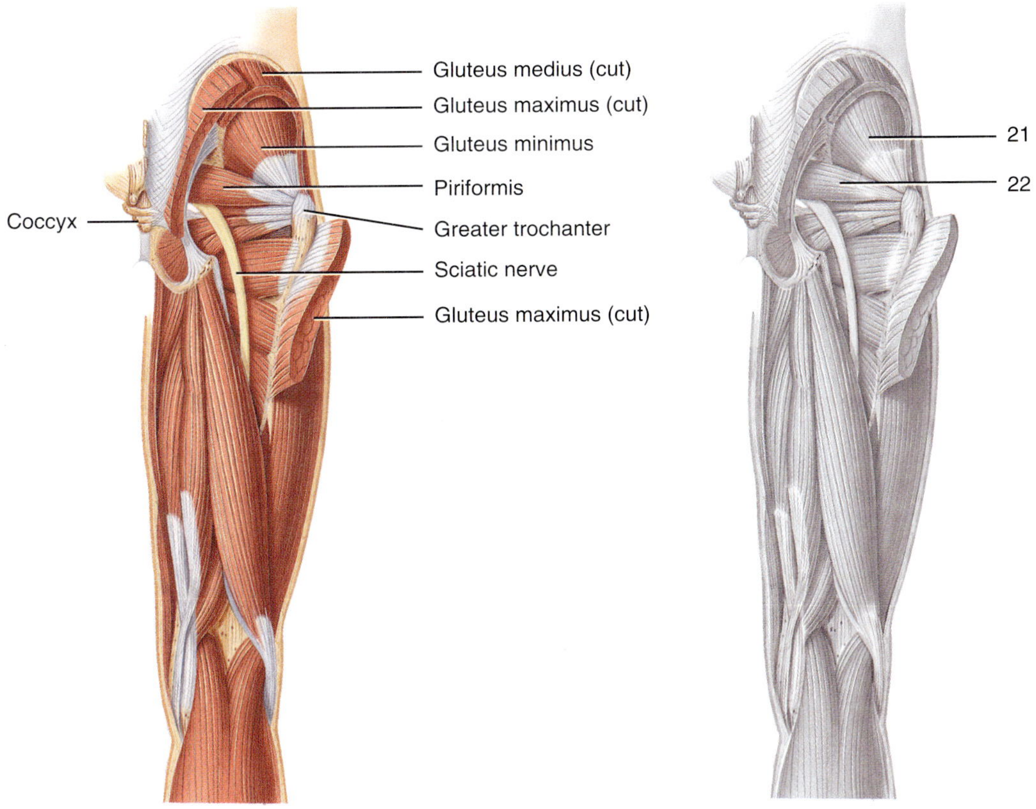

(d) Posterior deep view

- gluteus minimus
- piriformis

21 ______________

22 ______________

FIGURE 12.7 **Muscles of the thigh, *continued.***

8. Muscles of the Leg, Ankle, and Foot

Palpate the tibia of your leg. Find the anterior crest, and the lateral and medial borders of the tibia. Observe that the muscles anterior to the tibia are located lateral to the anterior crest of the tibia. The anterior and lateral superficial muscles are in order starting at the anterior crest just below the knee and moving laterally: tibialis anterior, extensor digitorum longus, and the peroneus longus. The superficial muscles of the posterior leg include the gastrocnemius and the soleus. The soleus is deep to the gastrocnemius.

- extensor digitorum longus
- flexor digitorum longus
- gastrocnemius (gas-trok-NEE-mee-us)
- fibularis (peroneus) longus
- soleus (SOLE-ee-us)
- tibialis anterior

1 ______________________

2 ______________________

3 ______________________

4 ______________________

5 ______________________

6 ______________________

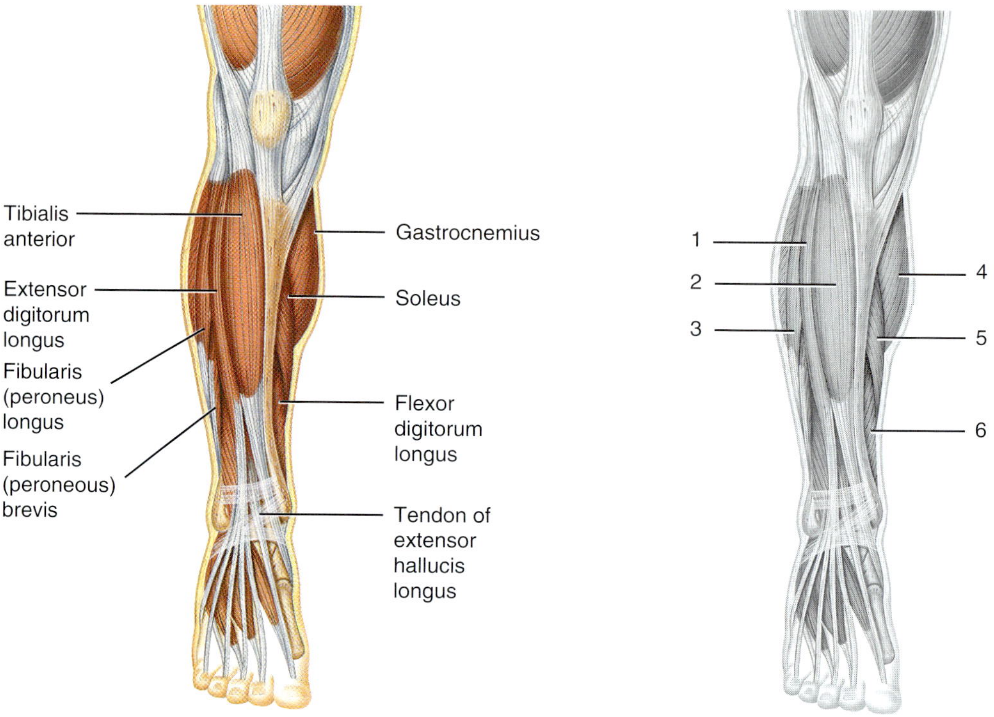

(a) Anterior superficial view

- extensor digitorum longus
- gastrocnemius
- fibularis (peroneus) longus
- soleus
- tibialis anterior

7 ______________________

8 ______________________

9 ______________________

10 ______________________

11 ______________________

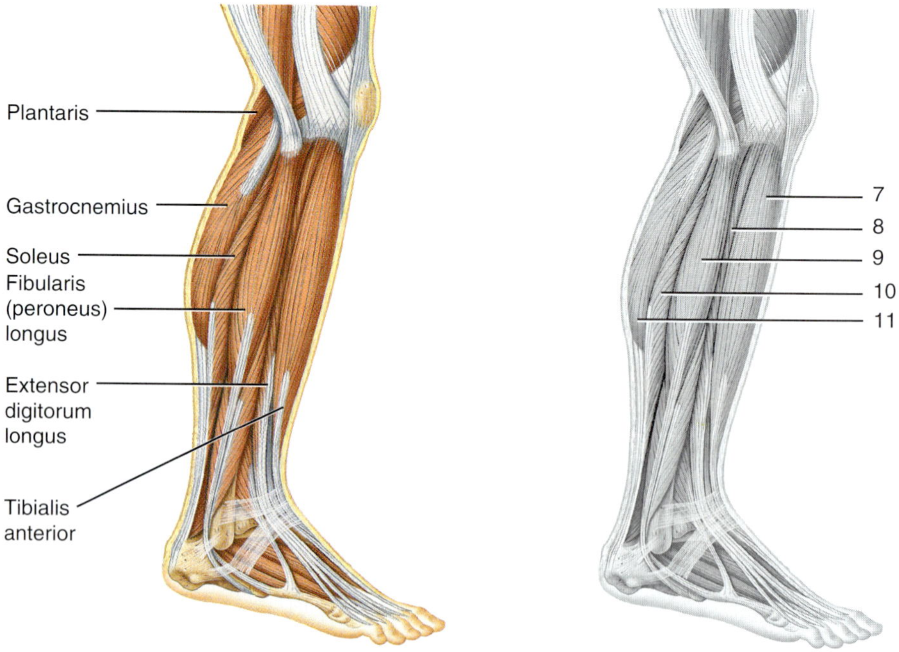

(b) Lateral superficial view

FIGURE 12.8 Muscles of the leg, ankle, and foot.

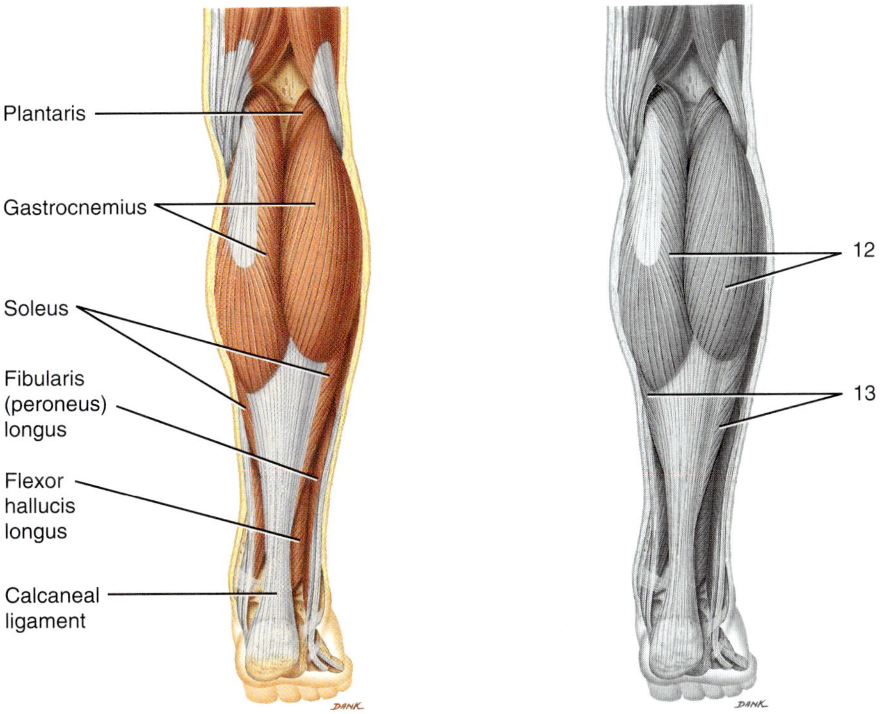

(c) Posterior superficial view

- gastrocnemius
- soleus

12 ____________________

13 ____________________

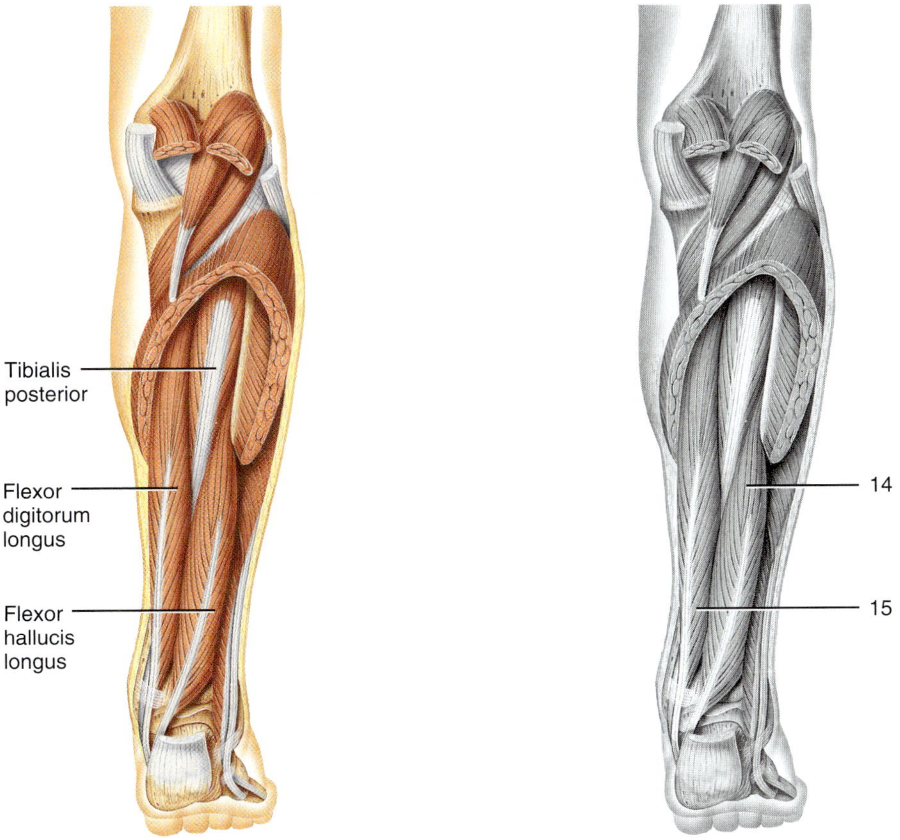

(d) Posterior deep view

- flexor digitorum longus
- flexor hallucis longus (HAL-a-kis)

14 ____________________

15 ____________________

FIGURE 12.8 **Muscles of the leg, ankle, and foot, *continued.***

TABLE 12.9 Muscles of the Leg, Ankle, and Foot

MUSCLE	LOCATION
Anterior and Lateral Superficial Muscles	
Tibialis anterior	Lateral to the anterior crest of the tibia
Extensor digitorum longus	Lateral to the tibialis anterior
Fibularis (peroneus) longus	Lateral to the extensor digitorum longus
Posterior Surface Muscles	
Gastrocnemius	Large superficial muscle on posterior leg
Soleus	Deep to gastrocnemius and posterior to the fibularis (peroneus) longus
Posterior Deep Muscles	
Flexor digitorum longus	Deep to soleus, medial muscle
Flexor hallucis longus (*hallucus* = big toe)	Deep to soleus, lateral muscle
Additional Muscles	

C. Skeletal Muscle Actions

When skeletal muscles contract, they pull their point of insertion toward their point of origin. For the muscles of facial expression, this moves the skin on the face and allows us to express emotion. For most other skeletal muscles, contraction results in movement of a bone at a joint. In the appendages, muscles that perform similar functions are surrounded by fascia, forming **compartments** that are served by the same major blood vessels and nerves.

If you refer to your textbook, you will notice that some skeletal muscles have many actions. For this exercise, we will only include the main action of a muscle that differentiates it or characterizes it as part of a contracting group. Some muscles cross two joints, and actions at both joints are included for these muscles.

ACTIVITY 3 Skeletal Muscle Actions

1 Use name, location, and/or origin and insertion to match the muscles in Tables 12.10–12.18 with the actions listed below each table. Refer to Figures 12.1–12.8 to review muscle location.

2 To reinforce your learning, locate the origin and insertion on an articulated skeleton, and pull the insertion toward the origin to stimulate muscle action.

3 Perform the action and try to palpate the muscle(s) on yourself.

1. Muscles of Facial Expression and Mastication

The muscles of facial expression move the skin of the face to convey a variety of emotions. Their origins are found in the superficial fascia beneath the skin and attached to skull bones, while their insertions are the skin of the face.

TABLE 12.10 Selected Muscles of Facial Expression and Mastication

MUSCLE	ORIGIN	INSERTION
Muscles of Facial Expression		
Frontalis	Galea (epicranial) aponeurosis	Skin superior to supraorbital margin
Occipitalis	Occipital bone and mastoid process of temporal bone	Galea (epicranial) aponeurosis
Orbicularis oris	Muscle fibers surrounding mouth	Skin at corner of mouth
Zygomaticus major	Zygomatic bone	Skin at angle of mouth and orbicularis oris
Zygomaticus minor	Zygomatic bone	Upper lip
Platysma	Fascia covering deltoid and pectoralis major	Mandible, muscles around angle of mouth, and skin of lower face
Orbicularis oculi	Medial wall of orbit	Skin around eyelids
Muscles of Mastication		
Masseter	Maxilla and zygomatic arch	Ramus and angle of mandible
Temporalis	Temporal and frontal bones	Coronoid process and ramus of mandible
Deep Muscles of Mastication		
Buccinator	Alveolar processes of maxilla and mandible	Orbicularis oris
Lateral pterygoid (external pterygoid)	Greater wing of sphenoid and lateral part of pterygoid process of sphenoid bone	Mandibular condyle; temporomandibular joint (TMJ)
Medial pterygoid (internal pterygoid)	Medial part of pterygoid process of sphenoid bone and maxilla bone	Ramus and angle of mandible

Skeletal Muscle Actions: Muscles of Facial Expression and Mastication

ACTION	MUSCLE
Muscles of Facial Expression	
Closes and purses lips	1.
Closes eye	2.
Pulls scalp posteriorly	3.
Raises corners of mouth (smiling)	4.
Raises eyebrows and wrinkles forehead	5.
Raises upper lips, exposing upper teeth	6. Zygomaticus minor
Tenses neck skin; depresses mandible; pouting	7.
Muscles of Mastication	
Depresses mandible (opening mouth) and moves it sideways	8. Lateral pterygoid
Presses cheeks inward to whistle and helps hold food between teeth while chewing	9.
Elevates and retracts mandible (2 muscles)	10.
	11.
Elevates and protudes mandible	12. Medial pterygoid

2. Muscles that Move the Head, Vertebral Column, and Abdominal Wall

Muscles on the anterior surface of the neck flex the head and neck, whereas muscles on the posterior surface of the neck extend the head and neck. The same division is seen with the muscles of the abdomen and back. Abdominal muscles flex the vertebral column, while the muscles of the back extend it. However, the transversus abdominis muscle cannot flex the vertebral column because it runs horizontally.

TABLE 12.11 Muscles that Move the Head, Vertebral Column, and Abdominal Wall

MUSCLE	ORIGIN	INSERTION
Anterior and Lateral Muscles that Move the Head and Vertebral Column		
Sternocleidomastoid	Sternum and clavicle	Mastoid process of temporal bone
Scalenes	Transverse processes of vertebrae C3 through C6	Ribs 1 and 2
Rectus abdominis	Pubic crest and symphysis	Cartilage of ribs 5–7 and the xiphoid process
External oblique	Ribs 5 through 12	Iliac crest and linea alba
Internal oblique	Iliac crest, inguinal ligament, and thoracolumbar fascia	Cartilage of ribs 9–12 and linea alba
Transverse abdominus	Iliac crest, inguinal ligament, lumbar fascia, and cartilage of ribs 7–12	Xiphoid process, linea alba, and pubis
Posterior Muscles that Move the Head and Vertebral Column		
Splenius capitis	Ligamentum nuchae and spinous processes of vertebrae C7 through T4	Occipital bone and mastoid process of temporal bone
Trapezius (superior portion only)	Occipital bone and spines of vertebrae C7 through T12	Clavicle, acromion (process), and spine of scapula
Erector spinae	Large group of muscles with origins on ribs, and cervical, thoracic, and lumbar vertebrae, and iliac crest	Skull, ribs, and cervical, thoracic, and lumbar vertebrae

Skeletal Muscle Actions: Muscles that Move the Head, Vertebral Column, and Abdominal Wall

ACTION	MUSCLE(S)
Extends head.	1.
Extends head when both muscles contract. Rotates head to same side as contracting muscle when only one muscle contracts.	2. Splenius capitus
Flexes head and elevates 1st and 2nd ribs when both muscles contract during deep inspiration.	3.
Flexes head (prayer muscle) when both muscles contract. Rotates head side to side (as in saying no) when one muscle contracts.	4.
Flexes vertebral column and compresses abdomen. Does not laterally flex vertebral column.	5.
Flexes vertebral column and compresses abdomen when both muscles contract and laterally flexes vertebral column when only one muscle contracts. (2 muscles)	6. 7.
Compresses abdomen only.	8. Transverse abdominis
Extends vertebral column and maintains erect posture when both muscles contract. Laterally flexes vertebral column when only one muscle contracts.	9.

3. Muscles that Act on the Thoracic Cage

Contraction of these muscles increases or decreases the diameter or length of the thoracic cage. These changes affect lung volume and result in inspiration or expiration. The major muscle of respiration is the diaphragm. Changes in thoracic cage diameter and its effects on respiration are discussed in the respiratory exercise.

TABLE 12.12 Muscles that Act on the Thoracic Cage

MUSCLE	ORIGIN	INSERTION
Scalenes	Transverse processes of vertebrae C3 through C6	Ribs 1 and 2
Pectoralis minor	Ribs 2–5	Coracoid process of scapula
External intercostal	Inferior border of rib above	Superior border of rib below
Internal intercostal	Superior border of rib below	Inferior border of rib above
Diaphragm	Xiphoid process of sternum, costal cartilages of inferior six ribs, and lumbar vertebrae	Central tendon

Skeletal Muscle Actions: Muscles that Act on the Thoracic Cage

ACTION	MUSCLE
Depresses ribs during forced expiration	1.
Elevates 3rd through 5th ribs during deep inspiration	2.
Elevates ribs 1 and 2 during deep inspiration	3.
Elevates ribs during deep inspiration	4.
Flattens, increasing length of thoracic cage, during normal inspiration	5.

4. Muscles that Move the Scapula

Movements of the scapula include elevation, depression, abduction, adduction, and rotation. Shrugging the shoulders or lifting an object over the head elevates the scapula. Depression of the scapula occurs when doing a pullup. Pushing up during a "push-up" abducts the scapula, and standing at attention adducts the scapula.

TABLE 12.13 Muscles that Move the Scapula

MUSCLE	ORIGIN	INSERTION
Pectoralis minor	Ribs 2–5	Coracoid process of scapula
Serratus anterior	Ribs 1–9	Vertebral border of scapula and inferior angle of scapula
Trapezius	Occipital bone, ligamentum nuchae, and spines of vertebrae C7–T12	Clavicle, acromion of scapula, and spine of scapula
Levator scapulae	Vertebrae C1–C5	Superior vertebral border of scapula
Rhomboid major	Spines of vertebrae T2–T5	Vertebral border of scapula inferior to spine
Rhomboid minor	Spines of vertebrae C7 and T1	Vertebral border of scapula superior to spine

Skeletal Muscle Actions: Muscles that Move the Scapula

ACTION	MUSCLE
Depresses and abducts scapula and rotates it downward	1. Pectoralis minor
Abducts scapula and rotates it upward (boxers muscle)	2.
Elevates scapula and rotates it downward	3.
Elevates and adducts scapula and rotates it downward (2 muscles)	4. Rhomboid major 5. Rhomboid minor
Superior portion elevates scapula, middle portion adducts scapula, inferior portion depresses scapula	6.

5. Muscles that Move the Arm at the Shoulder Joint

These muscles originate on the trunk and insert on the humerus. Contraction pulls the humerus toward the insertion, resulting in movement of the humerus at the shoulder joint. Because of the structure of the shoulder joint and the way these surround the humerus, contraction can cause the full range of motion possible at a synovial joint—flexion, extension, abduction, adduction, circumduction, and rotation. Muscles that insert on the anterior surface of the arm flex the arm while those on the posterior surface extend the arm. Muscles that insert on the lateral surface abduct the arm while those on the medial surface adduct the arm.

TABLE 12.14 Muscles that Move the Arm

MUSCLE	ORIGIN	INSERTION
Pectoralis major	Clavicle, sternum, and costal cartilages of 2nd–6th ribs	Greater tubercle and intertubercular sulcus of humerus
Latissimus dorsi	Ribs 9–12, spines of T7–T12 vertebrae, lumbar vertebrae, crests of sacrum and ilium	Intertubercular sulcus of humerus
Deltoid	Clavicle; acromion of scapula; and spine of scapula	Deltoid tuberosity of humerus
Teres major	Inferior angle of scapula	Intertubercular sulcus of humerus
Rotator Cuff Muscles: Deep muscles that move the arm and surround the shoulder joint like a sleeve cuff and help strengthen and stabilize the shoulder joint. Include the **subscapularis, supraspinitus, infraspinitus,** and **teres minor.**		

Skeletal Muscle Actions: Muscles that Move the Arm*

ACTION	MUSCLE
Extends arm at shoulder joint†	1.
Adducts and flexes arm at shoulder joint†	2.
Extends and adducts arm at shoulder joint (if arm is elevated over head, it brings it down)†	3.
Large muscle with 3 groups of fibers. Lateral portion abducts arm, anterior portion flexes arm,† posterior portion extends arm‡	4.

*Many of these muscles also medially or laterally rotate the arm.
†Also medially rotate the arm.
‡Also laterally rotate the arm.

6. Muscles that Move the Forearm at the Elbow Joint and the Radioulnar Joints

These muscles have their origin on the scapula or humerus and their insertion on the bones of the forearm. When these muscles contract, they move the forearm at the elbow joint and/or the joints between the radius and ulna. The muscles that have origins on the scapula can also move the arm at the shoulder joint.

Muscles of the appendages that perform similar functions often are surrounded by fascia forming compartments. Muscles in the **anterior compartment** of the arm, such as the biceps brachii and brachialis muscles, flex the forearm whereas those in the **posterior compartment,** the triceps brachii, extend the forearm.

Observe that the pronator teres has its origin on the medial surface and its insertion on the lateral surface, whereas the supinator has its origin and insertion on the lateral and medial surface, respectively. When these muscles contract, they change the position of the radius and ulna.

TABLE 12.15 Muscles that Move the Forearm

MUSCLE	ORIGIN	INSERTION
Biceps brachii	**Long head:** tubercle superior to glenoid cavity of scapula **Short head:** coracoid process of scapula	Radial tuberosity
Brachialis	Anterior surface of distal humerus	Ulnar tuberosity and coronoid process of ulna
Triceps brachii **Long head** **Lateral head** **Medial head**	**Long head:** inferior to glenoid cavity of scapula **Lateral head:** posterior humerus superior to radial groove **Medial head:** posterior humerus inferior to radial groove	Olecranon of ulna
Pronator teres	Medial epicondyle of humerus; coronoid process of ulna	Midlateral surface of radius
Supinator	Lateral epicondyle of humerus; proximal ulna	Proximal 1/3 of radius
Brachioradialis	Distal border of humerus	Superior to styloid process of radius

Skeletal Muscle Actions: Muscles that Move the Forearm

ACTION	MUSCLE
Extends forearm at elbow and extends arm at shoulder	1.
Flexes forearm at elbow	2.
Flexes forearm at elbow and flexes arm at shoulder	3.
Flexes forearm and pronotes and supinates forearm	4. Brachioradialis
Pronates forearm	5.
Supinates forearm	6.

7. Muscles that Move the Hand at Wrist and Fingers

Muscles originating on the forearm cross the wrist to insert on the hand or digits. The muscles of the **superficial anterior compartment** of the forearm are: flexor carpi radialis, palmaris longus, flexor carpi ulnaris, and flexor digitorum superficialis. These muscles are the flexors of the hand or digits, and originate on the medial epicondyle of the humerus. Muscles of the **superficial posterior compartment** of the forearm are: extensor carpi radialis longus, extensor carpi radialis brevis, extensor digitorum, and extensor carpi ulnaris. These muscles are extensors and originate on the lateral epicondyle of the humerus. Muscles near the lateral surface of the forearm abduct the wrist, whereas those near the medial surface adduct it.

TABLE 12.16 Muscles that Move the Hand and Fingers

MUSCLE	ORIGIN	INSERTION
Flexor carpi radialis	Medial epicondyle of humerus	2nd and 3rd metacarpals (insertion tendon is a guide for taking radial pulse)
Palmaris longus	Medial epicondyle of humerus	Flexor retinaculum and palmar aponeurosis
Flexor carpi ulnaris	Medial epicondyle of humerus; superior posterior surface of ulna	Pisiform, hamate, and base of 5th metacarpal
Flexor digitorum superficialis	Medial epicondyle of humerus, coronoid process of ulna, and anterior surface of radius	Middle phalanges of each finger
Extensor carpi radialis		
Longus	Lateral supracondylar ridge of humerus	2nd metacarpal
Brevis	Lateral epicondyle of humerus	3rd metacarpal
Extensor digitorum	Lateral epicondyle of humerus	Distal and middle phalanges of each finger
Extensor carpi ulnaris	Lateral epicondyle of humerus and posterior ulna	5th metacarpal
Abductor pollicis longus	Posterior, middle radius and ulna	1st metacarpal
Extensor pollicis longus	Posterior, middle ulna	Proximal phalynx of 1st digit

Skeletal Muscle Actions: Muscles that Move the Hand and Fingers

ACTION	MUSCLE
Flexes and abducts hand at wrist	1.
Flexes and adducts hand at wrist	2.
Weakly flexes wrist	3. Palmaris longus
Flexes hand and proximal and middle phalanges	4.
Extends and abducts hand at wrist (2 muscles)	5. 6.
Extends and adducts hand at wrist	7.
Extends hand and proximal, middle, and distal phalanges	8.
Abducts thumb	9.
Extends thumb	10.

8. Muscles that Move the Thigh at the Hip Joint

Muscles that move the thigh have origins on the pelvis or vertebrae and insertions on the femur or tibia. Muscles on the anterior surface of the thigh flex the thigh, whereas the lateral surface of the thigh also abduct. Muscles of the **medial compartment** are: adductor magnus, adductor longus, adductor brevis, pectineus, and gracilis. These muscles adduct and flex the thigh. Muscles on the posterior surface extend and/or abduct the thigh.

TABLE 12.17 Muscles that Move the Thigh*

MUSCLE	ORIGIN	INSERTION
Psoas major	Lumbar vertebrae transverse processes and bodies	Lesser trochanter of femur
Iliacus	Iliac fossa	Lesser trochanter of femur
Tensor fasciae latae	Iliac crest	Iliotibial tract (fascia)
Pectineus	Superior ramus of pubis	Between lesser trochanter and linea aspera
Adductor brevis	Inferior ramus of pubis	Proximal linea aspera of femur
Adductor longus	Pubic crest and pubic symphysis	Linea aspera of femur
Adductor magnus	Rami of ischium and pubis	Linea aspera of femur
Gracilis	Pulbic symphysis and pubic arch	Medial surface of anterior tibia
Gluteus maximus	Iliac crest, sacrum, coccyx	Gluteal tuberosity of femur and iliotibial tract
Gluteus medius	Ilium	Greater trochanter of femur
Gluteus minimus	Ilium	Greater trochanter of femur

*Many of these muscles are also involved in medial and lateral rotations of thigh.

Skeletal Muscle Actions: Muscles that Move the Thigh*

ACTION(S)	MUSCLES
Adducts and flexes thigh at hip joint (5 muscles)	1.
	2.
	3.
	4.
	5.
Flex thigh at hip joint only (2 muscles)	6. Psoas major
	7. Iliacus
Flex and abduct thigh at hip joint	8.
Extends thigh at hip joint only	9.
Abducts thigh at hip joint (2 muscles)	10. Gluteus medius
	11. Gluteus minimus

9. Muscles that Move the Leg at the Knee Joint

Muscles that move the leg have their origins on the pelvis or femur. Those with origins on the pelvis move the thigh at the hip joint and the leg at the knee joint, whereas those with origins on the femur only move the leg at the knee joint. Muscles of the **anterior compartment** of the thigh, the quadriceps femoris group, extend the leg. The rectus femoris muscle of this group also flexes the thigh. Muscles of the **posterior compartment** are the hamstring muscle group. These muscles flex the leg and extend the thigh. Notice that the sartorius spans both hip and knee joints, and has its origin near the lateral surface of the pelvis and its insertion near the medial surface of the tibia.

TABLE 12.18 Muscles that Move the Leg

MUSCLE	ORIGIN	INSERTION
Sartorius	Anterior superior iliac spine	Medial surface of anterior tibia
Quadriceps femoris		
Rectus femoris	Anterior inferior iliac spine	Patella (quadriceps tendon) and tibial tuberosity (patellar ligament)
Vastus lateralis	Greater trochanter and linea aspera	
Vastus medialis	Linea aspera of femur	
Vastus intermedius	Anterior and lateral surface of proximal femur	
Hamstrings		
Biceps femoris	Long head: Ischial tuberosity Short head: Linea aspera of femur	Head of fibula and lateral condyle of tibia Head of fibula and lateral condyle of tibia
Semitendinosus	Ischial tuberosity	Medial surface of proximal tibia
Semimembranosus	Ischial tuberosity	Medial condyle of tibia

Skeletal Muscle Actions: Muscles that Move the Leg

ACTION	MUSCLE
Extends leg at knee and flexes thigh at hip	1.
Extends leg at knee only (3 muscles)	2. 3. 4.
Flexes leg at knee and extends thigh at hip (3 muscles)	5. 6. 7.
Flexes leg at knee and flexes, abducts, and laterally rotates thigh at hip (allows us to flex and cross our legs)	8. Sartorius

10. Muscles that Move the Foot at the Ankle and Toes

Muscles of the **anterior compartment** of the leg include the tibialis anterior and extensor digitorum longus. These muscles dorsiflex the foot and also extend the toes if they insert on the phalanges. Muscles of the **posterior compartment** of the leg include the gastrocnemius, soleus, flexor digitorum longus, and flexor hallucis longus. These muscles plantarflex the foot and also flex the toes if they insert on the phalanges. Eversion of the foot is due to contraction of muscles near the lateral surface of the leg, whereas inversion is due to contraction of muscles near the medial surface of the leg.

D. Dissection of Cat Muscles

If you are dissecting a cat to observe skeletal muscles, refer to the appropriate accompanying dissection manual.

LAB SAFETY: *Use safety glasses and remember to properly dispose of any removed waste tissue as directed by your instructor. Always clean your dissection tools, tray, and lab surfaces as directed.*

TABLE 12.19 Muscles that Move the Foot and Toes

MUSCLE	ORIGIN	INSERTION
Tibialis anterior	Lateral condyle and body of tibia and interosseous membrane	1st metatarsal and first cuneiform (tarsal bone)
Extensor digitorum longus	Lateral condyle of tibia, anterior fibula, and interosseous membrane	Middle and distal phalanges of toes 2–5
Fibularis (peroneus) longus	Lateral condyle of tibia and head and body of fibula	1st metarsal and first cuneiform
Gastrocnemius	Lateral and medial condyles of femur	Calcaneus (calcaneal or Achilles tendon)
Soleus	Medial tibia and head of fibula	Calcaneus (calcaneal tendon)
Flexor digitorum longus	Posterior tibia	Distal phalanges of toes 2–5
Flexor hallucis longus	Inferior fibula	Distal phalanx of big toe

Skeletal Muscle Actions: Muscles that Move the Foot and Toes

ACTION	MUSCLE
Plantar flexes foot and flexes toes	1.
Plantar flexes foot and flexes leg at knee	2. Gastrocnemius
Plantar flexes foot only	3.
Plantar flexes and everts foot	4.
Dorsiflexes foot and extends toes	5.
Dorsiflexes and inverts foot	6. Tibialis anterior
Flexes big toe	7.

Name ______________________ Date ______________ Section ______________

EXERCISE 12

REVIEWING YOUR KNOWLEDGE

A. Criteria for Naming Muscles

Identify the criteria used to name each muscle. More than one criteria may apply to a muscle name.

a. orientation of muscle relative to body midline
b. muscle size
c. muscle shape
d. muscle action
e. number of origins
f. location
g. origin and insertion

______________________ **1.** vastus lateralis

______________________ **2.** zygomaticus

______________________ **3.** trapezius

______________________ **4.** adductor brevis

______________________ **5.** sternocleidomastoid

______________________ **6.** levator scapulae

______________________ **7.** serratus anterior

______________________ **8.** gluteus maximus

______________________ **9.** infraspinatus

______________________ **10.** erector spinae

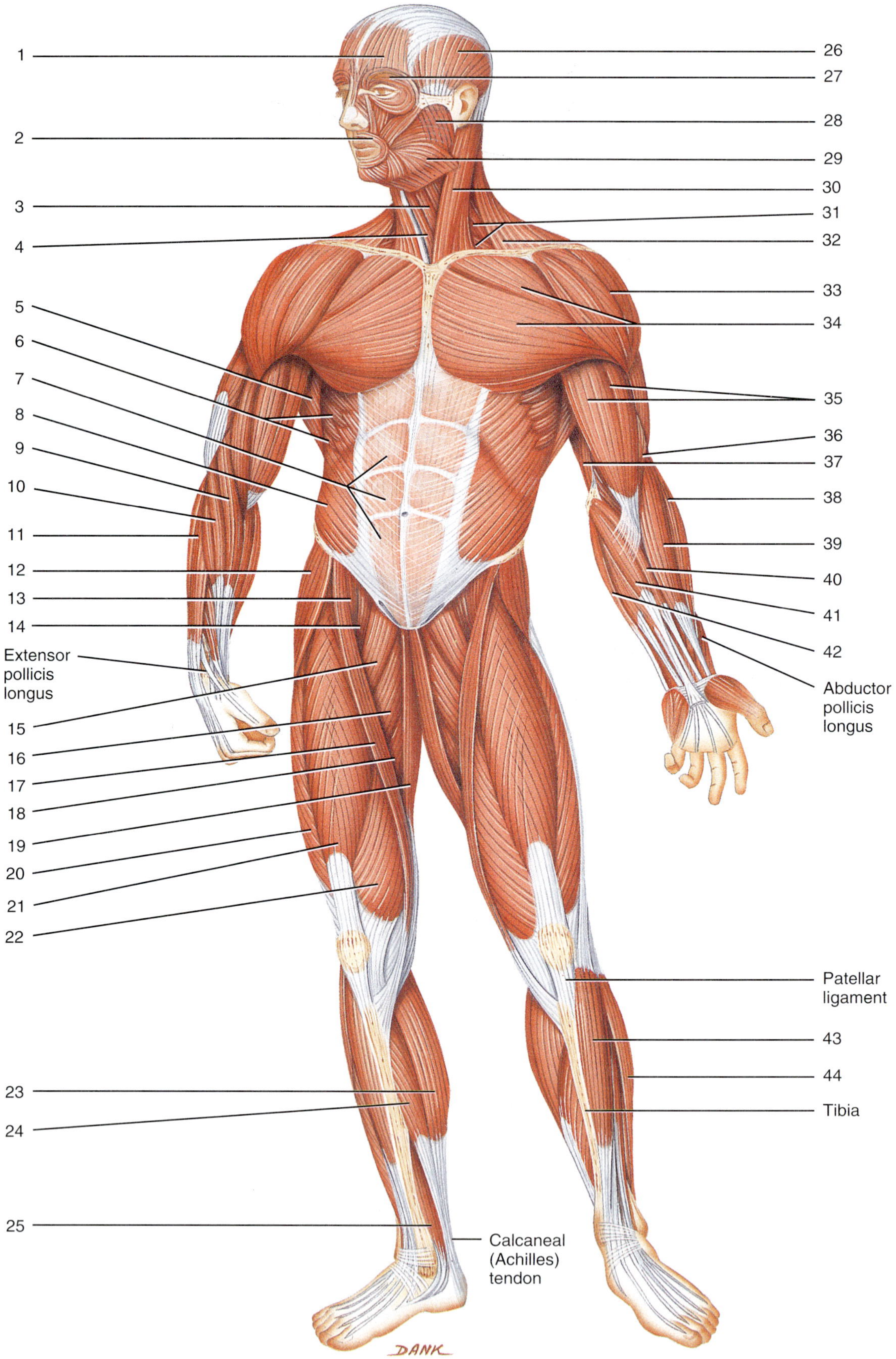

(a) Anterior view

FIGURE 12.9 Superficial skeletal muscles.

B. Muscle Location: Superficial Skeletal Muscles

Label the muscles in Figure 12.9.

1. ______________________
2. ______________________
3. ______________________
4. ______________________
5. ______________________
6. ______________________
7. ______________________
8. ______________________
9. ______________________
10. ______________________
11. ______________________
12. ______________________
13. ______________________
14. ______________________
15. ______________________
16. ______________________
17. ______________________
18. ______________________
19. ______________________
20. ______________________
21. ______________________
22. ______________________
23. ______________________
24. ______________________
25. ______________________
26. ______________________
27. ______________________
28. ______________________
29. ______________________
30. ______________________
31. ______________________
32. ______________________
33. ______________________
34. ______________________
35. ______________________
36. ______________________
37. ______________________
38. ______________________
39. ______________________
40. ______________________
41. ______________________
42. ______________________
43. ______________________
44. ______________________

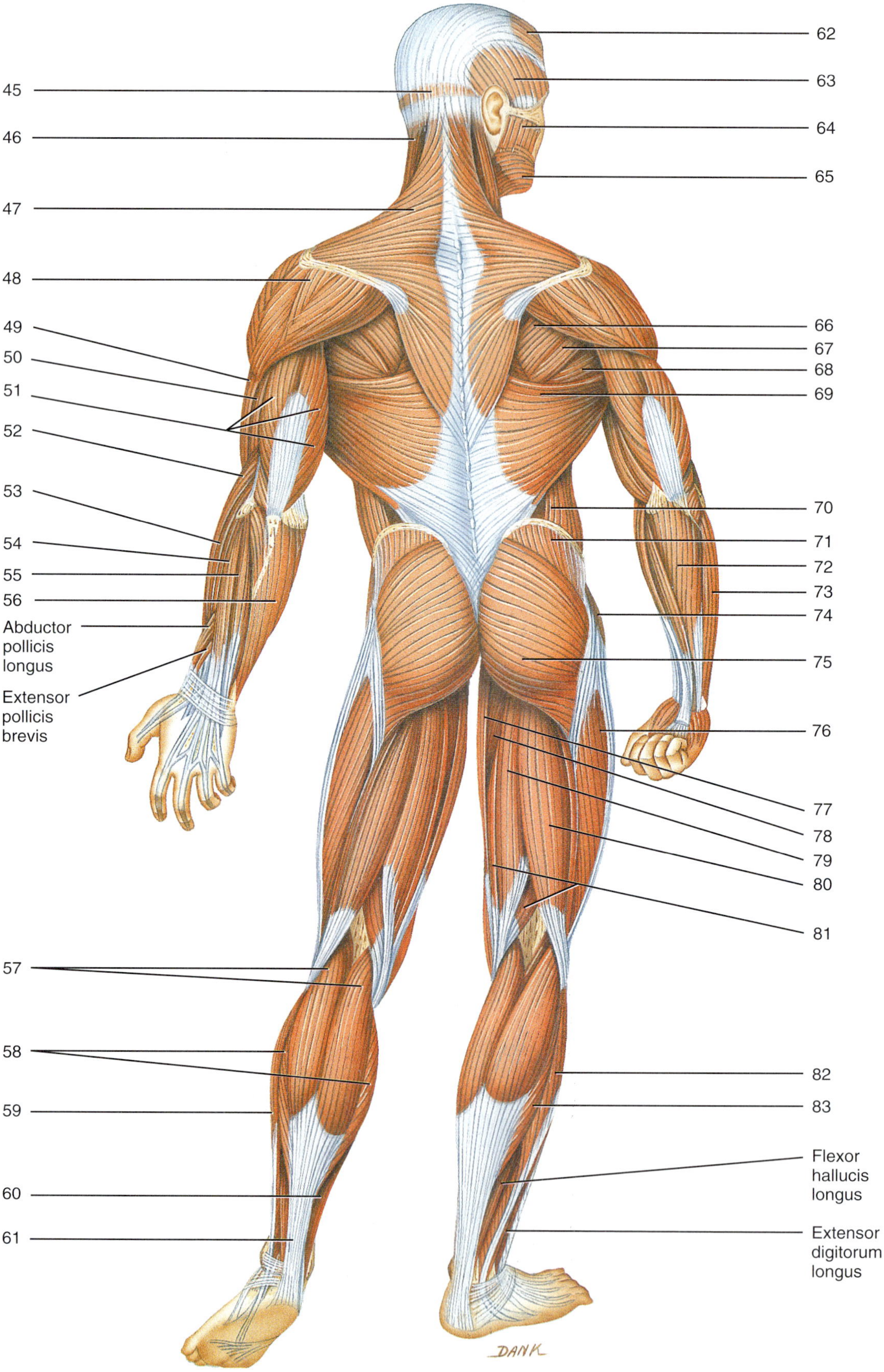

(b) Posterior view

FIGURE 12.9 **Superficial skeletal muscles,** ***continued.***

45. ______________________________

46. ______________________________

47. ______________________________

48. ______________________________

49. ______________________________

50. ______________________________

51. ______________________________

52. ______________________________

53. ______________________________

54. ______________________________

55. ______________________________

56. ______________________________

57. ______________________________

58. ______________________________

59. ______________________________

60. ______________________________

61. ______________________________

62. ______________________________

63. ______________________________

64. ______________________________

65. ______________________________

66. ______________________________

67. ______________________________

68. ______________________________

69. ______________________________

70. ______________________________

71. ______________________________

72. ______________________________

73. ______________________________

74. ______________________________

75. ______________________________

76. ______________________________

77. ______________________________

78. ______________________________

79. ______________________________

80. ______________________________

81. ______________________________

82. ______________________________

83. ______________________________

C. Muscle Function

Identify the muscles that perform each function. Note if muscle performs two functions, such as

Muscles of Facial Expression

1. ______________________ Smiling muscle
2. ______________________ Raises your eyebrows
3. ______________________ Tenses skin of neck
4. ______________________ Pulls scalp posterior
5. ______________________ Kissing muscle
6. ______________________ Closes eyelids

Muscles of Mastication

7. ______________________ Opens mouth (depresses mandible)
8. ______________________
9. ______________________ Closes mouth (elevates mandible)
10. ______________________
11. Buccinator ______________________ Compresses checks and aids in holding food between teeth

Muscles that Flex the Head

12. ______________________
13. ______________________

Muscles that Extend the Head

14. ______________________
15. ______________________

Muscles that Flex the Vertebral Column and Com-pressthe Abdomen

16. ______________________
17. ______________________
18. ______________________

Muscle that Compresses Abdomen only

19. ______________________

Muscle Group that Extends the Vertebral Column

20. ______________________

Muscles that Move the Scapula

21. ____________________

22. ____________________

23. ____________________

24. ____________________

25. ____________________

26. ____________________

Muscles that Flex the Arm ***(One of these muscles also flexes the forearm.)***

27. ____________________

28. ____________________

29. ____________________

Muscles that Extend the Arm

30. ____________________

31. ____________________

32. ____________________

Muscle that Abducts the Arm

33. ____________________

Muscles that Adduct the Arm

34. ____________________

35. ____________________

Muscles that Flex the Forearm

36. ____________________

37. ____________________

38. ____________________

Muscle that Extends the Forearm

39. ____________________

Muscles that Flex the Hand

40. ____________________

41. ____________________

42. ____________________

43. ____________________

Muscles that Extend the Hand

44. ____________________

45. ____________________

46. ____________________

47. ____________________

Muscles that Abduct Hand

48. ____________________

49. ____________________

50. ____________________

Muscles that Adduct Hand

51. ____________________

52. ____________________

Muscles that Flex the Thigh ***(One of these muscles also extends the leg.)***

53. ____________________

54. ____________________

55. ____________________

56. ____________________

57. ____________________

58. ____________________

59. ____________________

60. ____________________

61. ____________________

62. Sartorius

Muscles that Extend the Thigh (*Three of these muscles also flex the knee.*)

63. ______________________

64. ______________________

65. ______________________

66. ______________________

Muscles that Abduct the Thigh

67. ______________________

68. ______________________

69. ______________________

70. Sartorius

Muscles that Adduct the Thigh

71. ______________________

72. ______________________

73. ______________________

74. ______________________

75. ______________________

Muscle that Flexes Leg and Flexes, Abducts & Laterally Rotates Thigh at Leg

76. ______________________

Muscles that Extend the Leg

77. ______________________

78. ______________________

79. ______________________

80. ______________________

Muscles that Flex the Leg (*One of these also plantar flexes the foot.*)

81. ______________________

82. ______________________

83. ______________________

84. ______________________

85. Sartorius

Muscles that Plantarflex the Foot

86. ______________________

87. ______________________

88. ______________________

89. ______________________

Muscles that Dorsiflex the Foot

90. ______________________

91. ______________________

Rotator Cuff Muscles

92. ______________________

93. ______________________

94. ______________________

95. ______________________

Name ______________ Date ______________ Section ______________

EXERCISE 12

USING YOUR KNOWLEDGE

Identify the surface muscles on Figure 12.10.

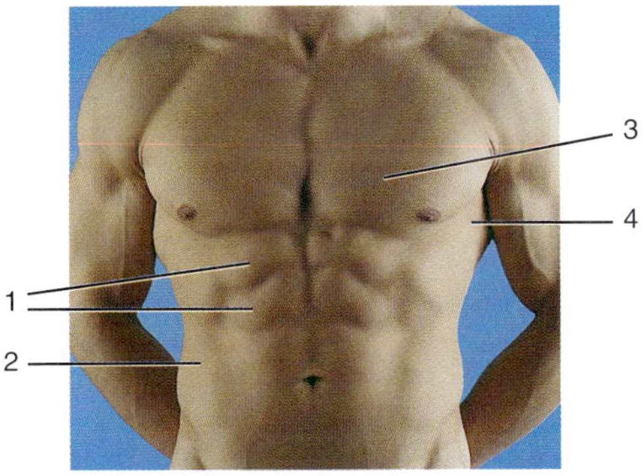

(a) Anterior view of the trunk

1. ______________

2. ______________

3. ______________

4. ______________

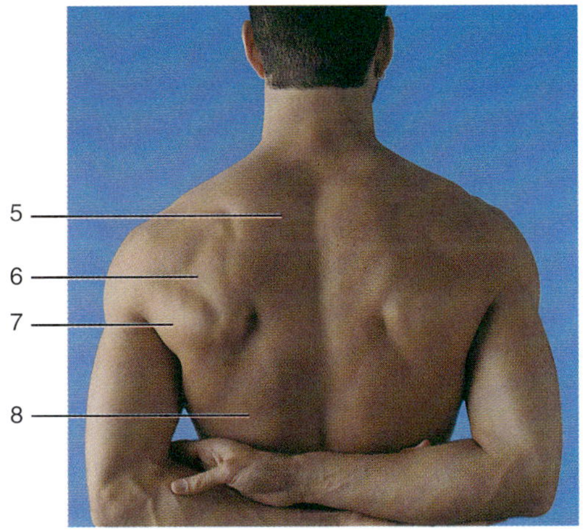

5. ______________

6. ______________

7. ______________

8. ______________

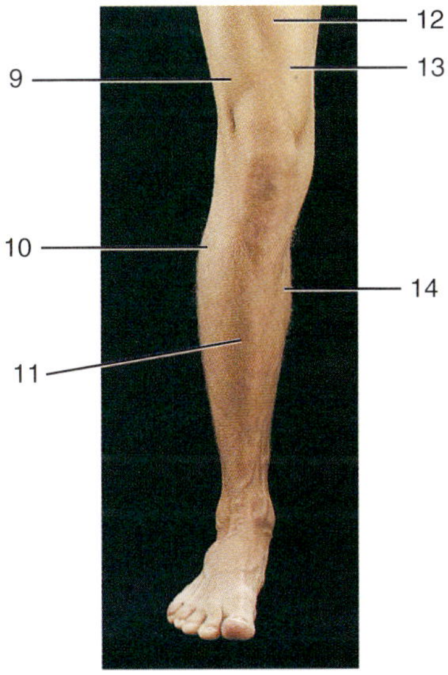

(c) Anterior view of the lower extremity

9. ______________

10. ______________

11. ______________

12. ______________

13. ______________

14. ______________

FIGURE 12.10 Surface anatomy, skeletal muscles.

Questions 15–20

15. Identify the major *thigh* and *leg* muscles you use when you *kick* a ball.

16. Identify the *forearm* muscles you use when you *turn* a key in a lock.

17. Identify the major *arm* muscles you use when you *lift* a glass to drink from it.

18. Identify the *neck* muscles you use when you *look both ways* to cross a street.

19. Identify the *abdominal* muscles you use when you do the *"twist"*.

20. Identify the *muscles of the head* that you use when you *whistle.*

EXERCISE 13

NERVOUS TISSUE

OUTLINE

OBJECTIVES

After completing this exercise, you should be able to:

- Describe the functions of the nervous system
- Name the two major divisions of the nervous system and their organs
- Explain the difference in function between neurons and neuroglia
- Identify neuron structures and describe their functions
- Describe the reception of a nervous impulse by a neuron
- Describe the generation and transmission of a nervous impulse to other neurons or target organs
- Understand and describe how neurons are classified structurally and functionally
- Identify unipolar, bipolar, and multipolar neurons on photomicrographs or prepared slides

MATERIALS

- models or charts of the nervous system
- models or charts of a neuron and neuroglia
- photomicrographs or prepared slides of astrocytes, motor neurons, dorsal root ganglia, cerebral cortex and teased, myelinated nerve fibers

Nervous tissue is found in the organs of the nervous system—the nerves, brain, and spinal cord, and contains cells that enable the nervous system to generate and transmit electrical signals called nerve impulses or action potentials.

A. Overview of Nervous System

The nervous system senses changes in our internal and external environments, coordinates and integrates this data, and initiates and transmits action potentials. It is organized into two basic components: the central nervous system (CNS) and the peripheral nervous system (PNS). The CNS, which consists of the brain and spinal cord, coordinates and integrates information received from sensory receptors and initiates and transmits impulses to neurons, muscles, or glands. The PNS contains an afferent division composed of sensory receptors and nerves, and an efferent division composed of motor nerves. Sensory receptors detect changes in the environment and transmit this information along sensory or afferent nerves to the CNS. Motor nerves transmit impulses from the CNS to target organs (neurons, muscles, or glands). The nervous system is streamlined to send rapid signals from cell to cell to maintain homeostasis and coordinate body organs and functions.

B. Structure of Nervous Tissue

Nervous tissue is located in the brain, spinal cord, and nerves, and is composed of two types of cells, neurons and neuroglia. **Neurons** conduct action potentials and are the structural and functional units of nervous tissue. **Neuroglia** (*neuro-* = nerve; *-glia* = glue) are cells that support, protect, furnish nutrients to, and augment the speed of neuron transmission.

1. Neuroglial Cells

Neuroglial cells are generally smaller and more abundant than neurons. Although they do not create action potentials, neuroglial cells have important roles in the nervous system. Of the six types of neuroglial cells, four are in the CNS and two are in the PNS. The four neuroglial cells in the CNS are: astrocytes, ependymal cells, microglia, and oligodendrocytes. **Astrocytes** (*astro-* = star; *-cyte* = cell) have many processes that make them look star-shaped. Their **perivascular** (*per* = around; *vascular* = vessel) **feet** wrap around and cover neurons and blood vessels to keep neurons in place. Astrocytes also guide neurons during development and control the composition of the chemical environment of the neurons by forming a **blood-brain barrier.** This barrier only allows certain substances to enter the nervous tissue at the blood vessel sites. **Oligodendrocytes** (*oligo-* = few; *dendro-* = tree) support the CNS neurons and have processes that form **myelin sheaths** around axons that increase the speed of nerve impulses. **Microglia** (*micro-* = small) are the phagocytes (*phago-* = to eat) of the CNS that engulf debris, necrotic tissue, and invading bacteria or viruses. **Ependymal cells** (*epen-* = above; *dym-* = garment) line all four ventricles (spaces or cavities) of the brain, as well as the central canal of the spinal cord. These cells form cerebrospinal fluid (CSF), and their cilia move the CSF through the ventricles. The two neuroglial cells in the PNS are Schwann cells and satellite cells. **Schwann cells** are flattened cells that wrap around the axons in the PNS. Many Schwann cells form the myelin sheath around one axon that increases nerve impulse speed and aids in the regeneration of PNS axons. **Satellite cells** have processes that are flattened and surround the neuron cell bodies located in ganglia in the PNS. They give support to these neurons and regulate their chemical environment.

TABLE 13.1 Neuroglial Cells

CELL TYPE	LOCATION	FUNCTION
1. ____________	CNS or PNS	Entire cell forms myelin sheath around a segment of an axon; helps regeneration of axons.
2. ____________	CNS or PNS	Lines 4 brain ventricles; forms and circulates CSF.
3. ____________	CNS or PNS	Engulfs invading microbes; clears debris; migrates to injured nerves.
4. ____________	CNS or PNS	Maintains environment around neurons; forms blood-brain barrier.
5. ____________	CNS or PNS	Covers sensory neuron cell bodies; maintains neuron environment.
6. ____________	CNS or PNS	Processes from cell form myelin sheaths around axons of neurons.

ACTIVITY 1 Neuroglial Cells

1 Complete Table 13.1 using the list of cells below. Under *location*, circle CNS or PNS.

- astrocyte
- ependymal cells
- microglia
- oligodendrocytes
- satellite cells
- Schwann cells

2 Label the neuroglial cells in Figure 13.1.

3 Pronounce the terms as you label Figure 13.1.

- astrocyte (AS-troh-cyte)
- ependymal cells (ee-PIN-dih-mahl)
- microglia (my-CROG-lee-a)
- oligodendrocytes (OL-ih-go-DEN-droh-sites)
- satellite cells
- Schwann cells (shh-WAN)

(a) CNS

1 ______________________

2 ______________________

3 ______________________

4 ______________________

(b) PNS

5 ______________________

6 ______________________

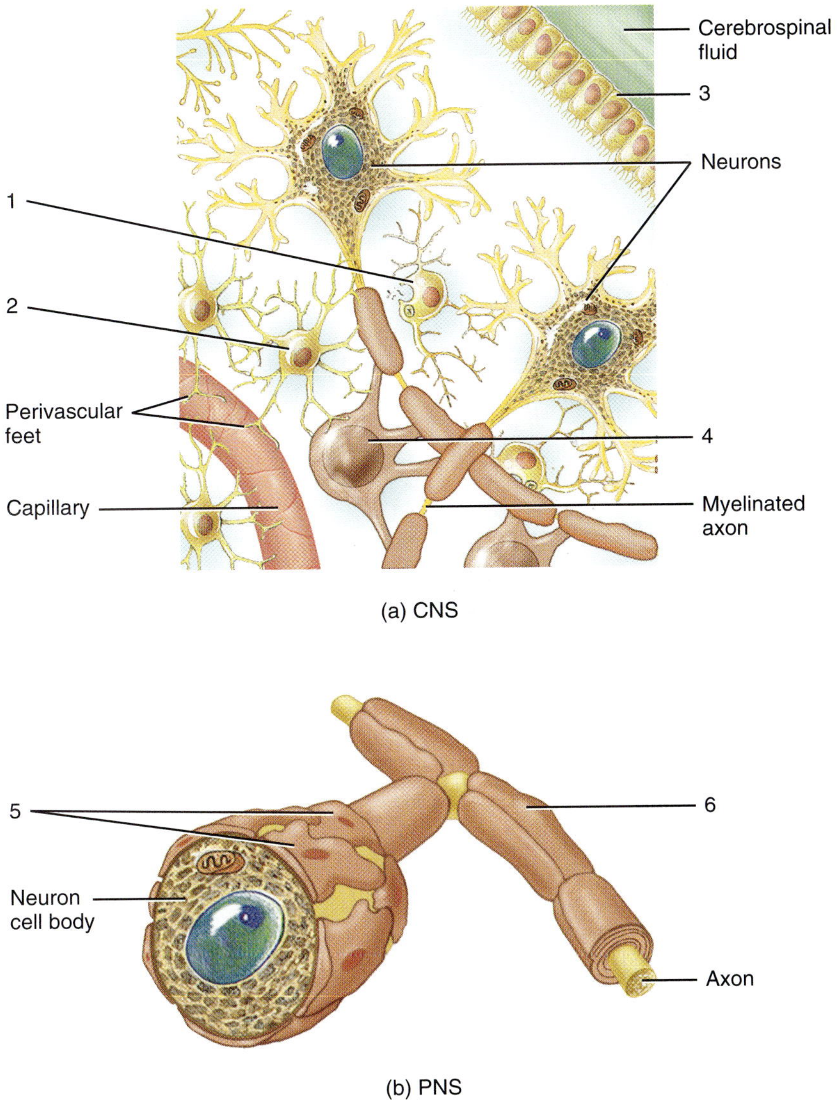

FIGURE 13.1 Neuroglial cells.

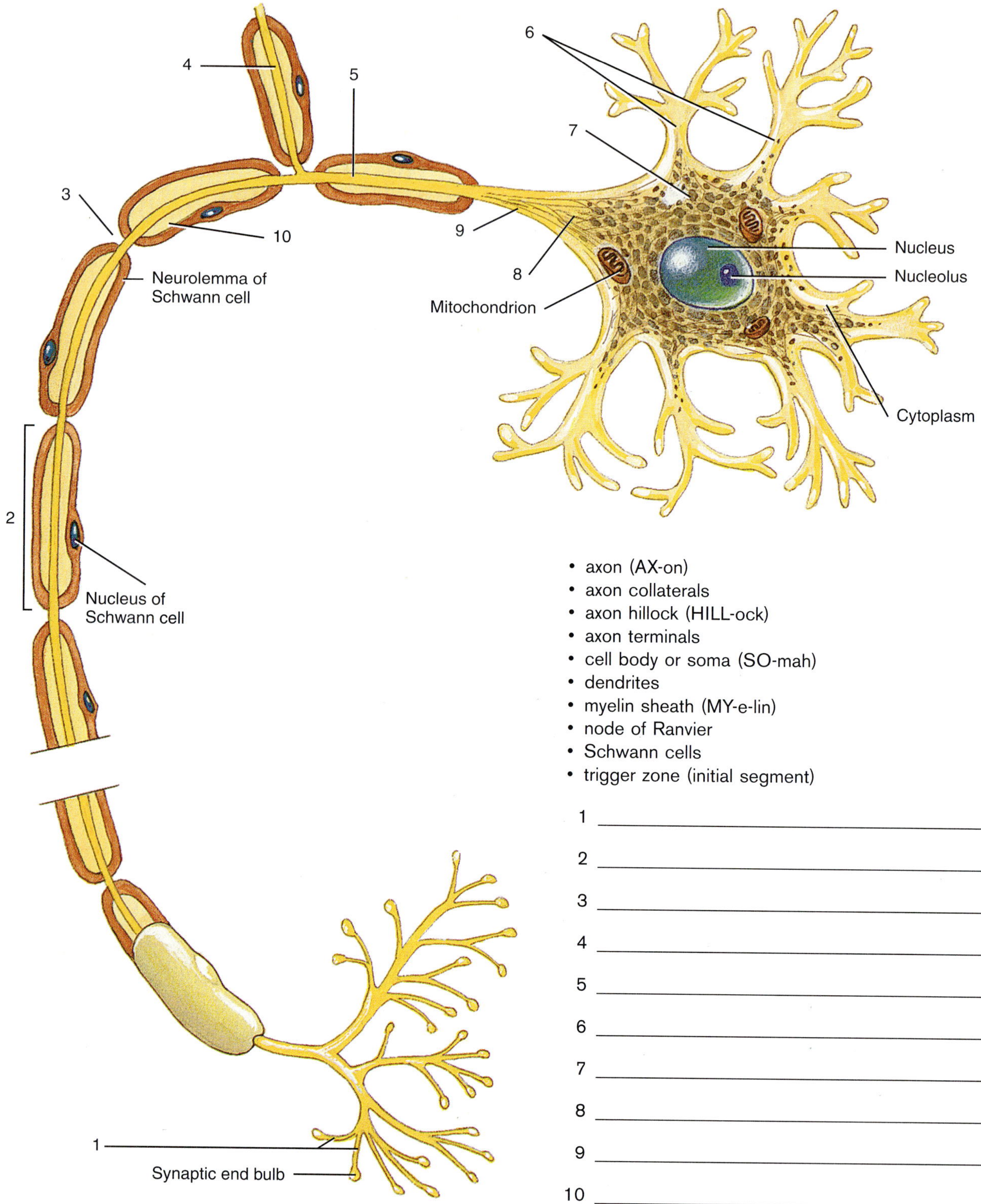

- axon (AX-on)
- axon collaterals
- axon hillock (HILL-ock)
- axon terminals
- cell body or soma (SO-mah)
- dendrites
- myelin sheath (MY-e-lin)
- node of Ranvier
- Schwann cells
- trigger zone (initial segment)

1 ______________________________

2 ______________________________

3 ______________________________

4 ______________________________

5 ______________________________

6 ______________________________

7 ______________________________

8 ______________________________

9 ______________________________

10 ______________________________

FIGURE 13.2 Parts of a motor neuron.

2. Structure of a Neuron

The longest cells in the body are **neurons** that can be over 3 feet long. Think about one neuron being long enough to reach from your spinal cord to the tips of your fingers or toes. There are three basic parts to any neuron: dendrites, a cell body, and an axon. Both the dendrites (*dendr-* = little trees) and the single axon are extensions of the nerve cell body called **processes. Dendrites** receive information from receptors or other neurons and send it as a change in membrane potential to the nerve **cell body** or **soma** (*soma* = body). Neuron cell bodies have most of the organelles present in other types of cells. There is usually a triangular or cone-shaped area of the cell body called the **axon hillock** (*hillock* = small hill). The **axon** (*axon* = axis) is a longer process than the dendrites that extends from the axon hillock. Changes in membrane potential travel to the axon hillock region where they are integrated to determine if an action potential will be initiated in the axon. The first part of the axon is known as the **trigger area** (initial segment), where the nerve impulse begins. The axon may be a single process, or it may have side branches called **axon collaterals.** Axons and axon collaterals conduct action potentials along their full lengths to end at fine processes called **axon terminals.** Neurotransmitter molecules are released from axon terminals and transmit signals across a synapse to other neurons or to effectors such as muscles or glands.

ACTIVITY 2 Structure of a Neuron

1 Identify and label the structures in Figure 13.2.

2 Pronounce the terms as you label Figure 13.2.

3 Identify and label the structures in Figure 13.3.

4 Examine a prepared slide of **astrocytes.**
- Using the low power objective, find an astrocyte and center it in the field of view.
- Using the high power objective, identify the **cell body** and **processes.**
- Note the size of the astrocytes.

5 Examine a prepared slide of **motor neurons.**
- Using the low power objective, find a large motor neuron and center it in the field of view.
- Using the high power objective, identify the **cell body, nucleus, dendrites, axon hillock,** and **axon.**
- Note the size of the motor neuron and the numerous small, dark-stained **neuroglial cells** near the neuron.

6 With your lab group compare the size of astrocytes and motor neurons.

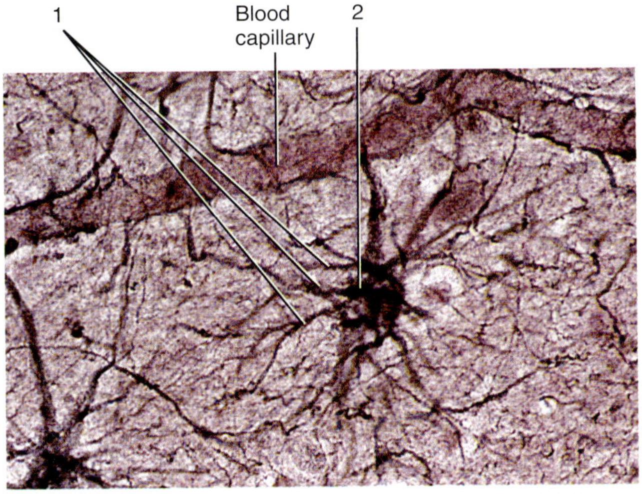

(a) Astrocyte LM 700x

- cell body
- processes

1 ________________

2 ________________

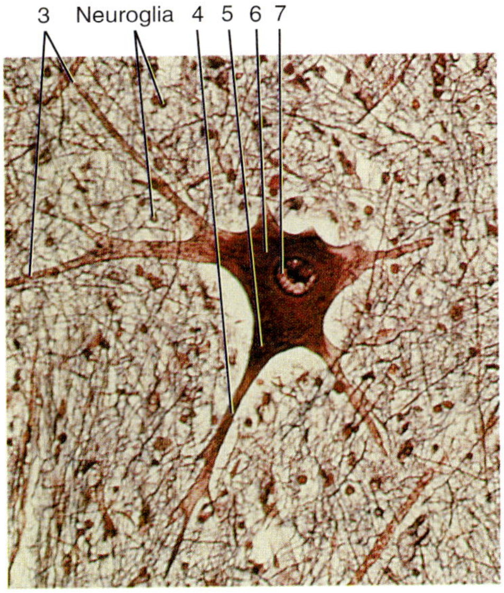

(b) Motor neuron LM 260x

- axon
- axon hillock
- cell body
- dendrites
- nucleus

3 __________ 6 __________

4 __________ 7 __________

5 __________

FIGURE 13.3 Photomicrographs of nervous tissue cells.

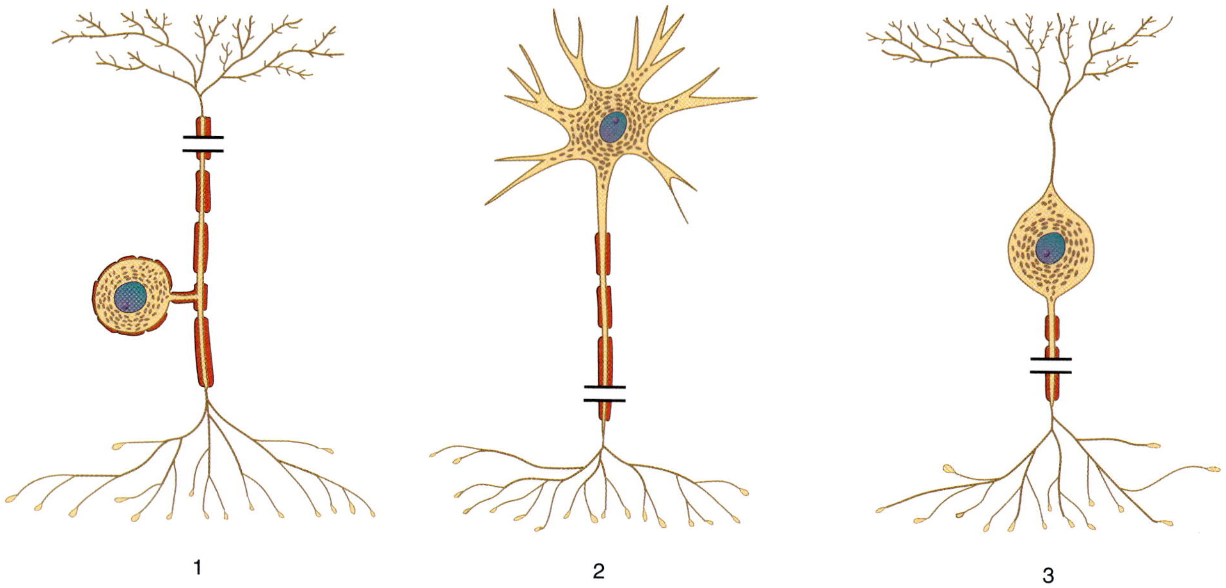

(a) Structural classification of neurons

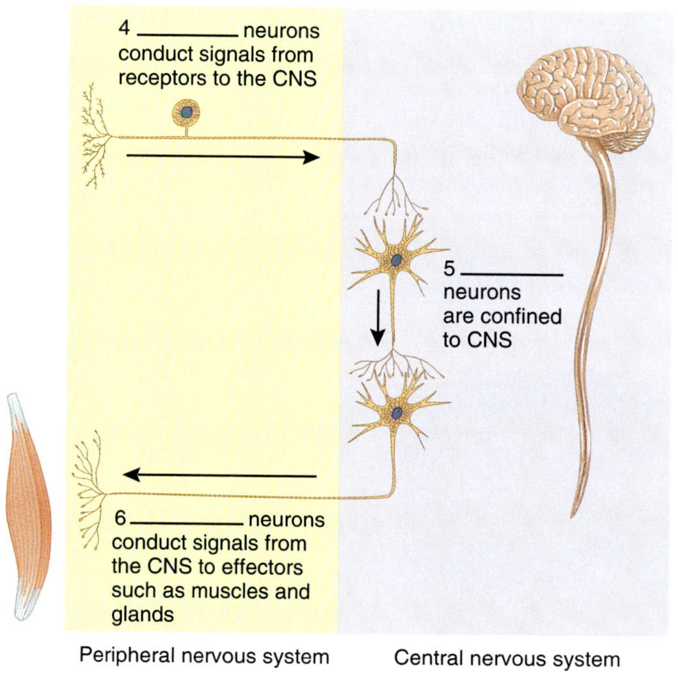

(b) Functional classification of neurons

(a) Structural classifications
- bipolar neuron
- multipolar neuron
- unipolar neuron

1 ______________________________

2 ______________________________

3 ______________________________

(b) Functional classifications
- interneuron (association neuron)
- motor neuron (efferent)
- sensory neuron (afferent)

4 ______________________________

5 ______________________________

6 ______________________________

FIGURE 13.4 Structural and functional classifications of neurons.

3. Structural Classification of Neurons

Neurons are classified both structurally and functionally. The number of processes that project from the cell body of the neuron determine its structural classification. The **multipolar neurons** have numerous processes with many dendrites and one axon. Motor neurons and interneurons (association neurons) are multipolar neurons and comprise most of the CNS neurons. **Bipolar neurons** have two processes, one dendrite and one axon, on either side of the cell body and are found in the special senses like the retina of the eye, the olfactory cells of the nose, and the inner ear. **Unipolar neurons** have only one process, an axon, leading to and from the neuron cell body. The dendrites are small and attach to the axon instead of the nerve cell body. Unipolar neurons are sensory neurons that bring sensory information from the skin, muscles, and organs to the spinal cord.

4. Functional Classification of Neurons

There are three classifications of neurons based on their functions: sensory, interneuron (association neuron), and motor neuron. Changes in the environment produce a stimulus that is detected by the receptors associated with the dendrites of a **sensory (afferent) neuron.** This neuron changes the stimulation into an action potential or nervous impulse which travels along the axon to the spinal cord. General sensory neurons are structurally unipolar neurons.

In the spinal cord, the axon of the sensory neuron synapses with either a motor neuron or an interneuron. The **interneuron (association neuron)** is structurally an unmyelinated multipolar neuron and comprises about 90% of the neurons in the CNS. In the spinal cord, the interneuron can synapse with a chain of interneurons sending the signal to the brain, and/or it can synapse with a **motor (efferent) neuron** that takes the impulse out of the spinal cord via a spinal nerve to an effector. Motor neurons are structurally multipolar neurons.

ACTIVITY 3 Structural and Functional Classifications of Neurons

1 Identify and label the neurons in Figure 13.4a and Figure 13.4b.

2 Identify and label the structures listed in Figure 13.5.

3 Examine prepared microscope slide of **dorsal root ganglia.**
- Using the low power objective, locate a neuron and place it in the center of the field of view.
- Identify the **neuron cell body, nucleus,** and **processes.**

4 Examine prepared microscope slide of **cerebral cortex.** Follow the same steps as above.

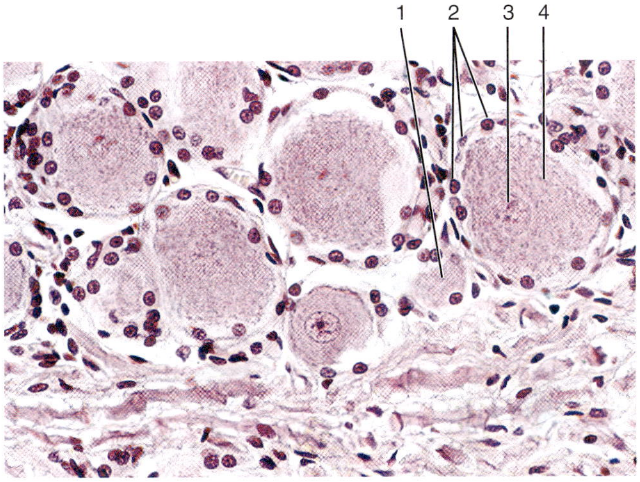

(a) Dorsal root ganglia, unipolar neurons LM 300x

- neuron cell body
- nucleus
- process
- satellite cell

1 ______

2 ______

3 ______

4 ______

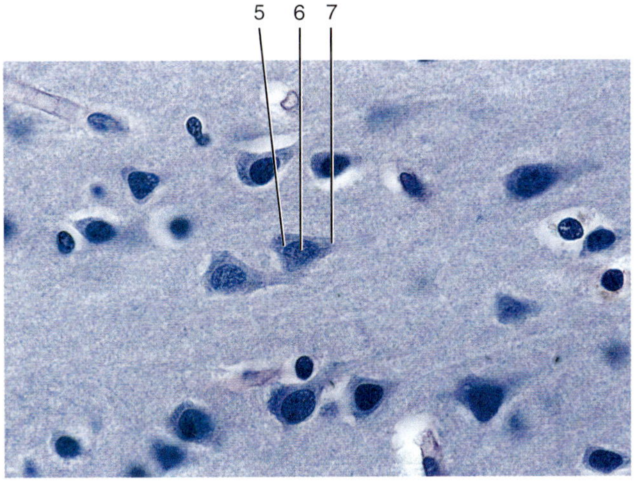

(b) Cerebral cortex, multipolar neurons LM 575x

- neuron cell body
- nucleus
- process

5 ______

6 ______

7 ______

FIGURE 13.5 Sectional views of the dorsal root ganglion and cerebral cortex.

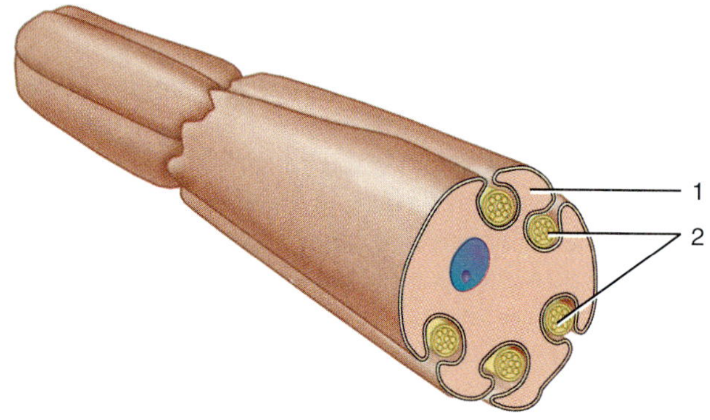

(a) Unmyelinated axons in PNS

(a)
- axons
- Schwann cell cytoplasm

1 ______________________

2 ______________________

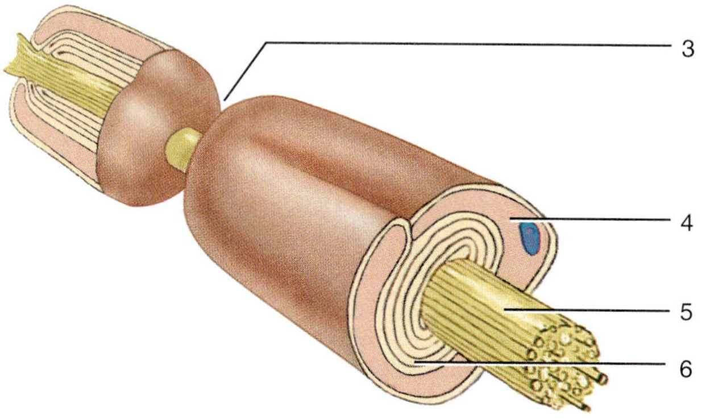

(b) Myelinated axons in PNS

(b)
- axon
- myelin sheath
- node of Ranvier
- Schwann cell cytoplasm

3 ______________________

4 ______________________

5 ______________________

6 ______________________

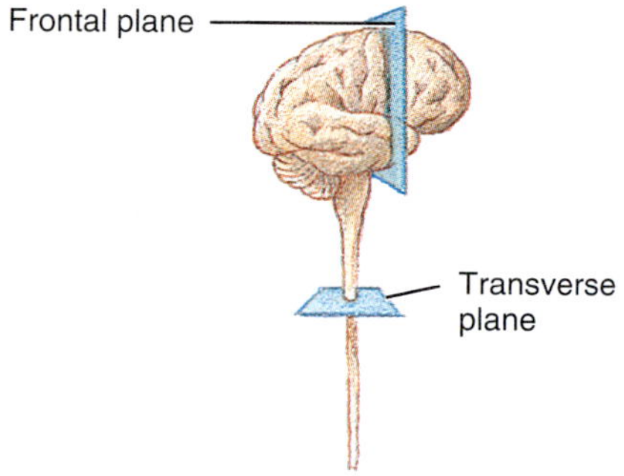

(c) and (d)
- gray matter in brain and spinal cord
- white matter in brain and spinal cord

7 ______________________

8 ______________________

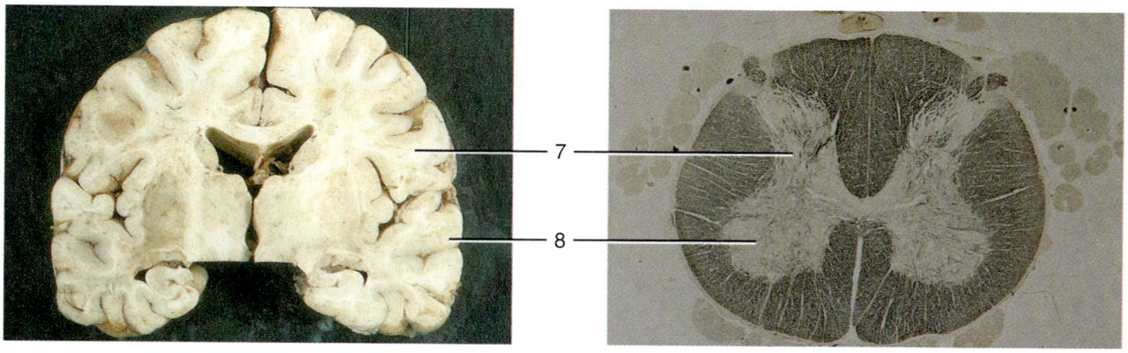

(c) Sectional view of brain

(d) Transverse view of spinal cord

FIGURE 13.6 Myelin sheaths, gray matter, and white matter.

5. Myelination of Axons

Two neuroglial cells, the **oligodendrocytes** (CNS) and the **Schwann cells** (PNS), form insulated wrappings called **myelin sheaths** around axons. As Schwann cells wrap around axons, their cytoplasm is pushed to the periphery and is called **neurolemma.** The multiple layers of myelin that surround the axons are composed of lipoprotein (about 80% lipids and 20% protein), similar to the make-up of plasma membranes. The high amount of lipid in the myelin sheath gives the axons a whitish appearance. Because babies and children do not have the complete myelin coverings encircling the axons, their need for dietary fat is different than that of an adult and is necessary for proper nervous system development. There is not a continuous myelin sheath around the axon, and gaps do exist between the cells. Gaps in the myelin sheaths are called **nodes of Ranvier** and are more numerous in the PNS than in the CNS. The myelin sheath provides protection and insulation for the axon, and also increases the speed of conductivity of the nervous impulse (action potential). Myelinated axons are also called myelinated fibers. The axons that are not myelinated are called **unmyelinated fibers.** They still have neuroglial cells, but only have a thin coating of the Schwann cell or oligodendricyte plasma membrane covering the axons. Unmyelinated fibers conduct impulses slower than myelinated fibers.

6. Gray and White Matter in the CNS

Myelin sheaths are white in color, giving nervous tissue with many myelinated axons a white color. Nervous tissue with few myelinated axons appears gray, the color of nervous tissue cells. Groups of myelinated axons in the CNS form **tracts** and are called **white matter.** The outer area or cortex of the brain is comprised of nerve cell bodies, their dendrites, axon terminals, and neuroglia and is called **gray matter** (not myelinated). There are also deeper areas within the brain that have isolated areas of gray matter that are called **nuclei** of the brain that also contain nerve cell bodies and their dendrites. Unlike the brain, the spinal cord has gray matter in a central H-shaped area made up of nerve cell bodies, dendrites, unmyelinated axons, axon terminals, and neuroglia.

ACTIVITY 4 Myelination of Axons, Gray Matter, and White Matter

1 Label the structures on Figure 13.6a, Figure 13.6b, and Figure 13.6c.

2 Pronouce the terms as you label the figures.

3 Label the structures in the photomicrograph of a teased myelinated nerve fiber in Figure 13.7.

4 Examine a microscope slide of a teased myelinated nerve fiber.
- Using the low power objective, locate a nerve fiber and place it in the center of the field of view.
- Using the high power objective, identify the **nodes of Ranvier, myelin sheath, axon,** and **neurolemma.**

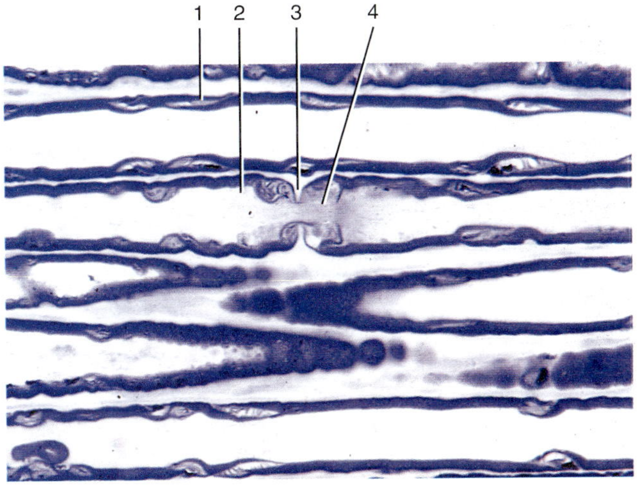

- axon
- myelin sheath
- neurolemma (ner-oh-LEM-ma)
- node of Ranvier

1 ____________

2 ____________

3 ____________

4 ____________

FIGURE 13.7 Teased myelinated nerve fiber.

Name ______________________ Date ______________ Section ________________

EXERCISE 13

REVIEWING YOUR KNOWLEDGE

A. Organization of Nervous System

Fill in the blanks with the correct term chosen from the following:

afferent	motor
effectors	peripheral
efferent	receptors

If you touch a hot stove with your hand, the sensory (1) ______________

in your hand send a signal of pain to the CNS through the (2) ______________

nerve fibers of the (3) ______________ nervous system. When the information

reaches the CNS and is processed, a/an (4) ______________ response

is sent through the (5) ______________ nerve fibers of the

PNS system to skeletal muscles that are (6) ______________.

B. Nervous Tissue Cells

Match the descriptions to nervous tissue cells. More than one cell type may apply to a description, and a cell type may be used more than once.

a. astrocyte
b. ependymal cells
c. microglia
d. neuron
e. oligodendrocytes
f. satellite cells
g. Schwann cells

______________________ **1.** Supporting cells of PNS

______________________ **2.** Supporting cells of CNS

______________________ **3.** Form myelin sheaths

______________________ **4.** Regulate chemical environment of neurons

______________________ **5.** Generate and transmit nerve impulses

______________________ **6.** Line cavities of brain and spinal cord; form and move CSF

______________________ **7.** Phagocytes that destroy debris, dead tissue, and pathogens

C. Structural Classification of Neurons

Match the descriptions listed below with the appropriate neuron type.

___ 1. Many processes associated with the cell body

___ 2. Has two cell processes

___ 3. One short process extends from cell body and divides

___ 4. Neuron is rare and is the sensory neuron in the eye and nose

a. multipolar neuron

b. bipolar neuron

c. unipolar neuron

D. Functional Classification of Neurons

Match the functional description of the neuron with its name. More than one neuron may fit a functional description.

a. interneuron
b. motor neuron
c. sensory neuron

______________ 1. Functional neuron type(s) that are structurally multipolar neurons.

______________ 2. Neuron type(s) whose cell body is in the spinal cord (CNS).

______________ 3. Neuron type(s) whose cell body is found in the PNS.

______________ 4. Functional neuron type(s) most prevalent in the CNS.

E. Gray and White Matter

Match the description to the appropriate term.

a. gray matter
b. white matter
c. myelinated fibers
d. unmyelinated fibers
e. nodes of Ranvier

___ 1. Contains myelinated fibers

___ 2. Contains neuron cell bodies and unmyelinated fibers

___ 3. These large diameter axons transmit impulses the fastest of all types of nerve fibers

___ 4. Nerve fibers that are gray in color

___ 5. Gaps in the myelin sheath

Name ______________________________ Date ______________ Section ________________

EXERCISE 13

USING YOUR KNOWLEDGE

A. Conduction of a Nervous Impulse

Write the following parts of a multipolar neuron in the correct order (1–8) of receiving and sending the nerve impulse.

____ **1.** axon

____ **2.** axon hillock

____ **3.** axon terminal

____ **4.** cell body

____ **5.** dendrites

____ **6.** second neuron or effector

____ **7.** synapse

____ **8.** trigger zone

B. Nervous Tissue and Diseases

Using your textbook or other references, identify the nervous tissue cell(s) that is(are) involved in each of the following diseases:

9. Multiple sclerosis

10. Epilepsy

EXERCISE 14

STRUCTURE AND FUNCTION OF THE BRAIN

OUTLINE

OBJECTIVES

After completing this exercise, you should be able to:

- Identify the major external and internal structures of the brain
- Describe the basic functions of the principal structures of the brain
- Name the three meninges and describe their similarities and differences
- Identify the four ventricles of the brain and describe their function
- Trace the cerebrospinal fluid circulation
- Compare the anatomy of the sheep brain with that of the human brain

MATERIALS

- human brain models and charts
- preserved human brain
- ventricular system model

Sheep Brain

- preserved sheep brains
- sheep brain models
- dissecting instruments and dissection trays
- disposable gloves and safety glasses

The human brain simultaneously conducts and coordinates a variety of incredible processes with which no computer is presently able to compete. Its expansive development distinguishes it from all other creatures. One of the largest organs in the human body, our brain, is responsible for our memory, intellect, ideas, and behavior. The brain is the center for cataloging sensory information, integrating this information with previously recorded information, and producing actions based on the results of the information synthesis.

A. Major Brain Regions

The brain is composed of four main regions: the brain stem, cerebellum (*cerebel-* = little brain), diencephalon (*di-* = through; *encephal-* = brain), and cerebrum (*cerebr-* = brain). The **brain stem** is connected to the superior part of the spinal cord, the **cerebellum** is posterior to the brain stem, and the **diencephalon** is superior to the brain stem in the center of the brain. The large **cerebrum** is the dominant brain structure with many folds and crevices enveloping the diencephalon.

ACTIVITY 1 Identification of Major Brain Regions

1 Label the terms in Figure 14.1.

2 Locate the structures on human brain models or charts.

3 Pronounce the terms as you point to them.

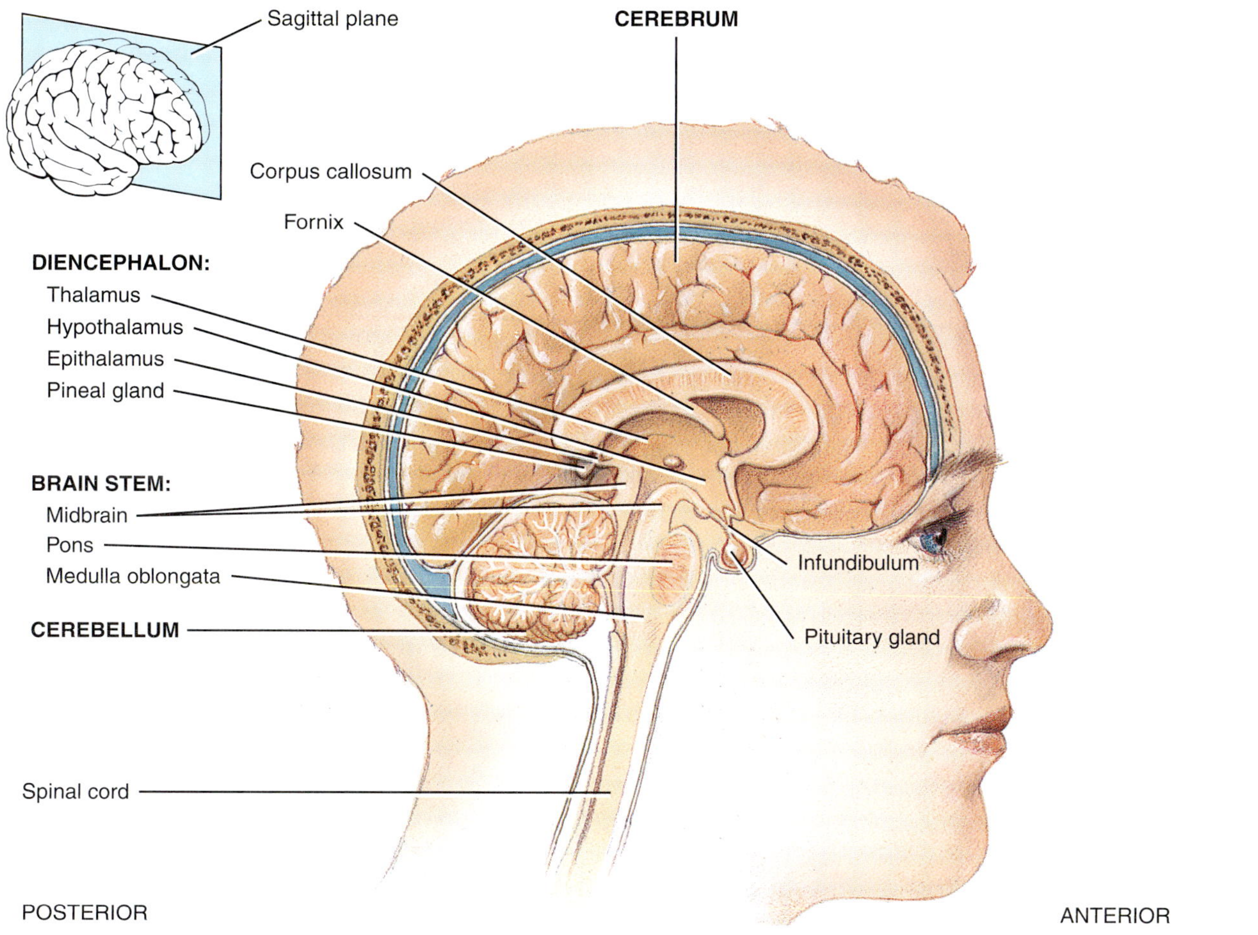

Sagittal section of brain, medial view

- brain stem
- cerebellum (cer-e-BELL-um)
- cerebrum (ce-REE-brum)
- diencephalon (dye-en-CEPH-a-lon)

1 ____________________

2 ____________________

3 ____________________

4 ____________________

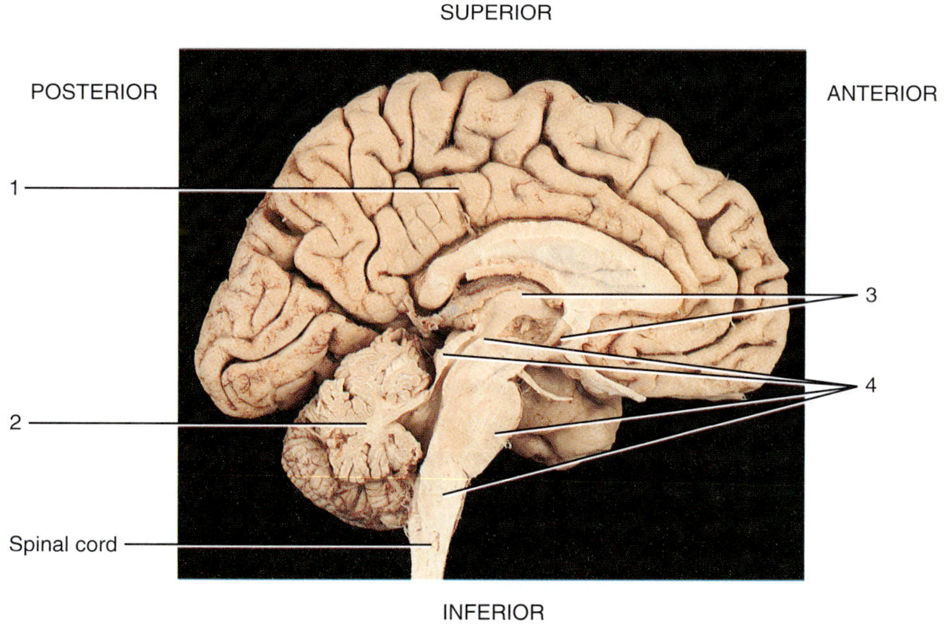

Sagittal section of brain, medial view

FIGURE 14.1 Four major brain regions.

B. The Brain Stem

The brain stem is comprised of three structures: the medulla (*medull-* = marrow) oblongata, the pons, and the midbrain.

1. Medulla Oblongata

The first brain structure, the **medulla oblongata,** is immediately superior to the spinal cord and is the most vital part of the brain because it houses the respiratory and cardiovascular control centers. The respiratory center controls rate and depth of breathing and the cardiovascular center is responsible for the rate and force of the heartbeat and blood pressure reflexes. Other reflex centers in the medulla are for coughing, vomiting, and sneezing.

2. The Pons

The **pons** is an expanded structure located superior to the medulla oblongata and anterior to the cerebellum, and has respiratory centers that assist the medulla oblongata in controlling breathing. The pons also relays information to the diencephalon and the cerebellum.

3. The Midbrain

The **midbrain** is a smaller area superior to the pons and inferior to the diencephalon, consisting of cerebral peduncles (*ped-* = foot) and the corpora quadrigemina (*corpora* = body; *quad-* = four; *gemin-* = twin; i.e., four twin bodies). The **cerebral peduncles** are white fibers that connect the upper and lower brain areas, and the **corpora quadrigemina** are composed of two superior colliculi (*colliculus* = small mound) and two inferior colliculi. The **superior colliculi** have reflex centers involved in eye, head, and neck movements with visual stimulation, whereas the **inferior colliculi** have reflex centers involved in auditory stimuli that result in head and trunk movements. The midbrain is observed best from a sagittal section, medial view. It spans from the dorsal to the ventral side of the brain.

ACTIVITY 2 The Brain Stem

1 Label the structures on Figure 14.2a and Figure 14.2b.

2 Identify the structures on a human brain model or chart.

3 Pronounce the terms as you point to them.

(a) Sagittal section
- brain stem
- cerebral peduncle
- corpora quadrigemina (cor-POR-a quad-ri-GEM-i-na)
- inferior colliculus (col-LIK-you-lus)
- medulla oblongata
- pons
- superior colliculus

1 ______________________

2 ______________________

3 ______________________

4 ______________________

5 ______________________

6 ______________________

7 ______________________

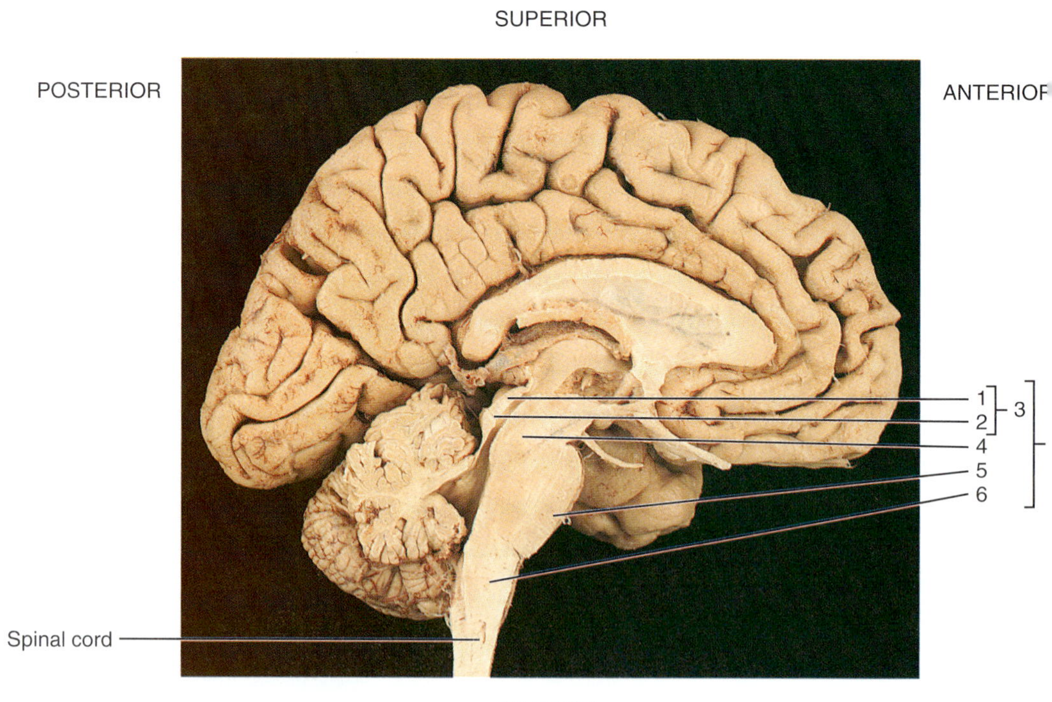

(a) Sagittal section, medial view

FIGURE 14.2a Brain stem.

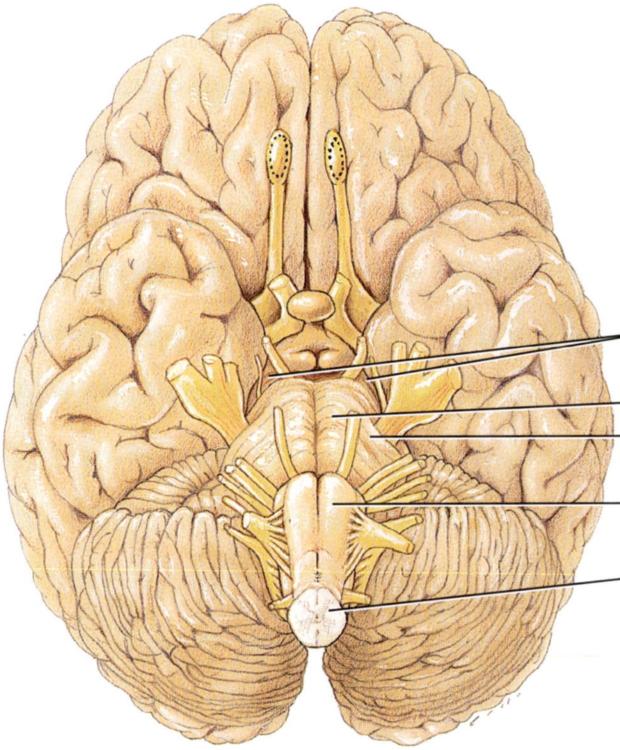

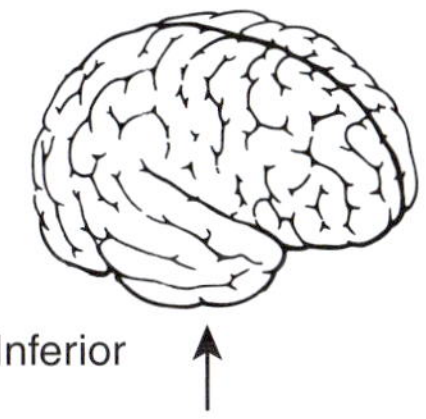

ANTERIOR

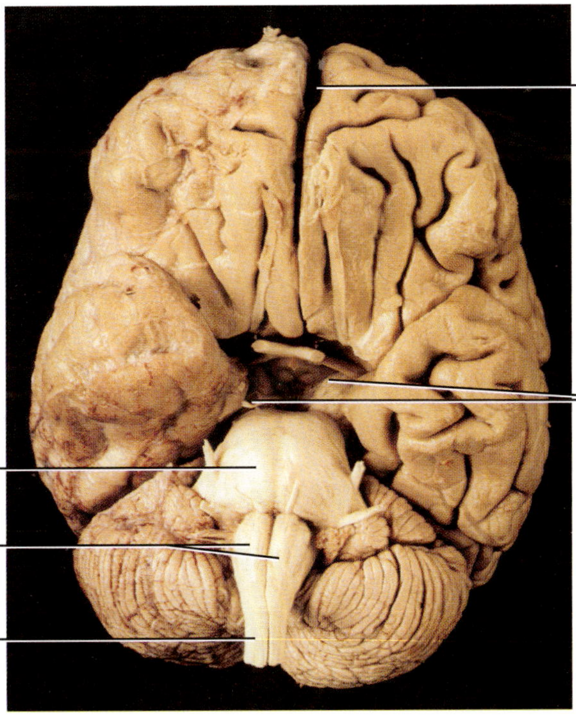

POSTERIOR

(b) Inferior view

(b) Inferior view
- medulla oblongata (meh-DEW-la ob-lon-GAH-tah)
- midbrain
- pons

8 ______________________

9 ______________________

10 ______________________

FIGURE 14.2b **Brain stem.**

C. The Cerebellum

The **cerebellum** (*cerebellum* = little brain) is second in size to the cerebrum, and is located inferior to it and posterior to the medulla and pons. There are two **cerebellar hemispheres** with a central area, the **vermis,** connecting them. When cut in sagittal section, the gray matter can be observed on the exterior, with the deep white matter called the **arbor vitae** (*arbor* = tree; *vitae* = living) appearing as branches of a tree. The outer layer of gray matter is called the **cerebellar cortex.** Like the cerebral cortex, the cerebellar cortex has folds to increase the surface area for more neuron cell bodies. The cerebellar folds are slender, pleated gyri or **folia** (*folia* = leaves) that look similar to pages in a book. The cerebellum regulates posture and balance and, in addition, smoothes and coordinates skilled skeletal muscle movements. The cerebellum is connected to the brain stem by the superior, middle, and inferior cerebellar peduncles (Figures 14.2b and 14.20). Do not confuse them with the cerebral peduncles.

ACTIVITY 3 Cerebellum Identification

1 Label the structures in Figure 14.3.

2 Identify these structures on a human brain model, picture, or chart.

3 Pronounce the terms as you point to them on the model.

(a) Posterior view
- cerebellar hemispheres (cer-e-BELL-ar)
- folia (FO-lia)
- vermis (VER-mis)

1 ____________________

2 ____________________

3 ____________________

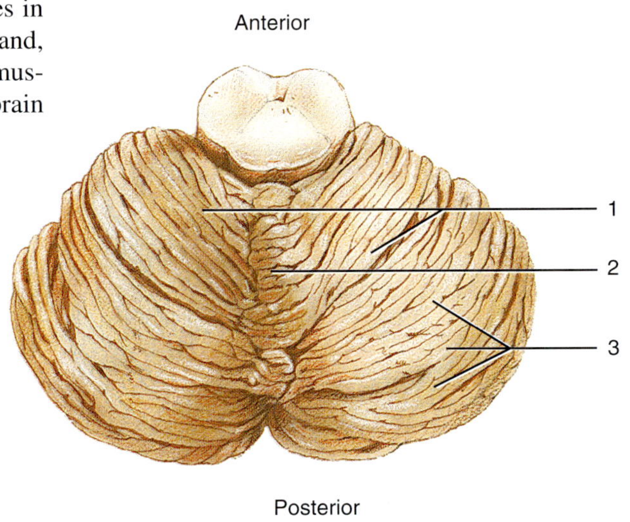

(a) Superior view

(b) Sagittal view
- arbor vitae (white matter)
- cerebellar cortex (gray matter)
- cerebral peduncle
- folia
- inferior colliculus
- medulla oblongata
- brain stem
- pons
- superior colliculus

4 ____________________

5 ____________________

6 ____________________

7 ____________________

8 ____________________

9 ____________________

10 ____________________

11 ____________________

12 ____________________

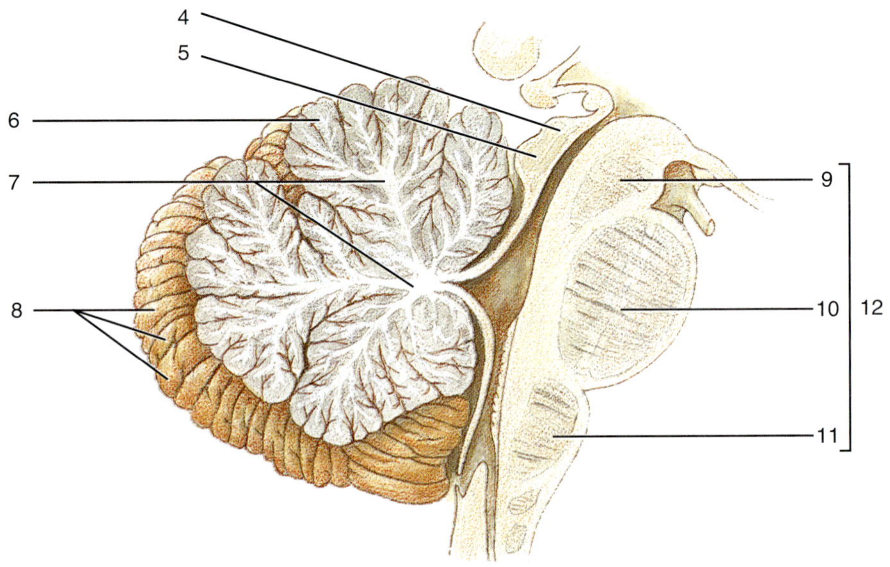

(b) Sagittal view

FIGURE 14.3 The cerebellum.

D. The Diencephalon

The **diencephalon** (*di-* = two; *-cephalon* = brain) is located in the brain's central area and has three main regions: the thalamus, the hypothalamus, and the epithalamus.

1. The Thalamus

The **thalamus** (*thala-* = inner chamber) is composed of paired, egg-shaped bodies centrally located in the diencephalon and comprising approximately 80% of this structure. Each cerebral hemisphere contains half of the thalamus, which is connected by a small bridge called the **intermediate mass.** The thalamus is the brain's "grand central relay station," because it is the principal relay station for sensory fibers and some somatic motor fibers. Sensory fibers that synapse in the thalamus are relayed to a particular area of the cerebral cortex to be interpreted, and other fibers relay messages to the somatic motor cortex. The thalamus also filters out unnecessary sensory information and is involved in consciousness, emotions, learning, and memory.

2. The Hypothalamus

The **hypothalamus** (*hypo-* = below) is located below the thalamus and is a quadrangular-shaped structure. The hypothalamus has important nuclei (nerve cell bodies) that control many body functions and homeostasis. Some of the major functions include integrating and controlling the pituitary gland and hormonal functions, autonomic functions, emotions and behavior, body temperature, eating and drinking.

The hypothalamus includes the infundibulum and mammillary bodies. The **infundibulum** (*infundibulum* = funnel) is a stalk that connects the pituitary gland to the hypothalamus. The **mammillary bodies** (*mammilla* = nipple), two small, round masses located just posterior to the infundibulum, are relay stations for smell and taste reflexes.

Other structures that are observed in this area are the optic chiasm and the pituitary gland. The **optic chiasm,** the area where the optic nerves cross, is anterior to the infundibulum. The **pituitary gland** looks like a large pea and is attached to the end of the infundibulum. The hypothalamus controls the pituitary gland.

3. The Epithalamus

The **epithalamus** (*epi-* = above) is superior and posterior to the thalamus and includes the **pineal** (*pineas* = pinecone) **gland** or **body,** a small endocrine gland that secretes the hormone melatonin.

ACTIVITY 4 The Diencephalon

1. Label the parts of the diencephalon in Figure 14.4a and Figure 14.4b. Refer to Figure 14.1 if necessary.
2. Identify the structures listed on the human brain model.
3. Pronounce the terms as you point to them.

(a) Sagittal section
- diencephalon
- hypothalamus (hypo-THAL-a-mus)
- pineal gland (in epithalamus) (pi-NEE-al)
- thalamus

1 ____________________

2 ____________________

3 ____________________

4 ____________________

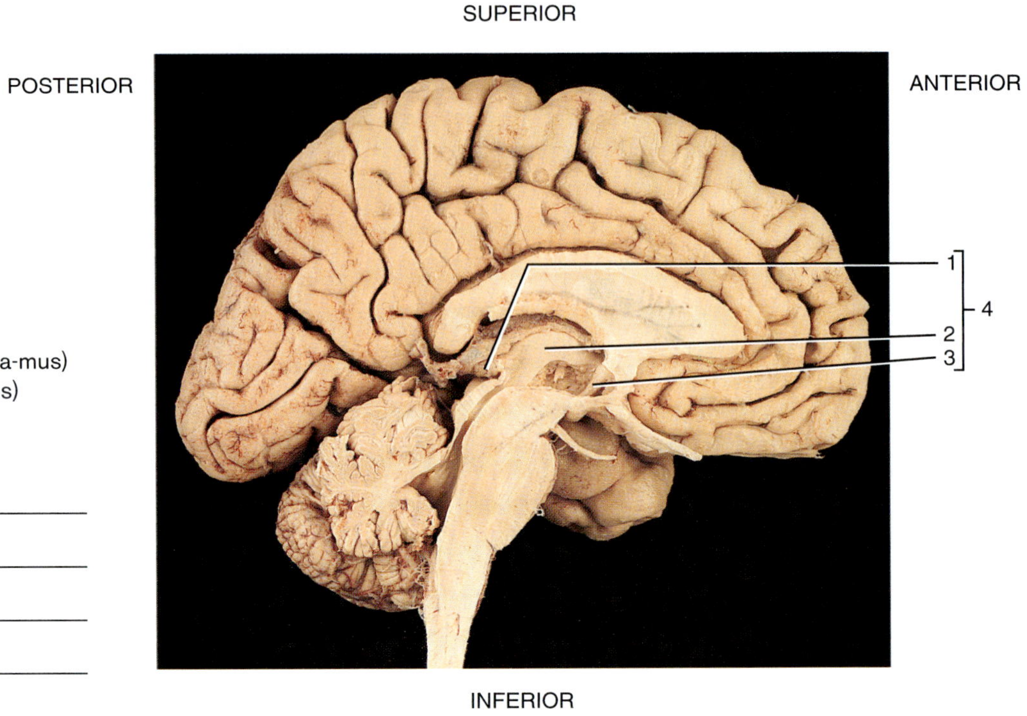

(a) Sagittal section, medial view

(b) Sagittal section of diencephalon, magnified
- hypothalamus
- infundibulum (in-fun-DIB-u-lum)
- intermediate mass of thalamus
- mammillary body (MAM-mil-lary)
- pineal gland
- thalamus (THAL-a-mus)

5 ____________________

6 ____________________

7 ____________________

8 ____________________

9 ____________________

10 ____________________

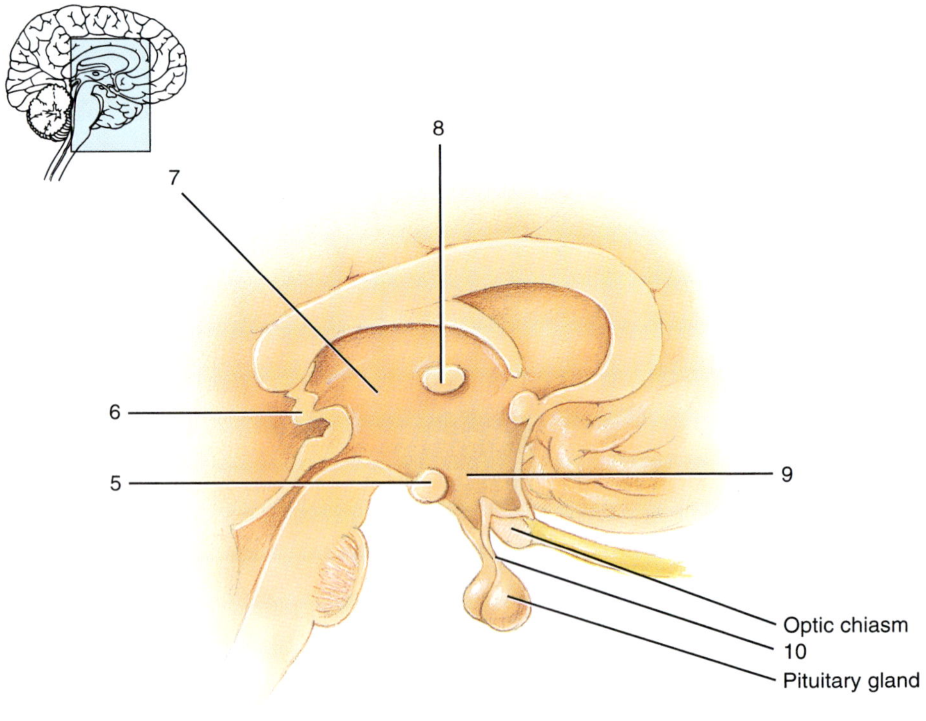

(b) Sagittal section, magnified

FIGURE 14.4 The diencephalon.

E. The Cerebrum

The **cerebrum** is made up of right and left **cerebral hemispheres** and is the largest and most complex division of the brain. The cerebrum is superior to and surrounds the diencephalon and part of the brain stem. Because all neurons going to and coming from the brain cross at various levels of the CNS, sensory neurons bring information from and motor neurons take information to the opposite side of the body. Due to the complexity of the cerebrum, this study is divided into four different sections with the functions listed under each section.

1. Organization of Cerebral Gray and White Matter

The three main regions of the cerebrum are the **cerebral cortex** (*cortex* = bark), **white matter,** and the deep **basal ganglia.** The **cerebral cortex** (also known as the cortical area) is the superficial gray matter on the exterior of the cerebrum composed of nerve cell bodies and dendrites. The **insula** is part of the cerebrum that lies deeper on the lateral sides of the brain. The cerebral cortex integrates sensory information, initiates motor output, and is also involved in emotions and intellectual processes. **Basal ganglia** (*ganglia* = knot) are areas of gray matter composed of paired nuclei (clusters of neuron cell bodies in the CNS) that are found deep within each cerebral hemisphere. The basal ganglia control automatic skeletal muscle movement and are involved with the limbic system or emotional brain.

White matter lies deep to the outer cortex and is comprised mostly of myelinated axons that give it the white appearance. These axons are organized into three kinds of fiber tracts in the cerebrum that are named according to the direction of the fibers. **Association fibers** transmit nerve impulses within the same hemisphere, whereas **commissural** (*commisura* = connection) **fibers** transmit nerve impulses between the two hemispheres. **Projection fibers** are ascending and descending tracts that project nervous impulses from inferior to superior brain areas or vice versa.

The corpus callosum is a prominent commissural fiber tract that is readily observable in midsagittal sections of the brain. The **corpus callosum** (*corpus* = body; *callosus* = hard) is the largest and best-known group of commissural fibers that connects the two cerebral hemispheres. The **fornix** looks like a group of commissural fibers, but is actually a tract of arched association fibers.

ACTIVITY 5 Organization of Gray and White Matter in Cerebrum

1. Label the structures in Figure 14.5a and Figure 14.5b using Figure 14.1 if needed.
2. Identify these structures on a human coronal section of brain or brain model.
3. Pronounce the terms as you point to them.

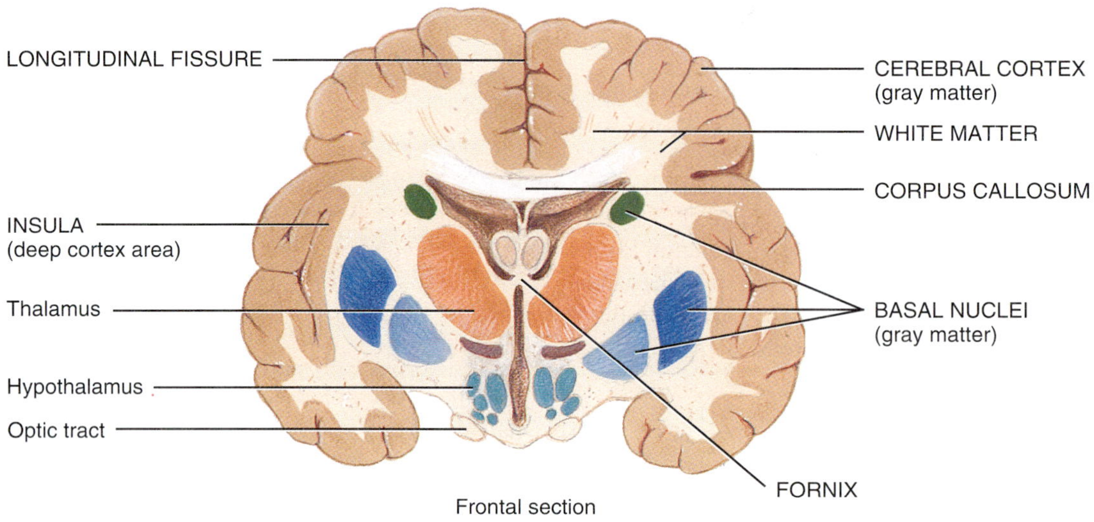

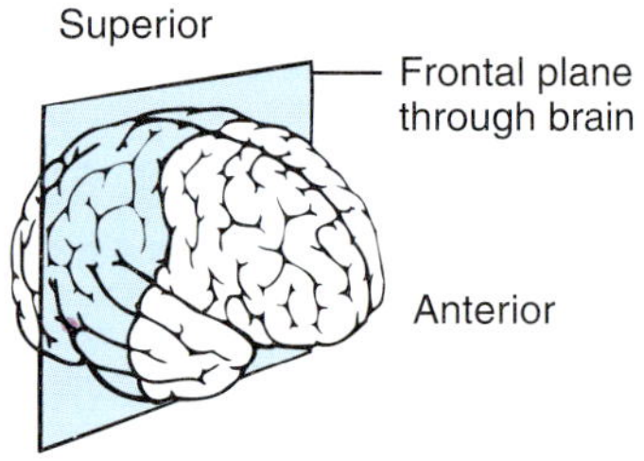

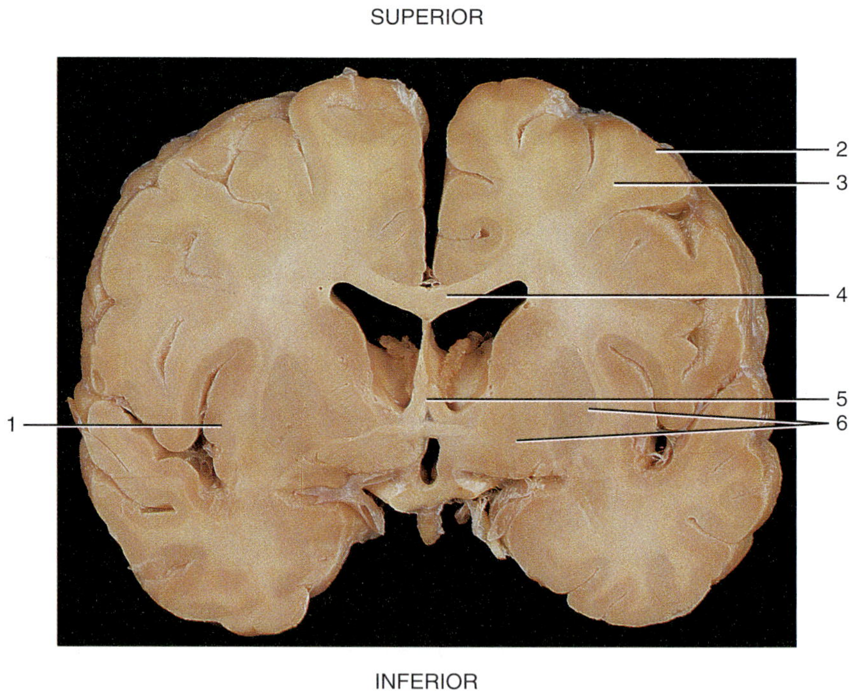

(a) Frontal section

(a) Frontal section
- basal nuclei (gray matter)
- cerebral cortex (gray matter)
- corpus callosum (white fibers)
- fornix (white fibers)
- insula (gray matter)
- white matter

1 ______________________ 4 ______________________

2 ______________________ 5 ______________________

3 ______________________ 6 ______________________

FIGURE 14.5a **Gray and white matter in the cerebrum.**

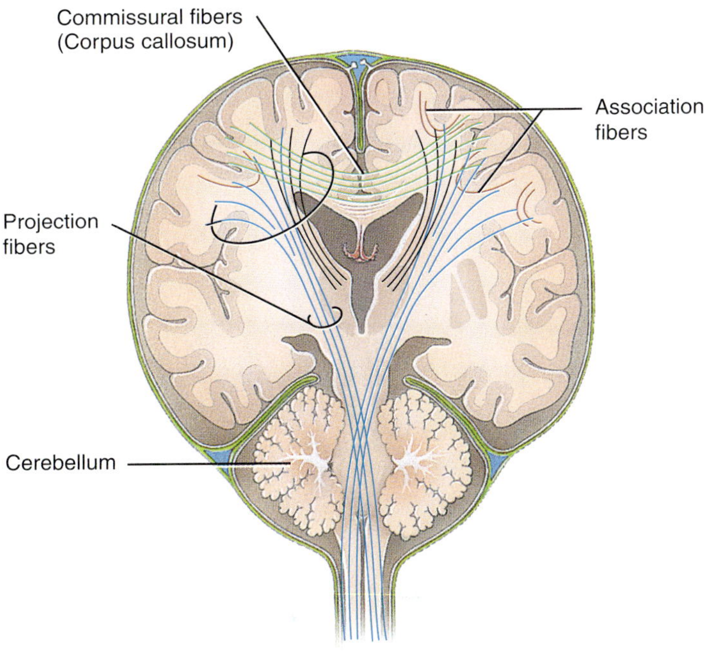

Frontal section

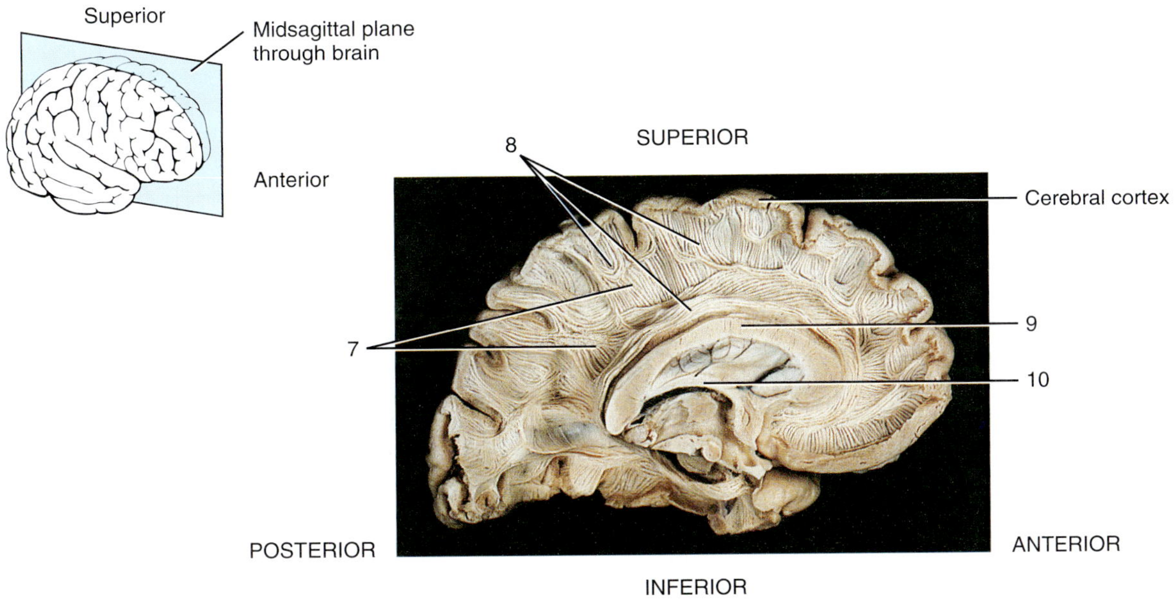

(b) Midsagittal section

(b) Sagittal section
- association fibers
- commissural fibers (corpus callosum)
- association fibers (fornix)
- projection fibers

7 ______________________________

8 ______________________________

9 ______________________________

10 ______________________________

FIGURE 14.5b **White fiber types.**

2. Surface Features of the Cerebrum

There are four lobes composing the exterior of the cerebrum that are mainly named for the overlying cranial bones. These lobes are the **frontal, parietal, occipital,** and **temporal lobes.** An inner lobe, the **insula,** lies deep to the lateral cerebral fissure and is not visible from the exterior.

Other obvious external anatomical features of the cerebrum include the following:

- **gyri** (*gyros* = circle; **gyrus,** singular)—Elevations or folds in the cerebral cortex; increase the surface area for neuron cell bodies
- **precentral gyrus**—elevation located just anterior to the central sulcus
- **postcentral gyrus**—elevation located just posterior to the central sulcus
- **sulci** (*sulcus* = furrow; **sulci,** plural)—Shallow grooves between elevations
- **central sulcus**—shallow groove separating the frontal lobe from the parietal lobe
- **lateral cerebral sulcus**—shallow groove separating the frontal and the temporal lobes
- **parieto-occipital sulcus**—shallow groove separating parietal and occipital lobes
- **longitudinal fissure**—deep groove separating the two cerebral hemispheres at the midline
- **transverse fissure**—deep groove separating the cerebrum from the cerebellum in the posterior/inferior part of the brain

ACTIVITY 6 External Features of the Cerebrum

1. Label the structures listed for Figure 14.6a, Figure 14.6b, and Figure 14.6c.
2. Identify these features on a brain model or chart.
3. Pronounce the terms as you point to them on a model.

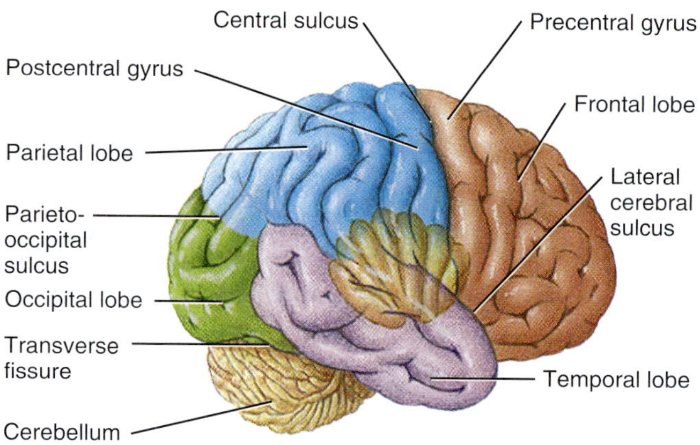

(a) Right lateral view
- central sulcus (SUL-cus)
- frontal lobe
- lateral cerebral sulcus
- occipital lobe
- parieto-occipital sulcus
- parietal lobe
- postcentral gyrus
- precentral gyrus
- temporal lobe
- transverse fissure (FISH-ur)

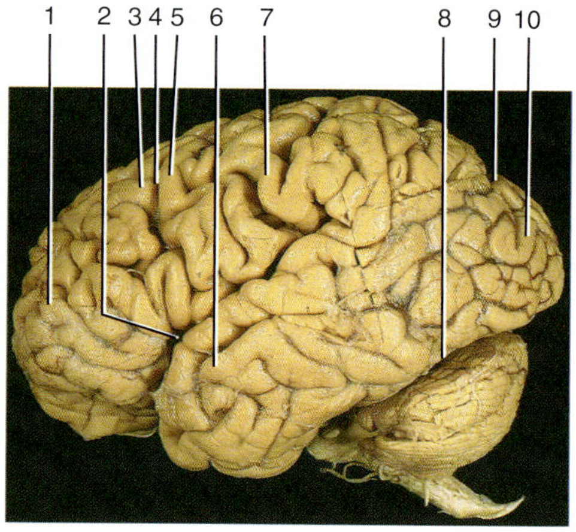

(a) Right lateral view

1 ______
2 ______
3 ______
4 ______
5 ______
6 ______
7 ______
8 ______
9 ______
10 ______

FIGURE 14.6 External features of the cerebrum.

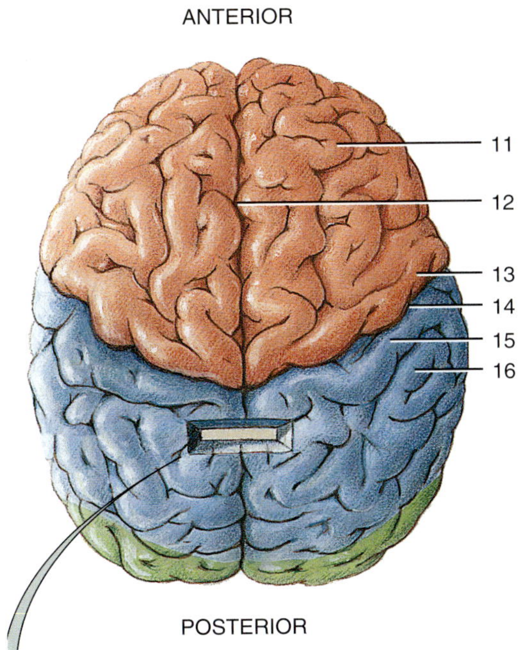

(b) Superior view

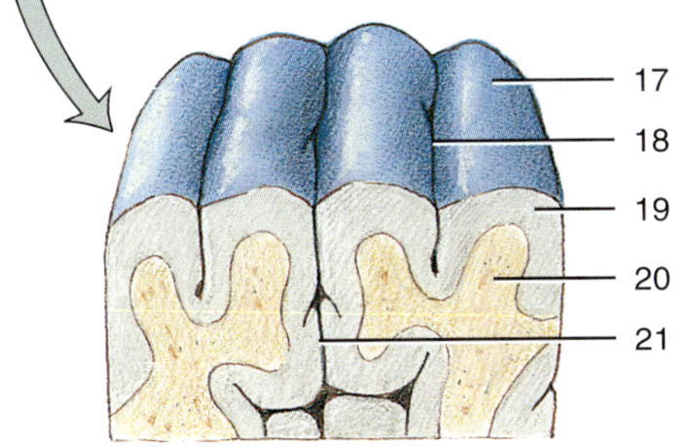

(c) Coronal section cut from cerebrum

(b) Superior view

- central sulcus
- frontal lobe
- longitudinal fissure
- parietal lobe
- postcentral gyrus
- precentral gyrus

11 ____________________

12 ____________________

13 ____________________

14 ____________________

15 ____________________

16 ____________________

(c) Coronal section cut from cerebrum

- gyrus
- sulcus
- white matter
- gray matter
- longitudinal fissure

17 ____________________

18 ____________________

19 ____________________

20 ____________________

21 ____________________

FIGURE 14.6 **External features of the cerebrum, *continued.***

3. Functional Areas of the Cerebral Cortex

The cerebral cortex is composed of three types of functional areas: motor, sensory, and association areas. **Sensory areas** receive and interpret impulses from sensory receptors while **motor areas** initiate impulses to skeletal muscles. **Association areas,** which perform complex integrative functions, receive and send information to multiple areas of the cortex via association fibers. The majority of the cortex is composed of association areas.

Motor Areas

- **primary motor cortex**—located in the precentral gyrus of each frontal lobe; initiates impulses to skeletal muscles
- **Broca's speech area**—located superior to the lateral sulcus and anterior to the primary motor cortex, usually in the left hemisphere; initiates impulses that result in speech

Sensory Areas

- **primary somatosensory cortex**—located in the postcentral gyrus of each parietal lobe; receives impulses from cutaneous receptors, proprioceptors, and determines body location stimulated
- **primary auditory area**—located in each temporal lobe across the lateral sulcus from the gustatory area; receives impulses from auditory receptors
- **primary gustatory area**—in each postcentral gyrus, just superior to the lateral sulcus; receives impulses from taste receptors
- **primary olfactory area**—located on the medial side of each temporal lobe; cannot be seen from the lateral view; receives impulses from olfactory receptors
- **primary visual area**—in the posterior occipital lobe; receives impulses from photoreceptors of eye

Selected Association Areas

- **Wernicke's area**—recognizes spoken words, translates words into thoughts, and possibly helps us sound out strange or new words
- **somatosensory, visual, and auditory association areas**—larger areas adjacent to the corresponding sensory cortex; integrate sensory information from sensory cortex with past experiences allowing us, for example, to identify objects by touch or to identify sound as music or speech

ACTIVITY 7 Functional Areas of Cerebral Cortex

1 Label the brain cortical area with its function in Figure 14.7.

2 Pronounce the terms as you point to the area on a human brain model.

- Broca's speech area
- primary auditory cortex
- central sulcus
- primary gustatory cortex (GUS-tah-tory)
- primary motor cortex (soh-ma-to-MO-tor)
- primary somatosensory cortex (so-ma-to-SEN-sory)
- primary visual cortex
- Wernicke's area

1 ____________________

2 ____________________

3 ____________________

4 ____________________

5 ____________________

6 ____________________

7 ____________________

8 ____________________

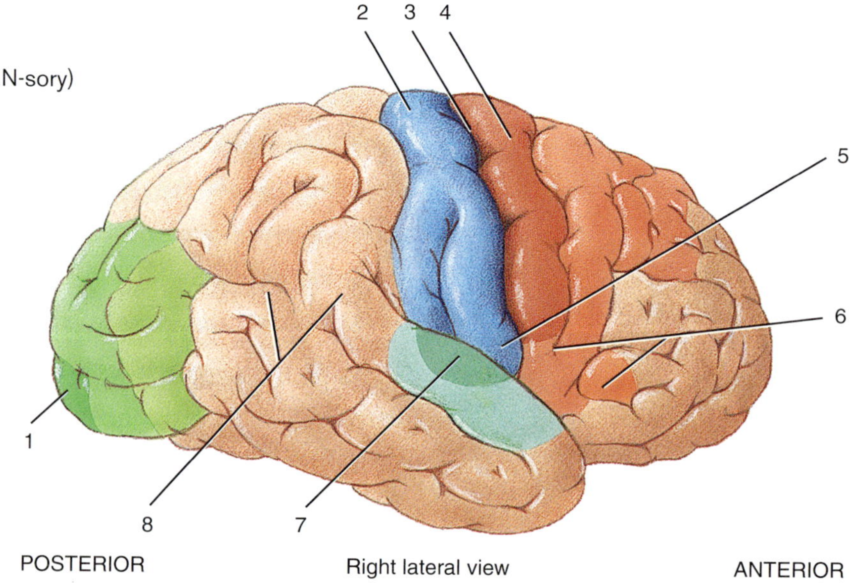

FIGURE 14.7 Functional areas of the cerebral cortex.

F. Protection of the Brain

The brain is protected both physically and chemically by cranial bones, the blood-brain barrier, the cranial meninges, and cerebrospinal fluid.

1. Cranial Meninges

There are three cranial meninges (connective tissue membranes): the dura mater, arachnoid mater, and pia mater. The **dura mater** (*dura* = hard; *mater* = mother) is the first meninx (singular) located deep to the cranial bones. It is comprised of two layers: the **periosteal layer,** which is a tough membrane attached to the cranial bones, and the **meningeal layer,** which is exterior to the arachnoid mater. The two dural layers split to form the **dural sinuses** that eventually drain cranial blood into the jugular veins. The **superior sagittal sinus,** located superior to the longitudinal fissure, is one of the main dural sinuses. The double-layered dura mater extends deep into the longitudinal fissure forming the **falx** (*falx* = sickle-shaped) **cerebri,** and into the transverse fissure, forming the **tentorium** (tent) **cerebelli.**

The **arachnoid** (*arachnoid* = spider-like) **mater** is the second meninx located deep in the dura mater. The **pia** (*pia* = delicate) **mater** is the thin, inner meninx. It hugs and overlays the cerebral cortex, following each gyrus and sulcus. Between the arachnoid and pia is the **subarachnoid** space.

ACTIVITY 8 Cranial Meninges

1 Label the structures on Figure 14.8.

2 Pronounce these terms as you label the figure.

3 Using a model, show where the falx cerebri and tentorium cerebelli would be found.

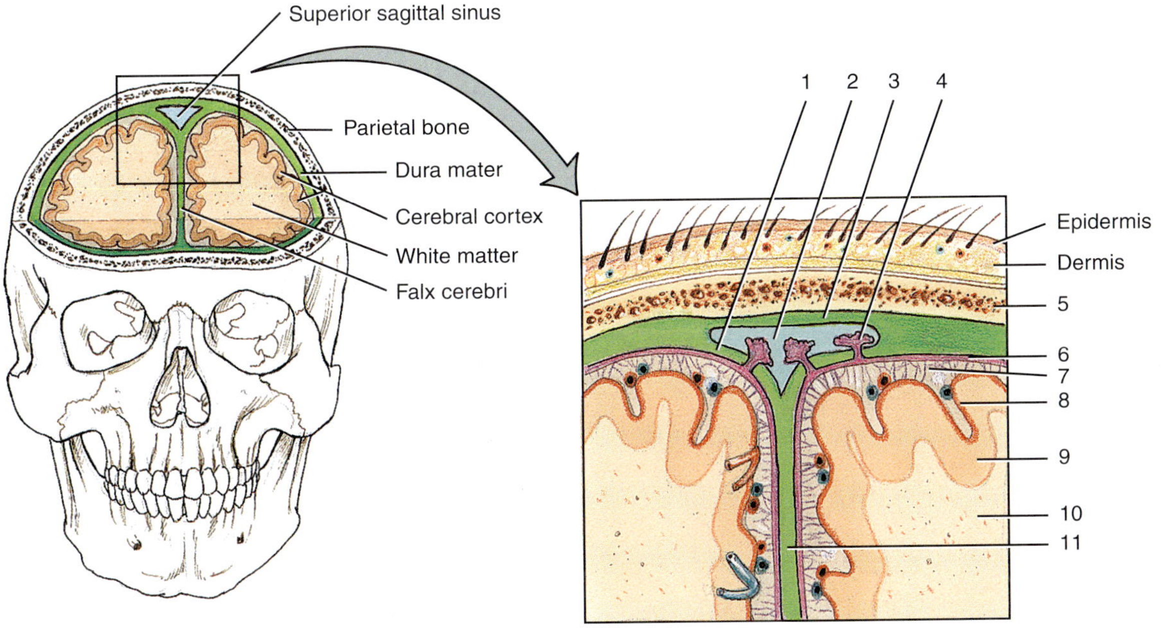

- arachnoid mater (a-RAK-noid MAH-ter)
- arachnoid villus (VIL-us)
- cerebral cortex (ce-REE-bral)
- falx cerebri (FAL-x ce-REE-bree)
- meningeal layer of dura mater (meh-NIN-gee-ul)
- parietal bone
- periosteal layer of dura mater (peri-OS-tee-ul)
- pia mater (PEE-ah)
- subarachnoid space (sub-a-RAK-noid)
- superior sagittal sinus (SAJ-jih-tahl)
- white matter

1 ______________ 7 ______________

2 ______________ 8 ______________

3 ______________ 9 ______________

4 ______________ 10 ______________

5 ______________ 11 ______________

6 ______________

FIGURE 14.8 Cranial meninges.

2. Cerebrospinal Fluid and Ventricles of the Brain

Cerebrospinal fluid (CSF) constantly bathes the brain and spinal cord with oxygen, nutrients, and vital chemicals. Although different in content, the cerebrospinal fluid is made from blood plasma that leaks out of the **choroid plexus** (*choroid* = membrane-like; *plexus* = pleated), specialized tiny blood vessels (capillaries), and passes through ependymal cells into four small brain cavities or ventricles. The ependymal cells have cilia that move the CSF in one direction. There are choroid plexuses in the roof of all four ventricles. A **lateral ventricle** is located in each **cerebral hemisphere** with a thin membrane, the **septum pellucidum** (*septum* = partition; *pellucid* = transparant), separating the two ventricles anteriorly. Each arched lateral ventricle has an **interventricular foramen** that opens medially into the third ventricle. The **third ventricle** is medially located between the paired masses of the thalamus and is narrower and smaller than the other ventricles. Connecting the third ventricle to the fourth ventricle is a thin tube, the **cerebral aqueduct** (*aqua* = water; *duct* = way; i.e., waterway). The **fourth ventricle** is located between the **pons** and the **cerebellum. Lateral** and **median apertures** or openings allow the CSF to flow from the fourth ventricle into the **subarachnoid space** surrounding the brain and the spinal cord. CSF also flows through the central canal of the spinal cord and back out into the subarachnoid space. Just as CSF enters the brain ventricles from the blood stream, it is returned to the blood by reabsorption through the **arachnoid villi** (tiny projections) located in the **superior sagittal sinus.**

ACTIVITY 9 CSF Circulation

1. Label the structures in Figure 14.9a and Figure 14.9b.
2. Identify these structures on a human brain model or chart.
3. Pronounce the terms as you point to them.
4. With your laboratory partner, trace a drop of CSF from its origin in a lateral ventricle through the other ventricles and subarachnoid space, and follow it until it is reabsorbed into the bloodstream.

(a) Right lateral view (ventricles superimposed)

- central canal of the spinal cord
- cerebral aqueduct (AH-que-duct)
- fourth ventricle
- interventricular foramen (in-ter-ven-TRIK-u-lur)
- lateral ventricles
- third ventricle

1 ______________________________

2 ______________________________

3 ______________________________

4 ______________________________

5 ______________________________

6 ______________________________

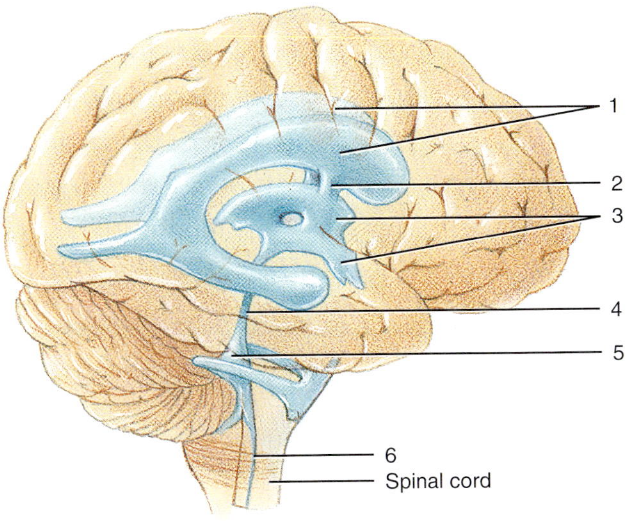

(a) Right lateral view (ventricles superimposed)

(b) Sagittal section of brain and spinal cord with CSF circulation

- arachnoid villus (a-RACH-noid VIL-us)
- central canal
- cerebral aqueduct
- choroid plexus (CHOR-oid PLEX-us)
- fourth ventricle
- lateral ventricle
- subarachnoid space (sub-ah-RAK-noid)
- superior sagittal sinus
- third ventricle

7 ______________________________

8 ______________________________

9 ______________________________

10 ______________________________

11 ______________________________

12 ______________________________

13 ______________________________

14 ______________________________

15 ______________________________

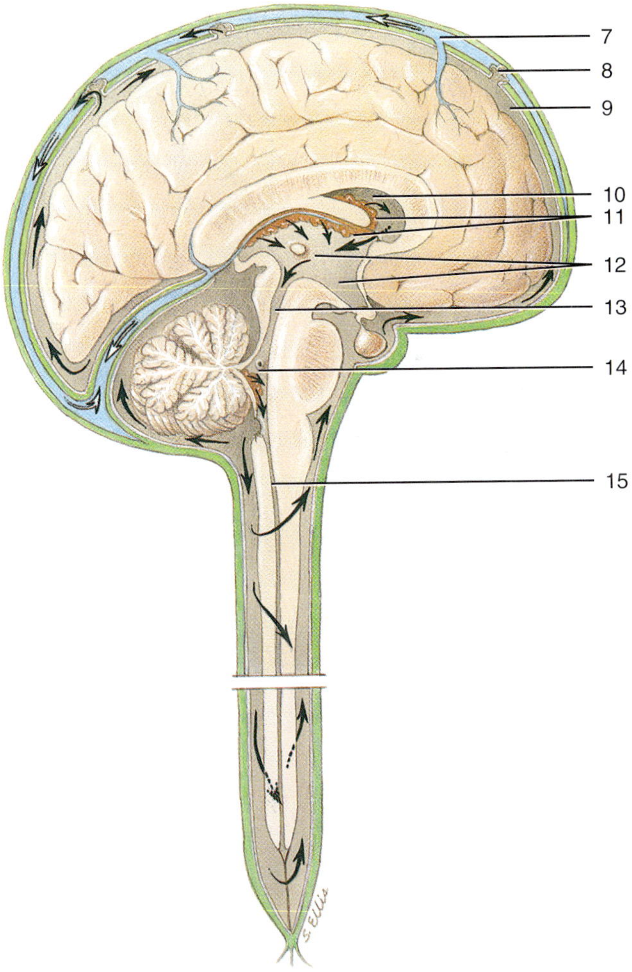

(b) Sagittal section of brain and spinal cord

FIGURE 14.9 **Ventricles of the brain and cerebrospinal fluid circulation.**

G. Sheep Brain Dissection

SAFETY PRECAUTION

- *Use disposable gloves, safety glasses, and a lab coat when handling preserved material.*
- *Wash hands after this lab activity.*
- *Follow your instructor's directions for cleaning dissection equipment and table tops.*
- *Consult instructor about saving or proper disposal of brains.*

Remember that preserved material does not look like a fresh specimen. Usually, more detail may be observed in a preserved brain because the tissue is firmer.

ACTIVITY 10 Dissection of Sheep Brain

1 Rinse the sheep brain to remove preservative.

2 Observe meninges and main brain regions.

- Examine the brain to see if the **dura mater** is present (tough, outer coat). If present, note the **falx cerebri** and **tentorium cerebelli.** Carefully remove the dura mater.
- Now look for the stringy, web-like **arachnoid mater** beneath and adhering to the dura mater. Deep to this membrane is the very thin **pia mater** that follows the contour of the gyri and sulci.
- Compare the sheep brain with the main external regions of the human brain (Fig. 14.1). Identify the **cerebrum, brain stem (medulla and pons),** and **cerebellum.**

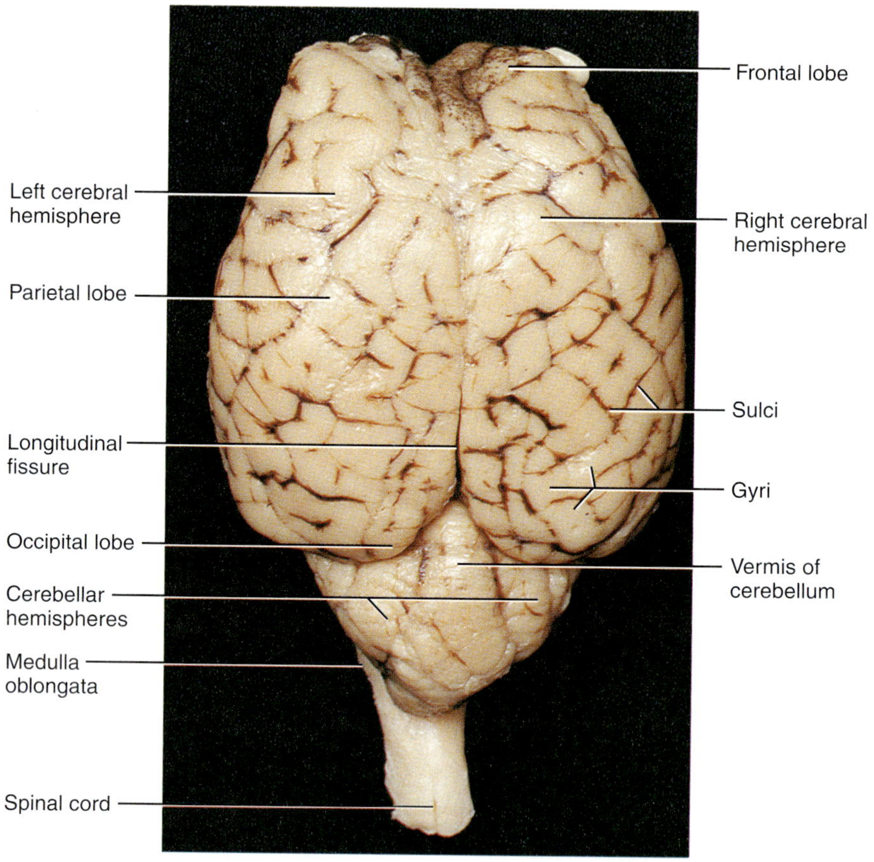

FIGURE 14.10 Superior view of the sheep brain.

3 Identify dorsal structures (Figure 14.10).
- With the dorsal side up, identify the **cerebral hemispheres, gyri, sulci, longitudinal fissure,** and **transverse fissure.**
- Note the four main **lobes** of the brain—**frontal, parietal, occipital,** and **temporal.**
- At the longitudinal fissure, gently separate the two parts and look down between them for the thick band of white fibers, the **corpus callosum.**

4 Identify ventral structures (Figure 14.11).
- Place the sheep brain ventral side up.
- Identify the **olfactory bulb, olfactory tract, optic nerve, optic chiasm,** and **optic tract.**
- Posterior to these structures, locate the *one* large **mammillary body.** How does the human mammillary body look different from the sheep? ________
- If present, identify the **infundibulum** and **pituitary gland.**
- Look at the three parts of the **brain stem**—the **midbrain, pons,** and **medulla oblongata.** How do these compare with the human brain? ____________

____

____

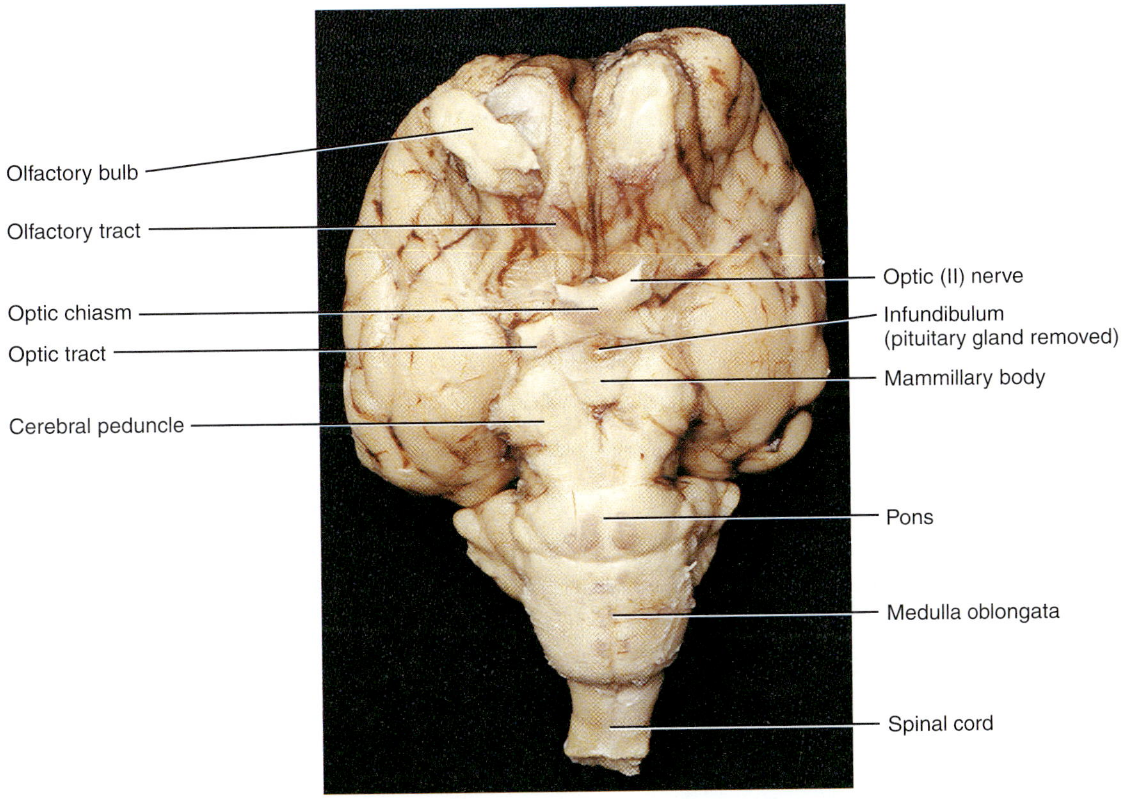

FIGURE 14.11 Inferior view of the sheep brain.

5 Identify dorsal structures (Figure 14.12).
- Carefully pull the cerebellum away from the cerebrum. Identify the **pineal body, superior colliculi,** and **inferior colliculi.**

6 Identify midsagittal section structures (Figure 14.13).
- Using a large, sharp knife or scalpel, carefully make a midsagittal section.
- Locate the **brain stem** components: the **medulla oblongata,** the **pons,** and the **midbrain.** Compare this with your human brain model.
- Identify the **arbor vitae** in the **cerebellum.** Does this structure look similar or different from the human brain? ______________________
- Note the **cerebral aqueduct** and the **fourth ventricle.**
- Identify the **thalamus, corpus collosum, septum pellucidum, fornix,** and **lateral ventricles.**

7 Observe coronal and transverse sections.
- Observe the coronal section your instructor may have as a demonstration. Note the **gray matter, white matter, longitudinal fissure, corpus callosum, thalamus, lateral ventricles,** and **third ventricle.**
- Observe the transverse or horizontal section your instructor may have as a demonstration. Identify the **gray matter, white matter,** and **ventricles.**

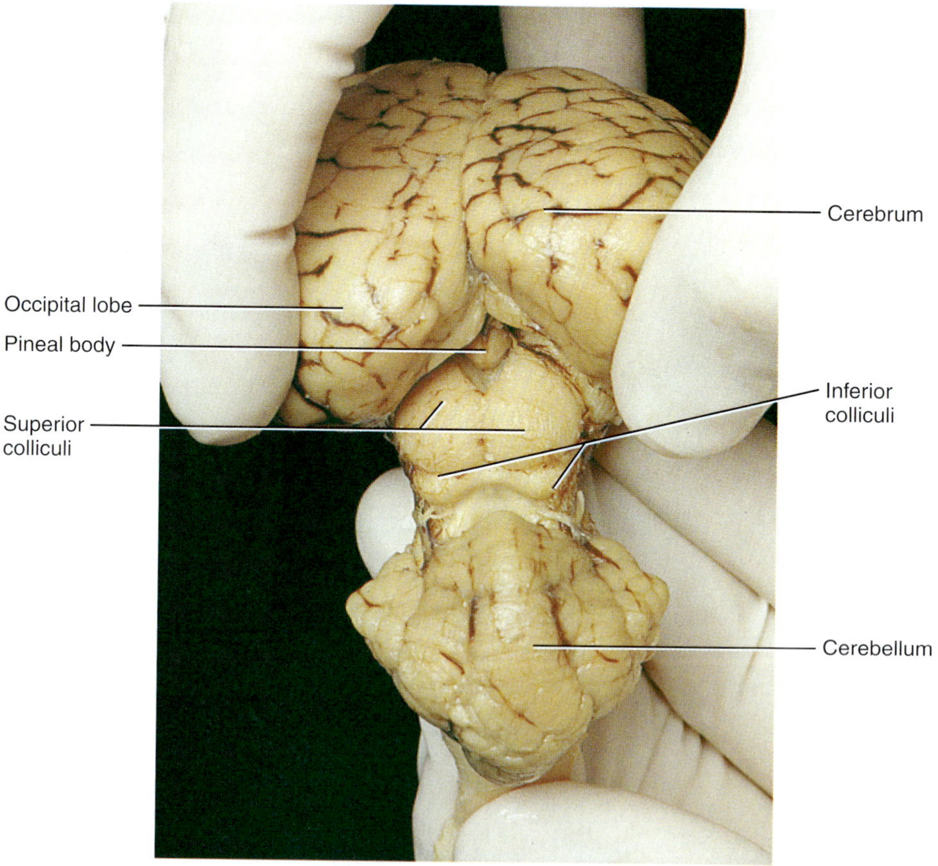

FIGURE 14.12 Posterior view of the sheep brain.

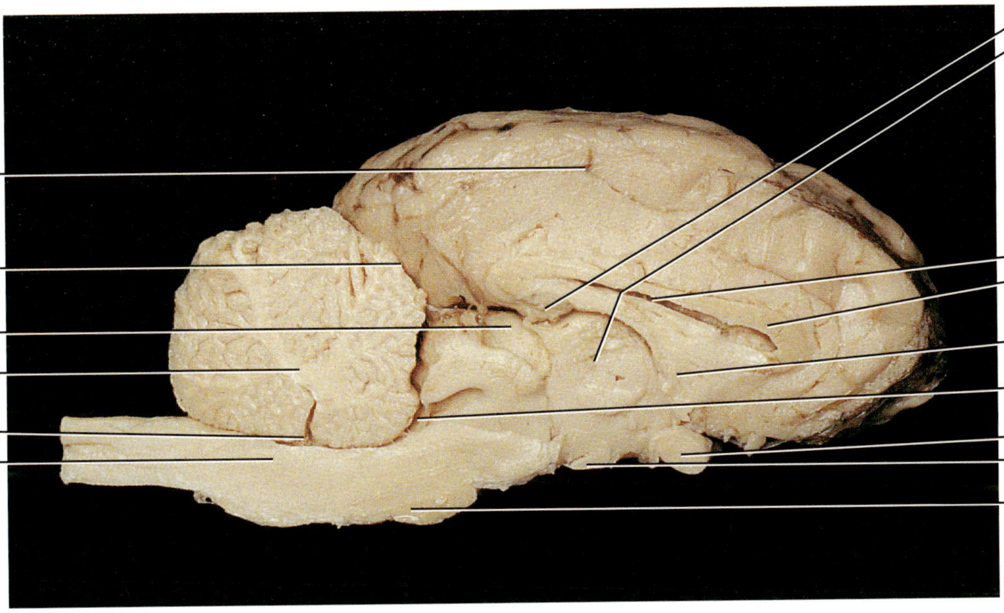

FIGURE 14.13 Midsagittal section of the sheep brain.

Name ______________________ Date ______________ Section ______________

EXERCISE 14

REVIEWING YOUR KNOWLEDGE

A. Structure of Brain Regions

Label the structures on Figure 14.14 in the spaces below.

1. ______________________
2. ______________________
3. ______________________
4. ______________________
5. ______________________
6. ______________________
7. ______________________
8. ______________________
9. ______________________
10. ______________________
11. ______________________
12. ______________________

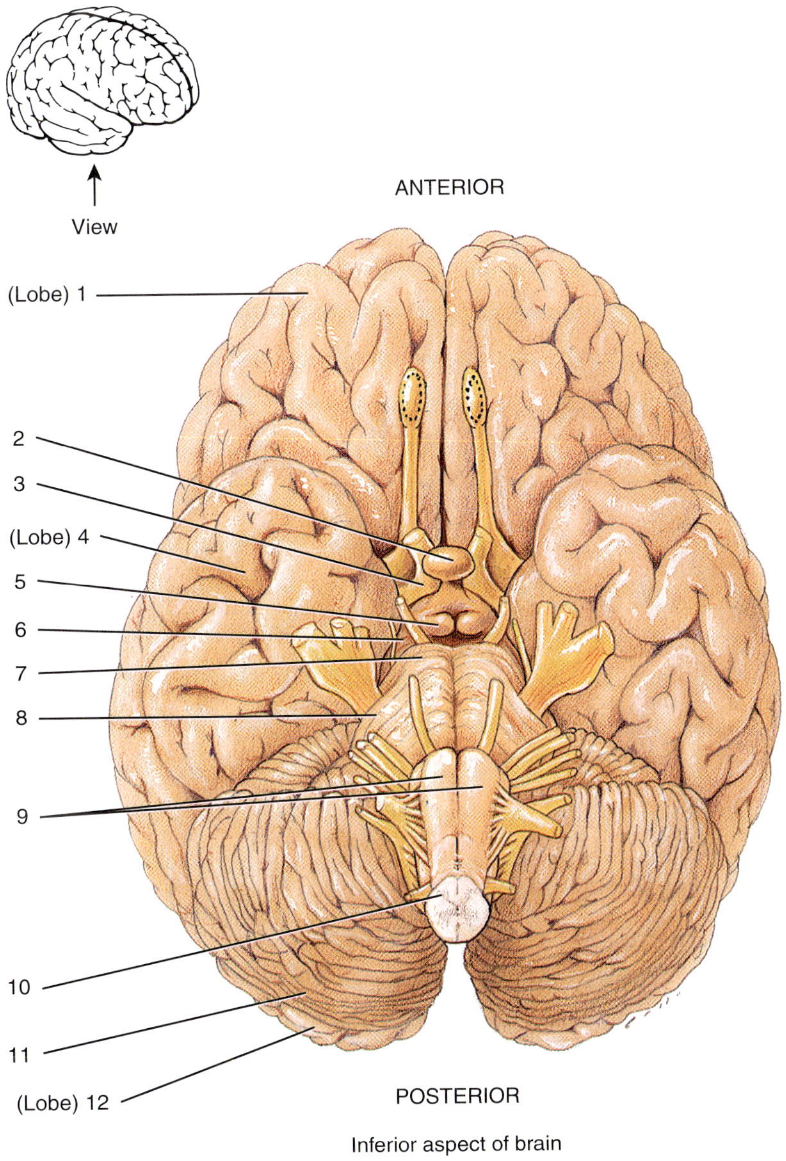

FIGURE 14.14 Ventral view of the human brain.

B. Cerebrospinal Fluid

Complete this exercise about the flow of cerebrospinal fluid (CSF) by filling in the blanks.

Fluid for the CSF is derived from the bloodstream. The sites of CSF formation are the (1), special tiny capillaries located in the walls of (2), (3), and (4). Cells that line the ventricles have cilia that move the CSF and are called (5). The two lateral ventricles are separated by a thin membrane called the (6). CSF flows by cilia movement from the two lateral ventricles through the interventricular foramen to the (7). From here, the CSF flows through the (8) into the fourth ventricle. The CSF leaves the fourth ventricle through three openings: the median aperture and two lateral apertures. CSF is now located in the (9) space around the brain, and circulates all around the cerebrum and cerebellum. CSF continues to flow down into the inner part of the spinal cord by flowing through the tiny (10) of the spinal cord, as well as around the exterior of the spinal cord in the (11) space. Because CSF is continually being made at the rate of about 20 mL/hr, it has to exit back into the bloodstream by being reabsorbed through the (12) that protrude into the dural venous sinuses. The venous sinus that is overlying the brain superiorly is called the (13).

1. ____________________

2. ____________________

3. ____________________

4. ____________________

5. ____________________

6. ____________________

7. ____________________

8. ____________________

9. ____________________

10. ____________________

11. ____________________

12. ____________________

13. ____________________

C. Functions of Brain Regions

Give the brain region for the functions described.

______________________ 1. Vital centers regulate heartbeat, breathing, blood pressure, vomiting, coughing.

______________________ 2. Smoothes and coordinates skilled skeletal muscle movement; also posture and balance or equilibrium.

______________________ 3. Secretes melatonin; sleep-wake cycle.

______________________ 4. Controls and integrates the ANS; regulates hormones, emotional behavior, temperature, eating, and drinking behavior.

______________________ 5. Interprets sensory input, controls skilled skeletal muscle movements, and is involved in emotional and intellectual processes.

______________________ 6. Helps control breathing; conducts impulses to and from the cerebellum, midbrain, and medulla.

______________________ 7. Relays all sensory input to the cerebral cortex; involved in skeletal muscle actions and memory processing.

______________________ 8. Coordinates visual and auditory reflexes.

______________________ 9. Coordinates gross, automatic muscle movements; also involved with limbic system.

______________________ 10. White fiber tracts communicating between hemispheres.

D. Location of Functional Areas of the Cerebral Cortex

Match the areas of the cerebral cortex with the location described.

A. Broca's speech area (motor)
B. primary auditory area
C. primary gustatory area
D. primary motor area
E. primary somatosensory area
F. primary visual area
G. Wernicke's area

______ **1.** precentral gyrus

______ **2.** postcentral gyrus

______ **3.** anterior to the primary motor cortex in frontal lobe

______ **4.** tip of occipital cortex

______ **5.** inferior end of postcentral gyrus near lateral cerebral sulcus

______ **6.** parietal lobe superior and posterior to lateral cerebral sulcus

______ **7.** posterior to gustatory cortex in superior part of temporal lobe; near the lateral cerebral fissure

Label Figure 14.15 with the functional areas of the cerebral cortex.
Color each complete area with a different color pencil.

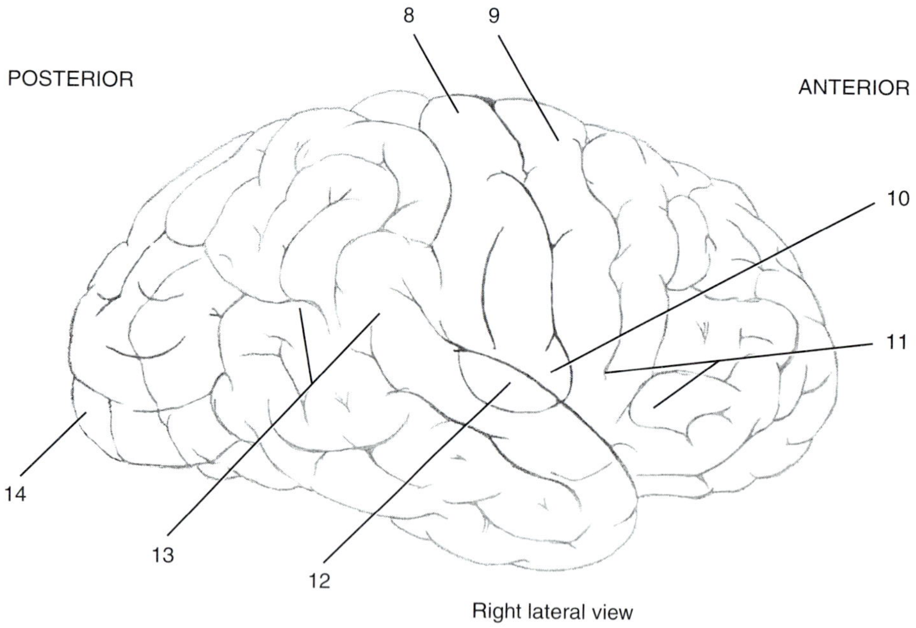

8. ____________________

9. ____________________

10. ____________________

11. ____________________

12. ____________________

13. ____________________

14. ____________________

FIGURE 14.15 Functional areas of the cerebral cortex.

Name ______________________ Date ______________ Section ______________

EXERCISE

14

USING YOUR KNOWLEDGE

A. Identifying Structures on a CT Scan of the Human Brain

Identify the structures in Figure 14.16, midsagittal view.

1. ______________________

2. ______________________

3. ______________________

4. ______________________

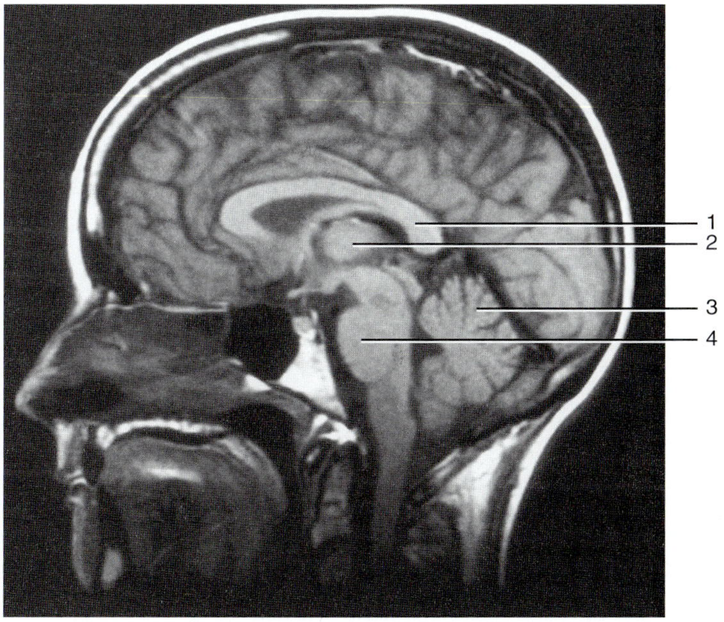

FIGURE 14.16 Midsagittal section of the human brain, CT scan.

B. Identifying Structures on a Human Brain

Identify the structures in Figure 14.17, a transverse section.

5. ______________________________

6. ______________________________

7. ______________________________

8. ______________________________

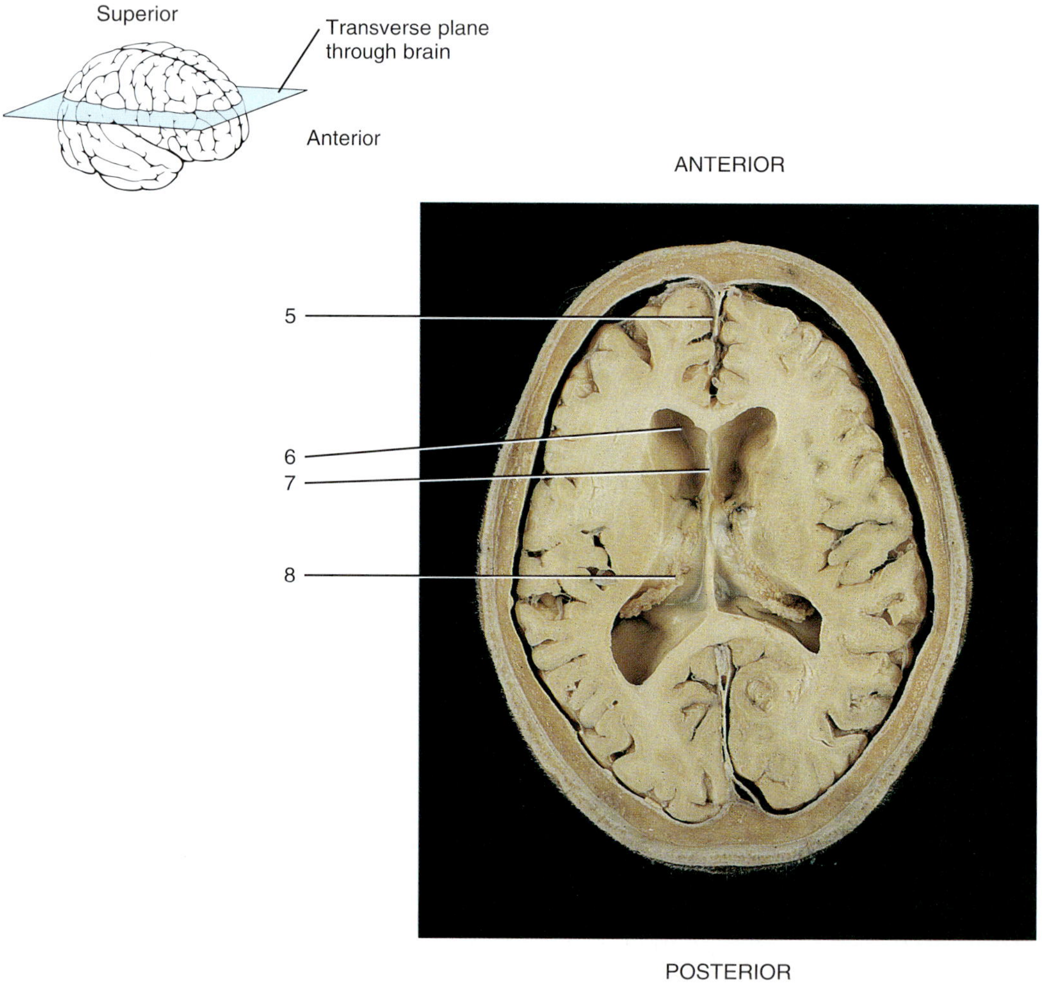

FIGURE 14.17 Human brain, transverse section.

C. Identifying Structures on the Brain of a Human Cadaver

Identify the structures in Figure 14.18, sagittal section.

9. ______________________________

10. ______________________________

11. ______________________________

12. ______________________________

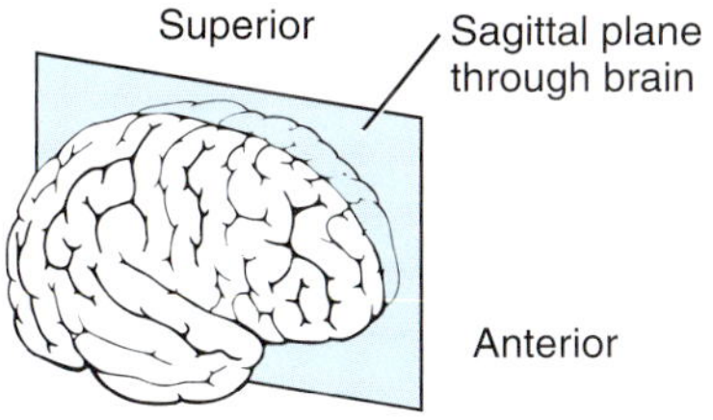

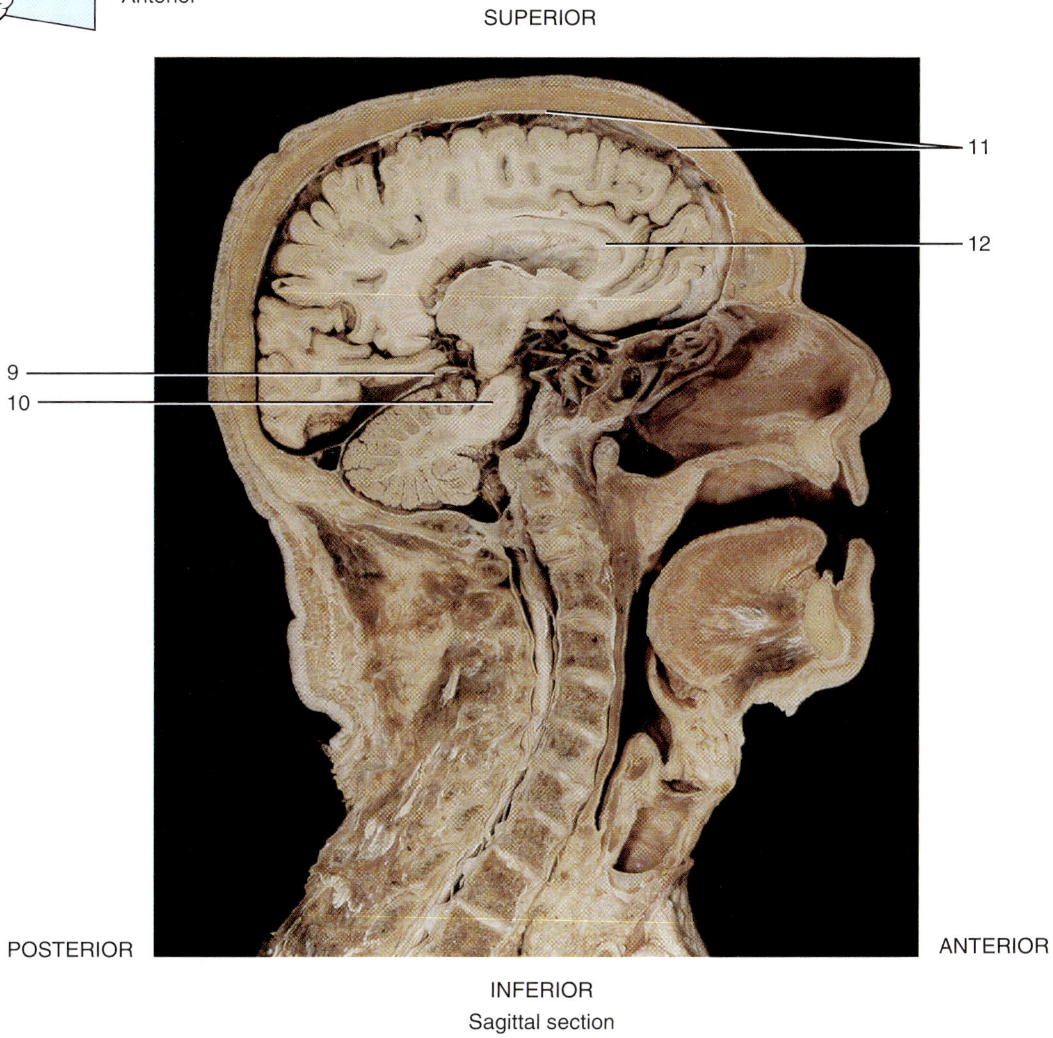

FIGURE 14.18 Human brain, sagittal section.

D. The Effects of Damage to the Brain

Match the brain injury to the appropriate change in function. Use Figure 14.19 to locate the area injured.

a. cessation of breathing
b. loss of equilibrium
c. loss of use of left arm
d. loss of vision

______ **13.** The effect of a blow to the back of the head that damages this area.

______ **14.** The effect of alcohol on this area.

______ **15.** The effect of a head injury (i.e. diving into a pool) that forces the dens into this area.

______ **16.** The effect of a stroke that damages this area.

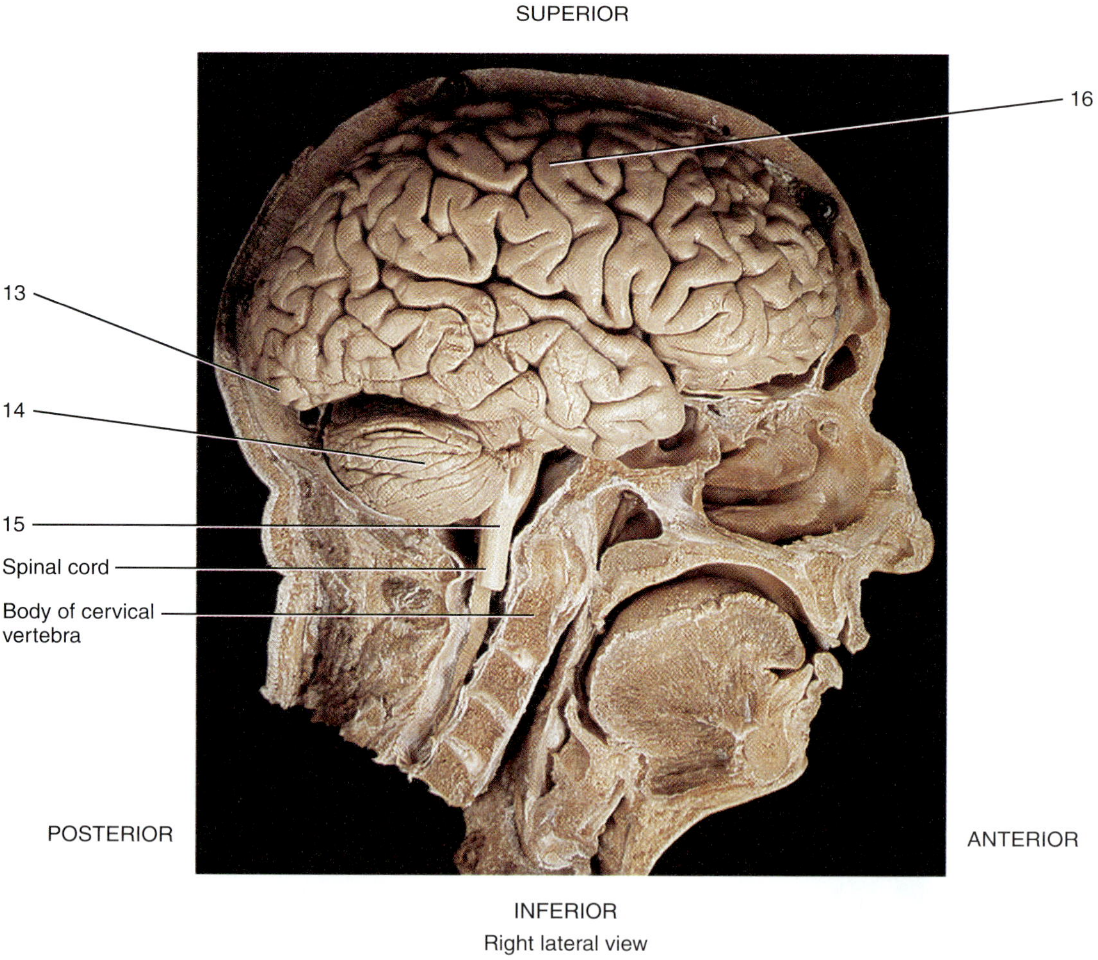

FIGURE 14.19 **Human brain, lateral view.**

E. Identifying Structures on a Human Cadaver Brain

Identify the structures in Figure 14.20, posterior view.

17. ______________________________

18. ______________________________

19. ______________________________

20. ______________________________

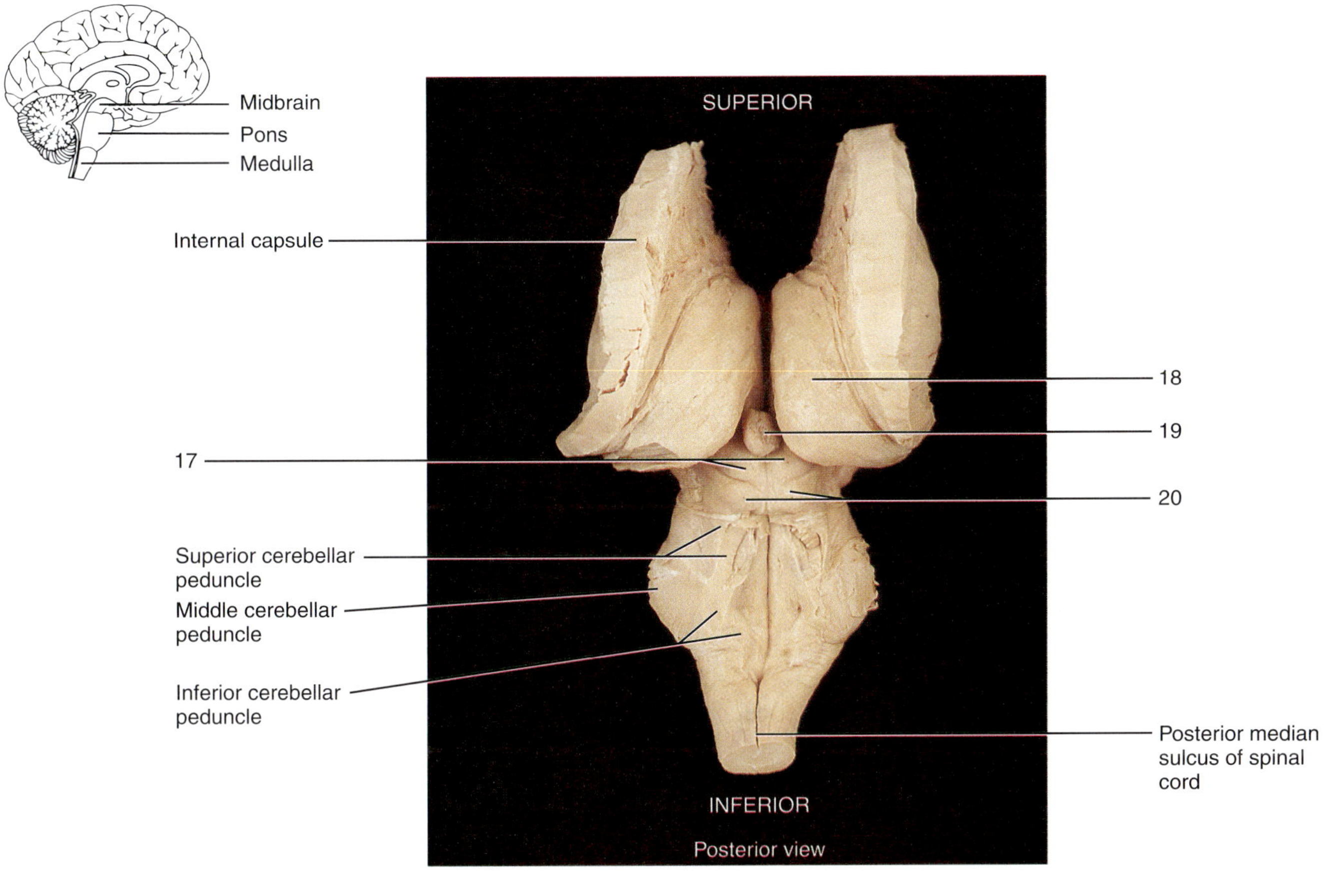

FIGURE 14.20 Human brain stem.

EXERCISE 15

ANATOMY OF THE SPINAL CORD

OUTLINE

OBJECTIVES

After completing this exercise, students will be able to:

- Describe the protective structures of the spinal cord
- Identify the external features of the spinal cord
- Identify the anatomical features of a spinal cord transverse section

MATERIALS

- Models or charts of the complete spinal cord, transverse section of the spinal cord, and vertebral column with spinal cord
- Prepared microscope slides or photomicrographs of spinal cord transverse section
- Preserved or fresh spinal cord with meninges (for demonstration)
- Dissection equipment and tray
- Disposable gloves

The spinal cord and the brain comprise the central nervous system. Being continuous with the brain, the spinal cord begins at the foramen magnum and terminates between vertebrae L1 and L2. It is suspended within the vertebral canal, an area formed by the vertebral foramen of the vertebral column. The spinal cord has two functions: (1) carrying sensory information to the brain and motor output to nerves and (2) mediating spinal reflexes. Spinal reflexes process sensory input from and convey motor output to the spinal nerves.

A. Protective Structures and Spinal Meninges

The **spinal cord** is protected by the bony vertebrae, adipose tissue, spinal meninges, and cerebrospinal fluid. Adipose tissue cushions the spinal cord and is found within the space between the vertebrae and the meninges, the **epidural space.** The three **meninges** (meninx, singular) or connective tissue membranes cover the spinal cord and are continuous with the cranial meninges that protect the brain. **Dura mater,** the outer meninx, is a tough, single-layered membrane that is deep to the epidural space and superficial to the spider web-like **arachnoid mater.** The inner meninx, the **pia mater** is delicate and hugs the spinal cord. Denticulate ligaments are lateral extensions of pia mater that fuse with arachnoid mater and secure the spinal cord. Between the pia and arachnoid mater is the **subarachnoid space** that contains **cerebrospinal fluid,** which also cushions the spinal cord.

ACTIVITY 1 Spinal Meninges

1 Label Figure 15.1 with the parts listed below.
2 Identify the spinal meninges on a spinal cord model or chart.
3 Pronounce the terms as you point to them.

- arachnoid mater with web-like projection
- dura mater
- epidural space
- pia mater
- subarachnoid space

1 ______________________

2 ______________________

3 ______________________

4 ______________________

5 ______________________

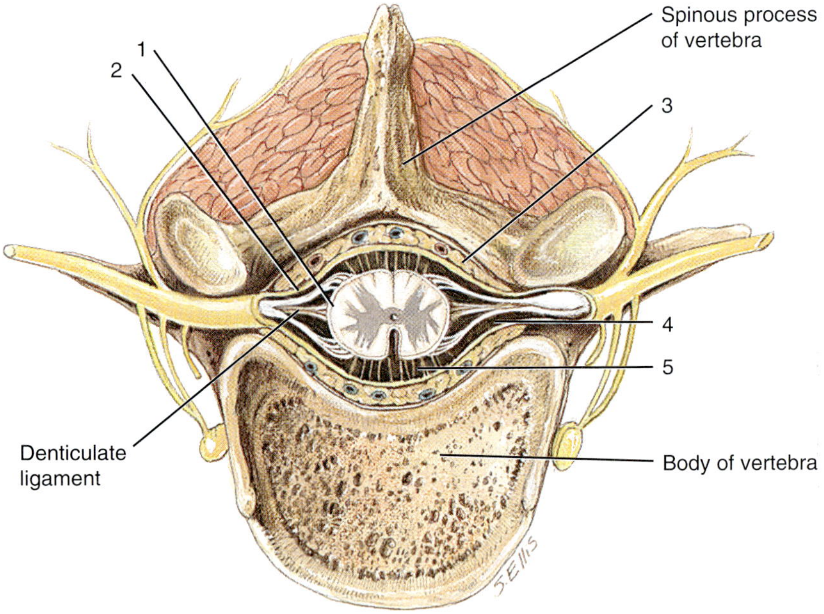

FIGURE 15.1 Spinal cord transverse section showing meninges.

B. External Features of the Spinal Cord

The long, cylindrical spinal cord has 31 pairs of spinal nerves attached to it, with each pair of spinal nerves arising from a different segment of the cord. The cord is wider in the cervical and lumbar regions forming two enlargements. The **cervical enlargement** is located at levels C3 or C4 through T1. This bulge designates the location of nuclei (collection of neuron cell bodies) for the upper extremities. The inferior **lumbar enlargement** is located at levels T9 through T12 and contains nuclei for the lower extremities. The spinal cord ends inferiorly as the **conus medullaris** between vertebrae levels L1 and L2. Nerves arising from the inferior portion of the spinal cord continue inferiorly as a group called the **cauda equina** (*cauda* = tail; *equin-* = tail), or "horse's tail." An extension of the pia mater continues past the conus medullaris as the **filum terminale** (*filum* = filament; *termin-* = terminal) and connects the spinal cord to the coccyx.

ACTIVITY 2 External Features of the Spinal Cord

1 Label Figure 15.2 with the parts listed below.

2 Identify these structures on a spinal cord model or chart.

3 Pronounce the terms as you point to them.

- cauda equina (CAU-da ee-QUI-na)
- cervical enlargement
- conus medullaris (CO-nus med-u-LAR-is)
- filum terminale (FI-lum ter-min-A-lee)
- lumbar enlargement

1 ______________________

2 ______________________

3 ______________________

4 ______________________

5 ______________________

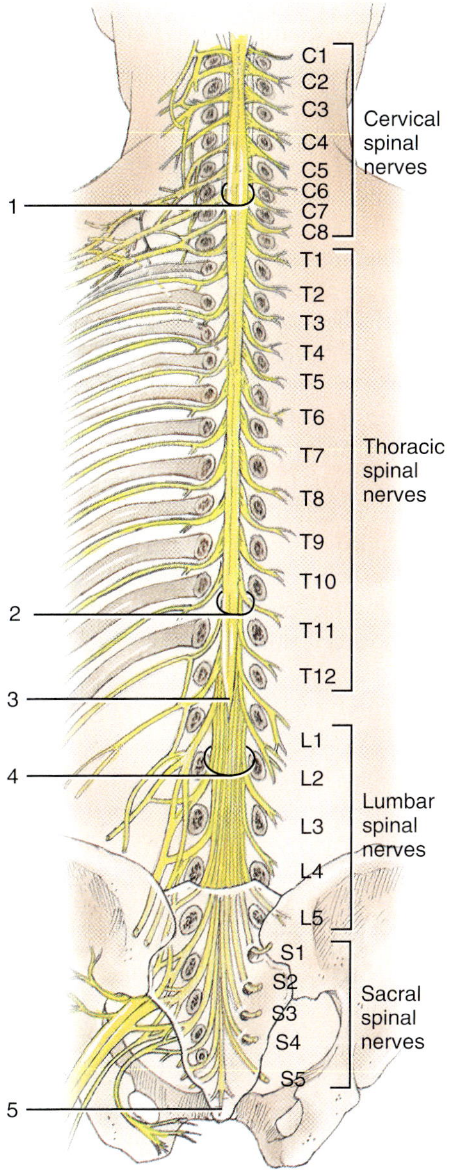

FIGURE 15.2 Longitudinal view of posterior spinal cord.

C. Transverse Section of the Spinal Cord

The most obvious parts of the spinal cord in cross section are the anterior median fissure, the posterior median sulcus, and the gray and white matter. The **anterior median fissure** is a wide, deep groove on the anterior surface of the spinal cord and the **posterior median sulcus** is a narrow groove on the posterior surface. The **gray matter** looks like a butterfly or a modified H and is more centrally located. The gray matter is divided into the anterior, lateral, and posterior gray horns and consists of nerve cell bodies and dendrites. Somatic motor neuron cell bodies are located in the **anterior gray horns,** whereas the **lateral gray horns** contain visceral motor neuron cell bodies. The **posterior gray horns** contain neuron cell bodies that receive impulses from sensory neurons. A **gray commissure** connects the right and left sides of the gray matter in the middle. The **central canal** is in the center of the gray commissure and contains cerebral spinal fluid. **White matter** surrounds the gray matter and forms the **anterior, lateral,** and **posterior white columns.** These columns or funiculi are made up of white, myelinated fibers (axons) that are either sensory or motor fibers.

Spinal nerves divide into the **posterior (dorsal) root** and **anterior (ventral) root.** Near the spinal cord, there is a bulge in the posterior (dorsal) root called the **posterior (dorsal) root ganglion.** The posterior (dorsal) root ganglion consists of somatic sensory neuron cell bodies that synapse onto motor nerve cell bodies in the anterior gray horn. The posterior (dorsal) root carries sensory fibers, whereas the anterior (ventral) root carries motor fibers. Because the sensory and motor roots merge to form the spinal nerve, these nerves are called **mixed nerves.**

ACTIVITY 3 Transverse Section of Spinal Cord

1. Label Figure 15.3 and Figure 15.4.
2. Identify these parts on a transverse section model or chart of spinal cord.
3. Pronounce these terms as you point to them.
4. Label the photomicrograph of a transverse section of spinal cord in Figure 15.5.
5. Examine a prepared slide of a transverse section of spinal cord.
   - Using the low power objective lens, identify the structures listed in Figure 15.5.
   - Using the high power objective, observe myelinated axons in the white matter and unmyelinated processes, neuron cell bodies, and neuroglia in the gray matter.

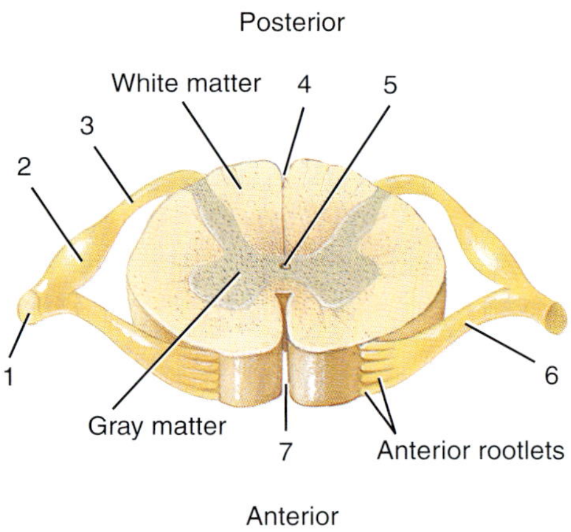

- anterior median fissure
- anterior (ventral) root
- central canal
- posterior (dorsal) root
- posterior (dorsal) root ganglion (GANG-li-on)
- posterior median sulcus
- spinal nerve

1 ______________________

2 ______________________

3 ______________________

4 ______________________

5 ______________________

6 ______________________

7 ______________________

FIGURE 15.3 Transverse section of spinal cord.

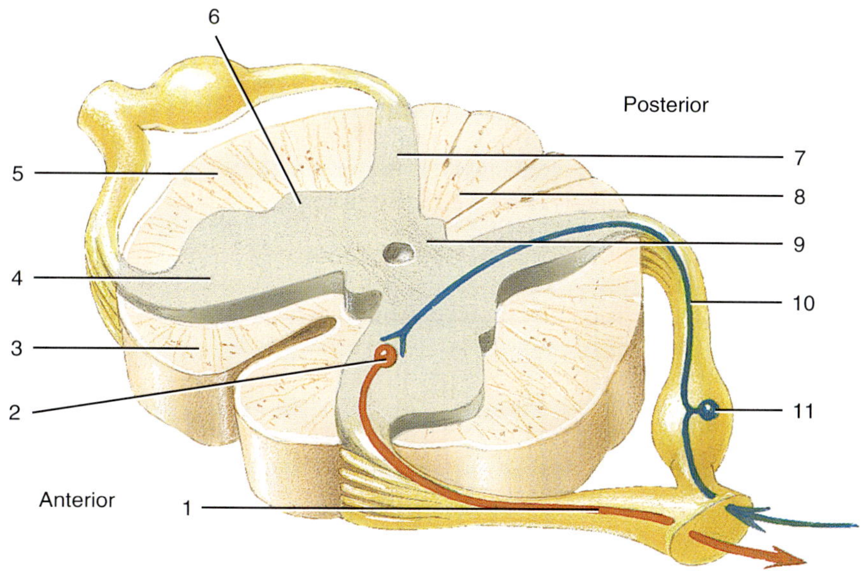

- anterior gray horn
- anterior white column
- axon of motor neuron
- axon of sensory neuron
- cell body of motor neuron
- cell body of sensory neuron
- gray commissure (COM-mis-sure)
- lateral gray horn
- lateral white column
- posterior gray horn
- posterior white column

1 ______________ 5 ______________ 9 ______________

2 ______________ 6 ______________ 10 ______________

3 ______________ 7 ______________ 11 ______________

4 ______________ 8 ______________

FIGURE 15.4 Transverse section of spinal cord with areas of gray and white matter.

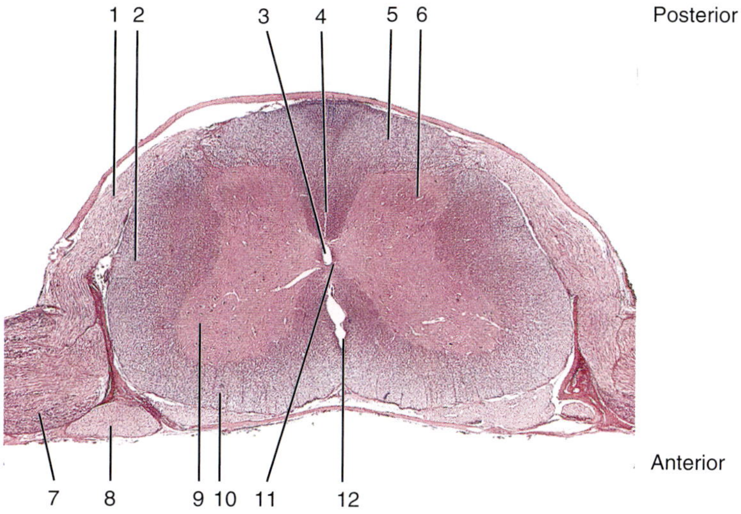

- anterior gray horn
- anterior median fissure
- anterior (ventral) root
- anterior white column
- central canal
- gray commissure
- lateral white column
- posterior (dorsal) root
- posterior (dorsal) root ganglion
- posterior gray horn
- posterior white column
- posterior median sulcus

1 ______________ 5 ______________ 9 ______________

2 ______________ 6 ______________ 10 ______________

3 ______________ 7 ______________ 11 ______________

4 ______________ 8 ______________ 12 ______________

FIGURE 15.5 Photomicrograph of spinal cord cross-section with spinal nerve.

D. Dissection of the Spinal Cord

Use either a preserved cow or sheep spinal cord or a fresh spinal cord from a butcher. Remember, if the specimen is preserved, it will be firmer and look different from a fresh specimen.

> **LAB SAFETY:** *Use safety glasses and remember to properly dispose of any removed waste tissue as directed by your instructor. Always wash your dissection tools, tray, lab surfaces and hands before leaving.*

ACTIVITY 4 Spinal Cord Dissection

1 Observe the posterior structures. Refer to Figure 15.6.
- After putting on your gloves, place the spinal cord in the dissection pan.
- Use a blunt probe or forceps to separate the **spinal meninges.**
- Identify the **dura** and **arachnoid mater.**
- Use a pointed dissection probe or pin to detach the **pia mater** from the spinal cord.
- Identify the **denticulate ligaments.**
- Peel back the meninges to uncover the **posterior (dorsal)** and **anterior (ventral) roots** of the spinal nerve. Locate the **rootlets.**
- Identify the **posterior (dorsal) root ganglion.**

2 Observe transverse section structures. Refer to Figure 15.4.
- Cut a 1/4 inch to 1/2 inch section from your spinal cord.
- Use Figure 15.5 as a reference for the transverse section.
- Identify the **anterior median fissure, posterior median sulcus, central canal, gray commissure, gray horns,** and **white columns.**

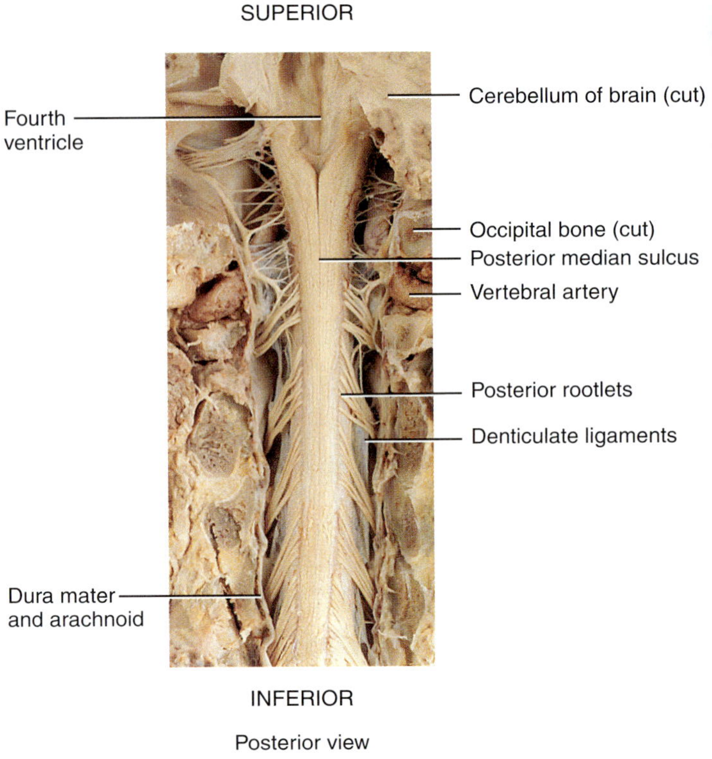

FIGURE 15.6 Photograph of posterior view of spinal cord with meninges and spinal nerve roots.

Name ______________________ Date ____________ Section ______________

EXERCISE 15

REVIEWING YOUR KNOWLEDGE

A. Meninges

Match the terms with the correct description.

___ **1.** Arachnoid mater

___ **2.** Denticulate ligament

___ **3.** Dura mater

___ **4.** Epidural space

___ **5.** Pia mater

___ **6.** Subarachnoid space

A. middle meninx; weblike
B. tough, outer meninx
C. space filled with adipose tissue
D. thin meninx intimate with spinal cord
E. contains cerebrospinal fluid
F. extension of pia mater attaching to dura

B. Identification of Spinal Cord Structures

Label the spinal cord structures in Figure 15.7.

1. ______________________________

2. ______________________________

3. ______________________________

4. ______________________________

5. ______________________________

6. ______________________________

7. ______________________________

8. ______________________________

9. ______________________________

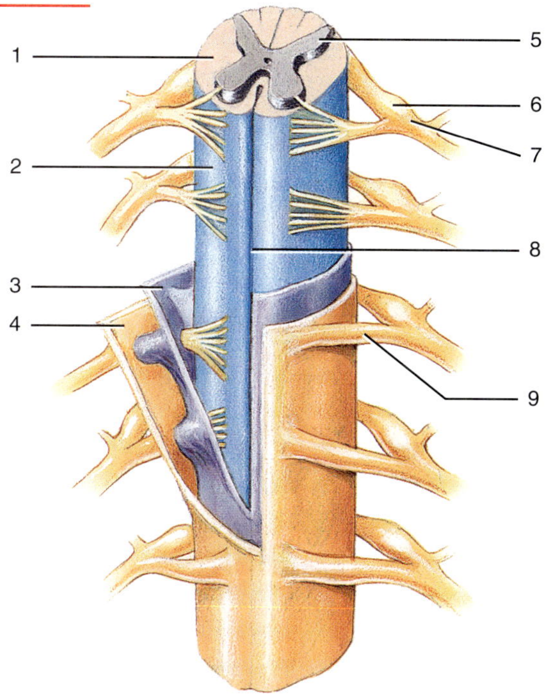

FIGURE 15.7 Anterior view of spinal cord with meninges and gray and white matter.

C. Spinal Cord Structures

Write the terms by the correct description.

anterior gray horn
anterior median fissure
anterior (ventral) root
cauda equina
central canal
cervical enlargement
conus medullaris
filum terminale
gray commissure
gray matter
lumbar enlargement
posterior (dorsal) root
posterior (dorsal) root ganglion
posterior gray horn
posterior median sulcus
white matter

______________________ **1.** contains neuron cell bodies that receive impulses from sensory neurons

______________________ **2.** contains neuron cell bodies and unmyelinated processes

______________________ **3.** shallow groove on dorsal side

______________________ **4.** connects right and left halves of gray matter in spinal cord

______________________ **5.** sensory branch entering spinal cord

______________________ **6.** tapered end of spinal cord

______________________ **7.** motor branch exiting spinal cord

______________________ **8.** contains sensory neuron cell bodies

______________________ **9.** collection of spinal nerves that arise from inferior end of spinal cord

______________________ **10.** contains myelinated axons

______________________ **11.** contains somatic motor neuron cell bodies

______________________ **12.** contains cerebral spinal fluid

______________________ **13.** bulge in spinal cord containing cell bodies of motor neurons supplying upper limb

______________________ **14.** wide, deep groove

______________________ **15.** extension of pia mater that attaches spinal cord to coccyx

______________________ **16.** bulge in spinal cord at T9–T12

Name ______________________ Date ______________ Section ______________

EXERCISE 15

USING YOUR KNOWLEDGE

A. Spinal Cord Structure

Label Figure 15.8.

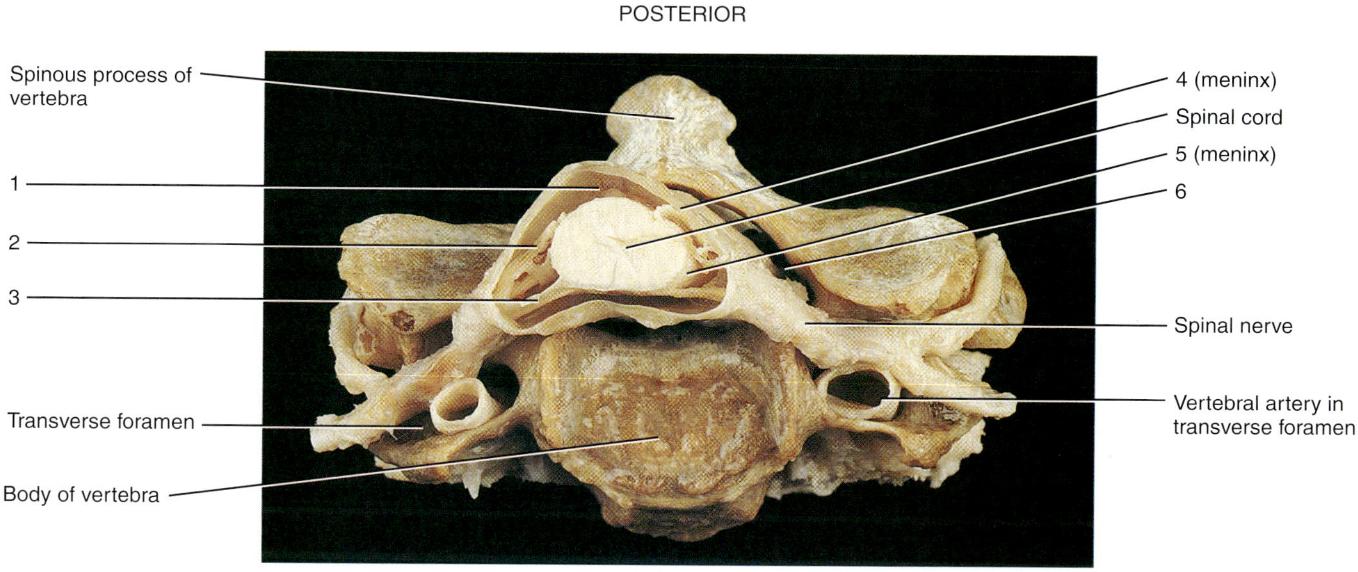

FIGURE 15.8 Photographic cross section of spinal cord and cervical vertebra.

1. ______________________
2. ______________________
3. ______________________
4. ______________________
5. ______________________
6. ______________________

B. Spinal Cord Questions

7. The polio virus can cause skeletal muscle paralysis by destroying neuron cell bodies. Identify the area of the spinal cord that is destroyed.

8. Shingles is a condition characterized by pain, discoloration of the skin, and eruption of skin blisters along a sensory nerve. It is caused by the herpes zoster virus, the same virus that causes chicken pox. Using your textbook or another source, identify the spinal cord structure to which herpes virus retreats after chicken pox. The virus remains dormant there until it is activated and causes a shingles outbreak.

9. Identify the structural class(es) of neurons whose cell bodies are present in the spinal cord—unipolar, bipolar, or multipolar.

10. Nerve fibers (axons) are classified according to diameter and presence or absence of a myelin sheath. Name the nerve fiber types (Type A, B, C) present in the (a) anterior (ventral) root (b) posterior (dorsal) root.

11. At what level of the spinal cord is a needle inserted to do a spinal tap? Explain why spinal taps are not done above this level.

C. Pathway of Sensory and Motor Impulses

Numbering 1–5, indicate the order of structures through which sensory impulses pass as they enter spinal cord and travel toward brain

____ **12.** posterior (dorsal) root ganglion

____ **13.** posterior (dorsal) root

____ **14.** posterior gray horn

____ **15.** white column

____ **16.** spinal nerve

Numbering 1–4, indicate the order of structures through which motor impulses pass as they descend from brain and leave spinal cord

____ **17.** spinal nerve

____ **18.** white column

____ **19.** anterior (ventral) gray horn

____ **20.** anterior (ventral) root

EXERCISE

17B

SOMATIC REFLEXES

OUTLINE

OBJECTIVES

After completing this exercise, you should be able to:

- Identify and describe the five components of a somatic reflex arc
- Describe how monosynaptic and polysynaptic reflex arcs differ
- Explain the significance of clinical testing of reflexes

MATERIALS

- reflex hammer (with rubber head)
- cross-section spinal cord model

Reflexes are rapid, involuntary motor responses to an environmental stimulus detected by sensory receptors. A nerve impulse travels from the receptor through a neural **reflex arc** pathway to an effector. If the motor response is contraction of skeletal muscle, the reflex is a **somatic reflex.** If the motor response involves cardiac muscle, smooth muscle, or glands, the reflex is an **autonomic (visceral) reflex.** Reflexes mediated by spinal nerves are called **spinal reflexes,** whereas reflexes mediated by cranial nerves are called **cranial reflexes.** Most reflexes help our bodies maintain homeostasis and therefore have a protective function.

A. Reflex Arcs

There are five components of a reflex arc:

1. **Sensory receptor.** If the stimulus to the sensory receptor is strong enough, an action potential is generated in the sensory neuron.
2. **Sensory neuron.** The sensory neuron propagates the action potential and synapses with neurons in the spinal cord or brain stem.
3. **Integrating center.** The integrating center is located within the gray matter of the CNS, and transfers information from the sensory neuron to the motor neuron. The integrating center of a **monosynaptic reflex arc** is a single synapse between a sensory and motor neuron. In a **polysynaptic reflex arc,** the integrating center consists of multiple synapses involving one or more interneurons (association neurons) between a sensory and a motor neuron.
4. **Motor neuron.** The motor neuron carries the action potential initiated by the integrating center to the effector.
5. **Effector.** An effector can be a skeletal muscle (somatic reflex), cardiac muscle, smooth muscle, or glands (somatic reflex). A **reflex** is the response of the effector to stimulation by the motor neuron of the reflex arc.

Reflex arcs that involve sensory receptors, sensory nerve fibers, motor neurons, and effectors all on the same side of the body are **ipsilateral. Contralateral** reflex arcs involve sensory receptors and neurons on one side of the body and motor neurons and effectors on the opposite side.

ACTIVITY 1 Reflexes

1 Identify whether the reflexes in Table 17B.1 are somatic reflexes or autonomic reflexes, and whether a spinal nerve or a cranial nerve mediates it.

2 Label Figure 17B.1 with your lab group.

3 Answer discussion questions about Figure 17B.1 with your lab group.

4 Using the cross-section spinal cord model, trace the pathway of the reflex arc illustrated in Figure 17B.1.

DISCUSSION QUESTIONS: REFLEX ARC

1 Is the reflex arc in Figure 17B.1 monosynaptic or polysynaptic?

2 Is the reflex arc in Figure 17B.1 ipsilateral or contralateral?

TABLE 17B.1 Types of Reflexes

REFLEX ACTION	SOMATIC OR AUTONOMIC REFLEX	SPINAL NERVE REFLEXES OR CRANIAL NERVE REFLEXES
Plantar flexion of foot when Achilles tendon is stretched		
Salivation in response to lemon juice on tongue		
Blinking in response to touching the cornea		
Flexing of arm in response to touching a hot object		

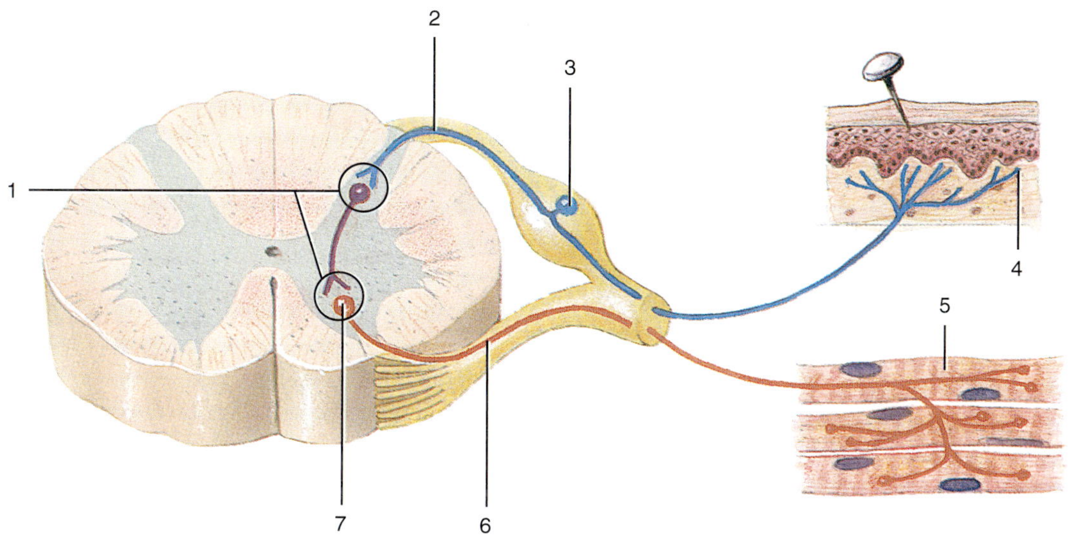

- effector
- integrating center
- motor neuron cell body
- motor neuron axon
- sensory neuron cell body
- sensory neuron axon
- sensory receptor

1 ____________________
2 ____________________
3 ____________________
4 ____________________
5 ____________________
6 ____________________
7 ____________________

FIGURE 17B.1 Reflex arc components.

B. Reflex Testing

A series of reflex tests are used clinically to evaluate the nervous system and to diagnose an abnormality or dysfunction.

1. Patellar Reflex (Knee Jerk)

The **patellar reflex** is the extension of the knee that occurs when the patellar tendon is stretched. The components of the **patellar reflex arc** are:

- Sensory receptors: **Muscle spindles** located in the quadriceps femoris muscle group. Tapping the patellar tendon stretches this muscle group and stimulates muscle spindles (stretch receptors), initiating nerve impulses in axons of sensory neurons.
- Sensory Neuron: Sensory axons carry nerve impulses to the integrating center (gray matter) in the spinal cord.
- Integrating Center: The **monosynaptic integrating center** (two neurons, one synapse) is located in the anterior gray horn of the spinal cord. The sensory axon synapses with and initiates nerve impulses in the motor neuron that innervates the quadriceps femoris muscle group.
- Motor neuron: Axons of the motor neuron travel in the femoral nerve to the quadriceps femoris muscle group.
- Effector: Quadriceps femoris muscle group (agonists) contracts and extends the leg when stimulated.

The sensory neuron associated with the monosynaptic stretch reflex arc is also a component of a **polysynaptic reflex arc** that has three neurons and two synapses. This reflex arc inhibits the motor neuron to the antagonist muscle group and results in its relaxation. This is referred to as **reciprocal innervation**—stimulation of contraction in agonistic muscles with simultaneous inhibition of antagonistic muscles.

ACTIVITY 2 Testing the Patellar Reflex

1 Label the patellar reflex arc and reciprocal innervation in Figure 17B.2.

2 Test the patellar reflex.

- Have the subject sit on the edge of a table or a tall lab chair with his/her knee off the table or chair and the leg dangling and relaxed.
- Palpate the patella and the tibial tuberosity; the patellar tendon, the insertion of the quadriceps femoris, is between these two structures. To be sure you have found the tendon, have the subject isometrically flex the quadriceps muscles, but not move the leg while you palpate the tendon.
- Gently but firmly tap the patellar tendon with the tapered end of a reflex hammer.
- Although the grading is subjective, grade the extension of the leg: Results: ______________________

  0 = no response (hyporeflexive)
  +1 = little response (hyporeflexive)
  +2 = normal response
  +3 = above normal response
  +4 = exaggerated reflex (hyperreflexive)
- Now ask the subject to clasp both hands in front of the chest and isometrically pull in opposite directions. This action leads to an enhancement of spinal reflexes causing a reinforced patellar reflex.
- While s/he is pulling, strike the patellar tendon again and observe the distance of leg movement this time.
- Reinforced patellar reflex results: ______________

3 Answer discussion questions about the patellar reflex with your lab group.

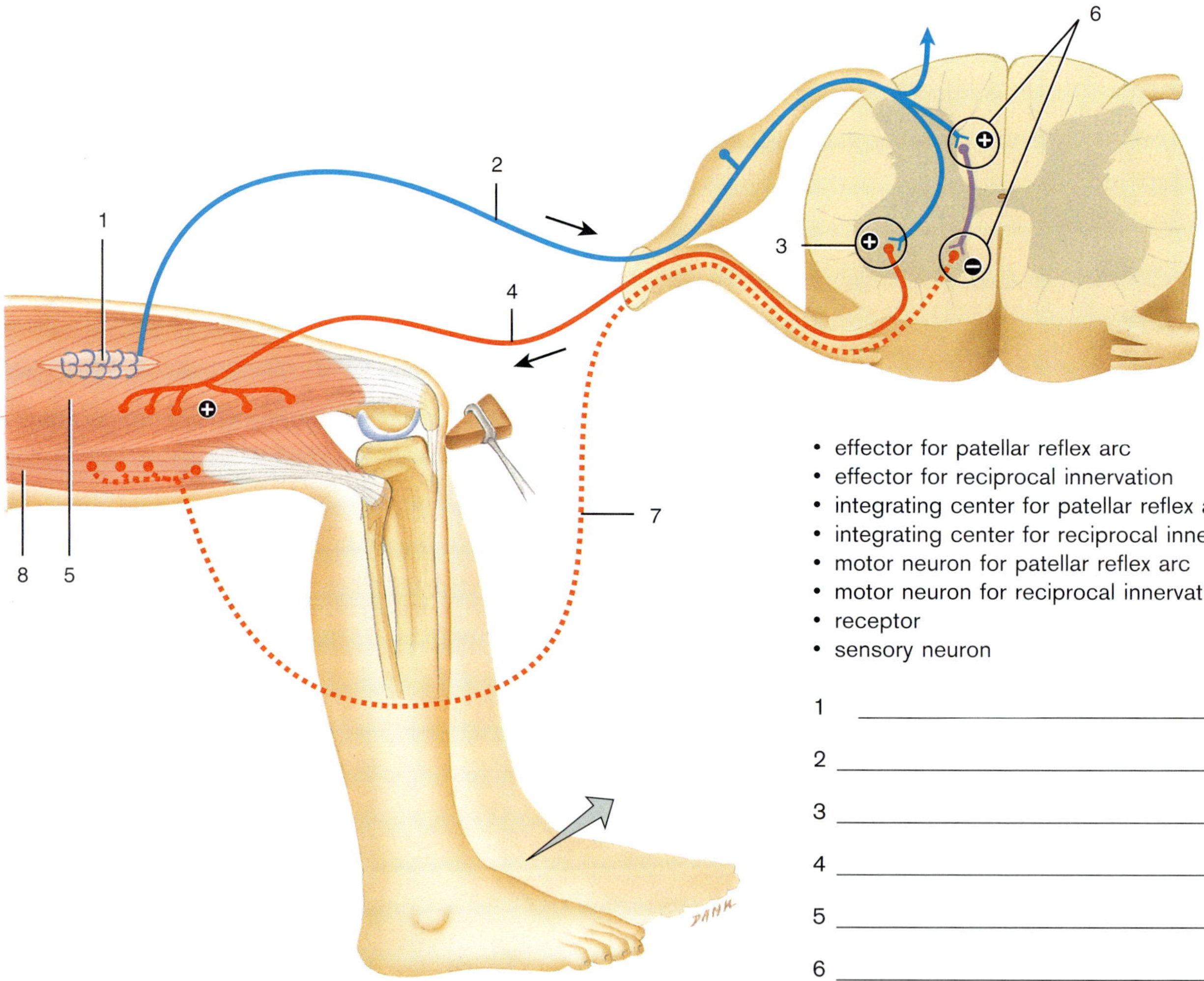

- effector for patellar reflex arc
- effector for reciprocal innervation
- integrating center for patellar reflex arc
- integrating center for reciprocal innervation
- motor neuron for patellar reflex arc
- motor neuron for reciprocal innervation
- receptor
- sensory neuron

1 ______________________

2 ______________________

3 ______________________

4 ______________________

5 ______________________

6 ______________________

7 ______________________

8 ______________________

FIGURE 17B.2 Patellar reflex arc.

DISCUSSION QUESTIONS: PATELLAR REFLEX

1 Is the patellar reflex ipsilateral or contralateral?

2 During the patellar reflex, are the motor neurons supplying the hamstrings stimulated or inhibited?

3 Describe the effect that clasping and pulling the hands has on the patellar reflex compared with the first patellar reflex.

2. Biceps Reflex (Biceps Jerk)

The **biceps reflex** is the contraction of the biceps brachii muscle that occurs when the biceps tendon is stretched. Although the biceps brachii flexes the forearm, in this test you may only see the contraction or tension in the biceps brachii muscle because the forearm is resting on the table.

ACTIVITY 3 Testing the Biceps Reflex (Biceps Jerk)

1 Test the biceps reflex.
- Have the subject stand with an arm completely relaxed and hanging down at the side.
- Ask the subject to isometrically contract the biceps brachii so you can palpate the tendon in the antecubital fossa.
- After locating the tendon, have the subject relax and place your thumb over the tendon.
- Gently but firmly tap your thumb with the tapered end of the reflex hammer.
- Biceps reflex results: ______________________
- If the reflex is absent, have the subject clench his/her teeth and try the reflex test again.
- Reinforced biceps reflex results: ______________

2 Answer the discussion questions with your lab group.

DISCUSSION QUESTIONS: BICEPS REFLEX

1 Name the nerve that carries the sensory and motor axons for this reflex arc.

2 Name the antagonistic muscles that are inhibited by reciprocal innervation.

3. Triceps Reflex (Triceps Jerk)

The triceps reflex is the contraction of the triceps brachii muscle that occurs when the triceps brachii tendon is stretched.

ACTIVITY 4 Triceps Reflex (Triceps Jerk)

1 Test the triceps reflex.
- Have the subject stand with an arm completely relaxed and hanging down at the side.
- Palpate the triceps tendon (superior to olecranon process) as the subject isometrically contracts the triceps muscles.
- Keep your finger on the tendon and have the subject bend the arm across the front of the body.
- Have the subject support the arm by holding it in his/her other hand.
- Use the tapered end of the reflex hammer to tap the triceps tendon.
- Triceps tendon reflex results: ________________
- If the reflex is absent, have the subject clench his/her teeth and try the reflex again.
- Reinforced triceps tendon results: ______________

2 Answer the discussion questions with your lab group.

DISCUSSION QUESTIONS: TRICEPS REFLEX

1 Name the nerve that carries the sensory and motor axons for this reflex arc.

2 Name the antagonistic muscles that are inhibited by reciprocal innervation.

4. Achilles Reflex (Ankle Jerk)

The response of this reflex is plantar flexion when the Achilles (calcaneous) tendon is tapped with the reflex hammer.

ACTIVITY 5 Achilles Reflex (Ankle Jerk)

1 Test the achilles reflex.
- Have the subject keep one foot on the floor and place the knee of the other leg on a chair with the foot dangling over the edge.
- Ask the subject to slightly dorsiflex the foot to stretch the tendon a little, but be relaxed.
- Tap the calcaneal tendon with the tapered end reflex hammer and observe the response of the foot.
- Calcaneal reflex results: ______________________

2 Answer the discussion questions with your lab group.

DISCUSSION QUESTIONS: ACHILLES REFLEX

1 Name the nerve that carries the sensory and motor neurons for this reflex arc.

2 Name the antagonistic muscles that are inhibited by reciprocal innervation.

5. Plantar Flexion

This test stimulates the cutaneous receptors and involves the brain in addition to the spinal cord. In adults, **plantar flexion** and flexed (curled) toes occurs when the plantar surface of the foot is stroked. A reaction of dorsiflexion with extended flared toes (Babinski's sign) is seen in infants because all the nerve fibers are not myelinated. The Babinski's sign is abnormal in adults.

ACTIVITY 6 Plantar Flexion

1 Test the plantar flexion reflex.
- Have the subject seated with a foot propped up and relaxed.
- Using the metal end of the reflex hammer, stroke the plantar surface of the foot starting at the heel, extending up the lateral side of the foot, and crossing over to the great toe area.
- Plantar flexion results: ______________________

2 Name the nerve tested ______________________.

Name ______________________ Date ______________ Section ________________

EXERCISE 17B

REVIEWING YOUR KNOWLEDGE

A. Reflex Arc

1. Name the five components of a reflex arc in order.

a. ______________________________________

b. ______________________________________

c. ______________________________________

d. ______________________________________

e. ______________________________________

2. How many neurons are in a monosynaptic reflex arc? ______ How many synapses are in the integrating center? ______

3. How many neurons are in a polysynaptic reflex arc? ______ How many synapses are in a polysynaptic reflex arc containing two interneurons in the integrating center? ______

4. Which type of neuron does the sensory neuron synapse with in a monosynaptic reflex arc? ______

5. Which type of neuron does the sensory neuron synapse with in a polysynaptic reflex arc? ______

B. Reflex Tests

Name the nerve that is tested in each of the following reflexes.

6. Achilles reflex ______________

7. Biceps reflex ______________

8. Patellar reflex ______________

9. Plantar flexion reflex ______________

10. Triceps reflex ______________

11. Is a Babinski's sign normal in adults? ______

C. Reflexes

1. Define reflex.

2. Describe the difference between a somatic and visceral reflex.

3. Describe the difference between a cranial and spinal reflex.

4. Describe the difference between an ipsilateral and contralateral reflex arc.

5. Define reciprocal innervation.

Name ______________________ Date ______________ Section ______________

EXERCISE 17B

USING YOUR KNOWLEDGE

A. Flexor and Crossed Extensor Reflex

You are walking along the beach barefoot and step on a sharp object with your right foot. You immediately flex the right leg and balance yourself by extending the left leg. Label the following neurons in Figure 17B.3.

1. Sensory neuron
2. Interneuron sending impulses up and down the spinal cord
3. Interneuron synapsing with motor neurons
4. Motor neuron causing flexion
5. Motor neuron causing extension

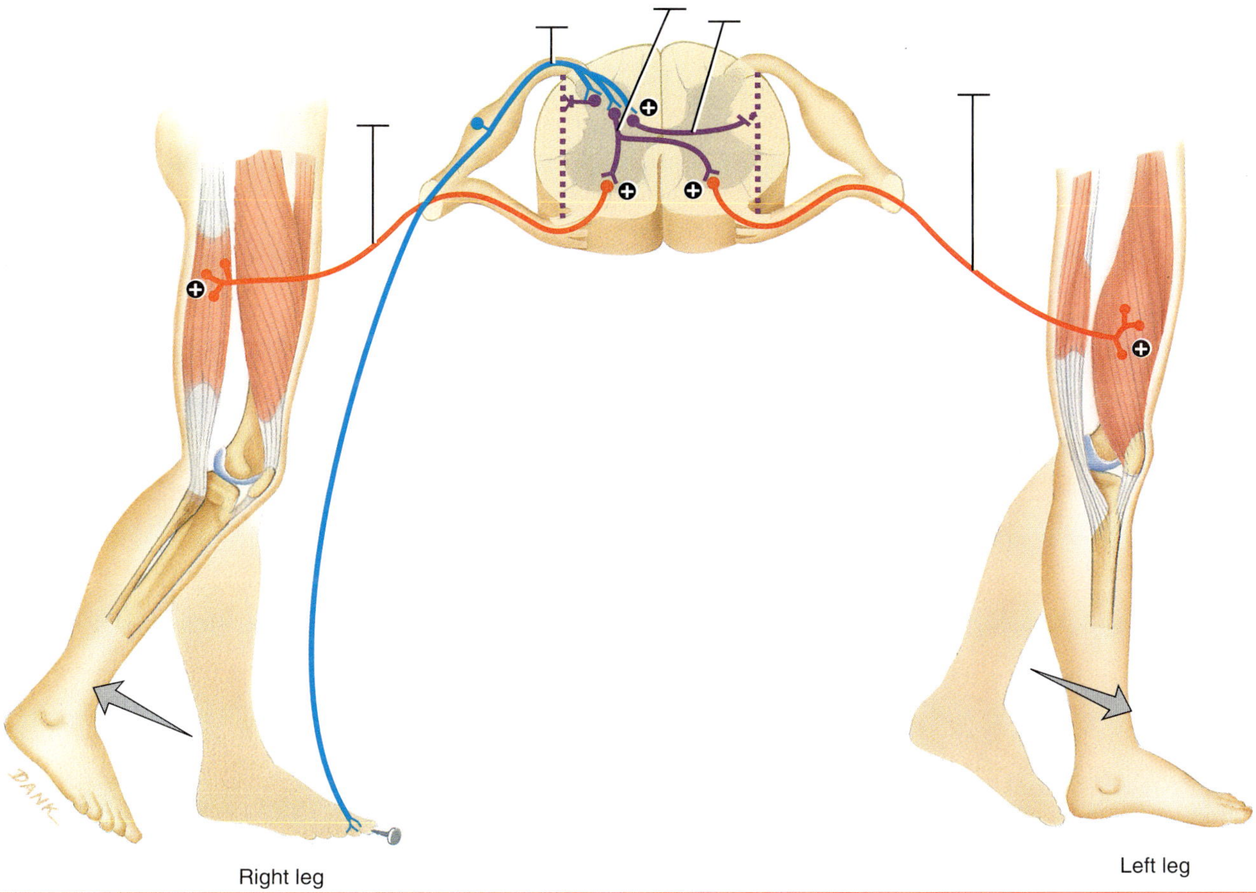

FIGURE 17B.3 Flexor and crossed extensor reflex arc.

For the reflex arc in Figure 17B.3, name the:

5. Nerve carrying pain sensory information from right foot ______________

6. Nerve carrying motor information causing right leg flexion ______________

7. Nerve carrying motor information causing left leg extension ______________

8. Agonistic muscles for right leg flexion ______________

9. Agonistic muscles for left leg extension ______________

C. Modification of Reflex Activity

10. Reflex activity can be modified by the cerebral cortex. For example, you are baking a roast in the oven. As you are moving the roast from the oven to the counter, hot juices splash you. Reflex activity would cause you to drop the pan, but you hold on to it. Explain how the cerebral cortex overrides the reflex.

EXERCISE

19B

SPECIAL SENSES

OUTLINE

MATERIALS

The Eye and Vision

- eye models or charts
- compound microscope, lens paper, prepared slides of an eyeball
- dissection equipment and trays, cow eyes, and gloves
- Snellen eye chart, ophthalmoscope, metric ruler

Note: The materials for Hearing and Equilibrium, Smell, and Taste precede their respective sections B, C, and D.

OBJECTIVES

After completing this exercise, you should be able to:

The Eye and Vision

- Identify the accessory structures of the eye and the structures of the eyeball
- Identify the three principle layers of the retina
- Perform visual tests that are used to determine myopia, hyperopia, presbyopia, and astigmatism

The Ear, Hearing, and Equilibrium

- Identify the structures of the external, middle, and internal ear
- Identify the major structures of the cochlea, vestibule, and semicircular canals
- Perform tests that are used in determining the cause of hearing loss
- Perform tests that exhibit the function of the receptors for dynamic and static equilibrium

The Nose and Olfaction

- Identify the location of receptors for olfaction
- Examine the structure of the receptors for olfaction
- Determine time of adaptation for olfactory receptors

The Taste Buds and Gustation

- Identify the location of receptors for taste
- Examine the structure of the receptors for taste
- Observe the influence of smell and texture on taste

A. The Eye and Vision

1. Accessory Eye Structures

Accessory structures of the eye include the **eyebrows,** eyelids or **palpabrae, eyelashes,** and the following structures:

conjunctiva—thin, protective mucous membrane that covers the anterior eye and folds to cover the inner eyelid

- **palpebral conjunctiva**—membrane that covers the inner surface of the eyelid
- **bulbar conjunctiva**—membrane that covers the anterior part of the white of the eye

lacrimal apparatus (*lacrim-* = tears)—group of structures that produces and drains tears

- **lacrimal gland**—produces and secretes tears onto eye surface
- **lacrimal canals**—two medial ducts that drain the tears from the eyes
- **lacrimal sac**—enlarged area receiving tears from lacrimal canals
- **nasolacrimal duct**—receives tears from lacrimal sac and drains into the nasal cavity

extrinsic eye muscles—6 skeletal muscles that insert on the exterior of the eyeball and move the eye

- **superior, inferior, medial,** and **lateral rectus**—4 muscles that are parallel to the long axis of the eyeball
- **superior** and **inferior oblique**—attach to eyeball at an angle

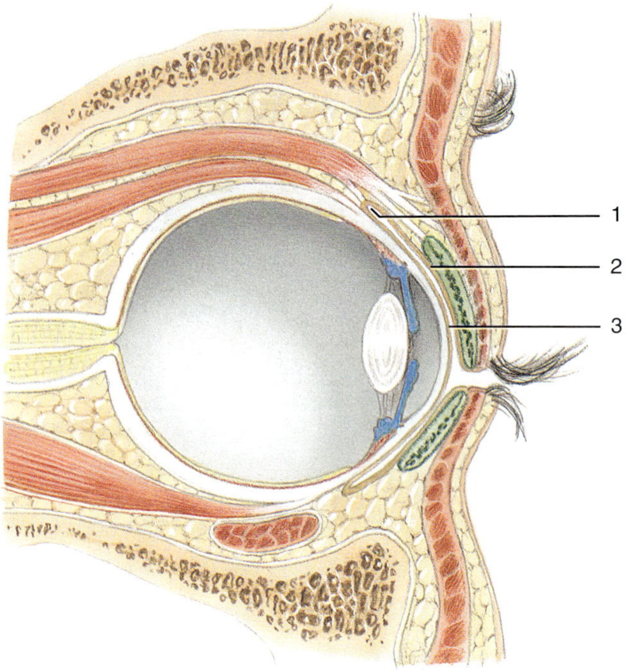

(a) Lateral view of eyeball

- bulbar conjunctiva (con-junk-TIE-va)
- conjunctival fold
- palpebral conjunctiva (PAL-puh-bral)

1 ______________________

2 ______________________

3 ______________________

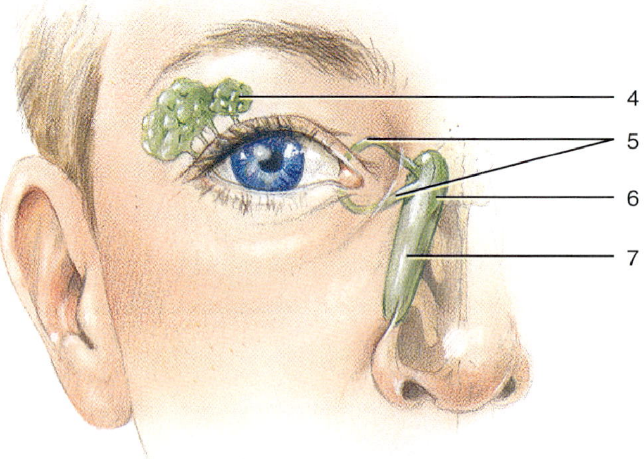

(b) Lacrimal apparatus

- lacrimal canals (LAK-rih-mal)
- lacrimal gland
- lacrimal sac
- nasolacrimal duct

4 ______________________

5 ______________________

6 ______________________

7 ______________________

FIGURE 19B.1 Accessory structures of the eye.

ACTIVITY 1 Accessory Structures of the Eye

1 Label the parts of the conjunctiva in Figure 19B.1a and structures of the lacrimal apparatus in Figure 19B.1b.

2 Label the extrinsic eye muscles in Figure 19B.2.

3 Identify all the accessory structures of the eye, including all parts of the lacrimal apparatus, on an eye model or chart and pronounce the terms as you point to them.

4 Identify the extrinsic eye muscles on an eye model or chart and pronounce the terms as you point to them.

5 Determine how each muscle moves the eye by observing where it inserts on the eye and how the eye would move if the insertion is moved toward the origin.

6 Write the function of each extrinsic eye muscle in Table 19B.1. Choose one of the following eye movements for each muscle: *moves eye superiorly, inferiorly, medially, laterally, superiorly and laterally, or inferiorly and laterally.*

TABLE 19B.1 Function of the Extrinsic Eye Muscles

EXTRINSIC EYE MUSCLE	FUNCTION
Inferior oblique	
Inferior rectus	
Lateral rectus	
Medial rectus	
Superior oblique	
Superior rectus	

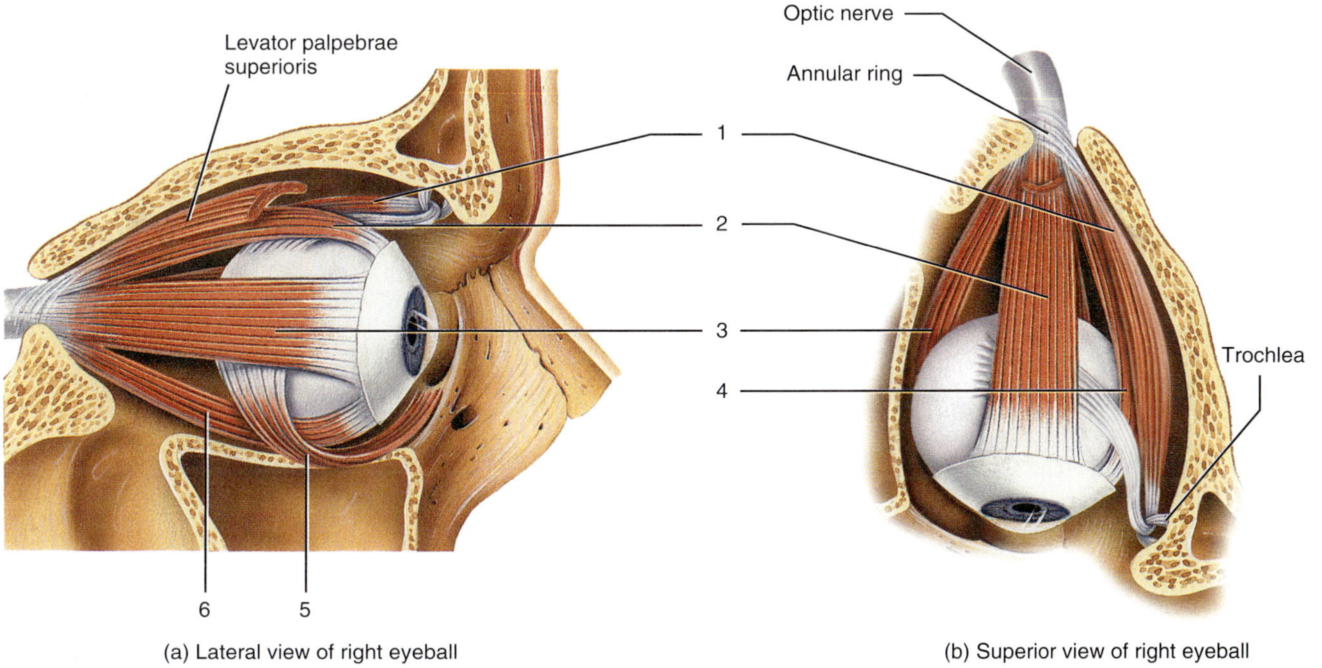

- inferior oblique
- inferior rectus
- lateral rectus
- medial rectus
- superior oblique
- superior rectus

1 ______________________

2 ______________________

3 ______________________

4 ______________________

5 ______________________

6 ______________________

FIGURE 19B.2 Extrinsic eye muscles.

2. Structure of the Eyeball

The wall of the eyeball has three layers: the outer fibrous tunic, the middle vascular tunic, and the inner retina.

Fibrous tunic—composed of the cornea and sclera

- **cornea**—transparent anterior portion that covers the iris and pupil
- **sclera** (*scler-* = hard)—white of the eye; comprises the majority of the eyeball
- **scleral venous sinus** (canal of Schlemm)—opening found at the junction of the cornea and sclera

Vascular tunic—composed of the iris, ciliary body, and choroid

- **iris**—most anterior portion made of circular smooth muscle; controls the pupil size
  pupil—opening in the middle of the iris
- **ciliary body**—begins at the junction of the cornea and sclera; consists of the ciliary muscle and ciliary processes
  ciliary muscle—circular smooth muscle that changes the lens shape
  ciliary processes—folds that protrude from the ciliary body toward the lens; attach to suspensory ligaments that attach to the lens
  ora serrata (*serra-* = jagged or serrated)—the jagged interface between the ciliary muscle and retina
- **choroid**—the most posterior part that lines most of the interior of sclera

Retina—starts at the ora serrata and continues posteriorly, lining the interior of the choroid

- **pigmental layer**—outer portion of the retina
- **neural layer**—inner portion that contains photoreceptors and associated neurons

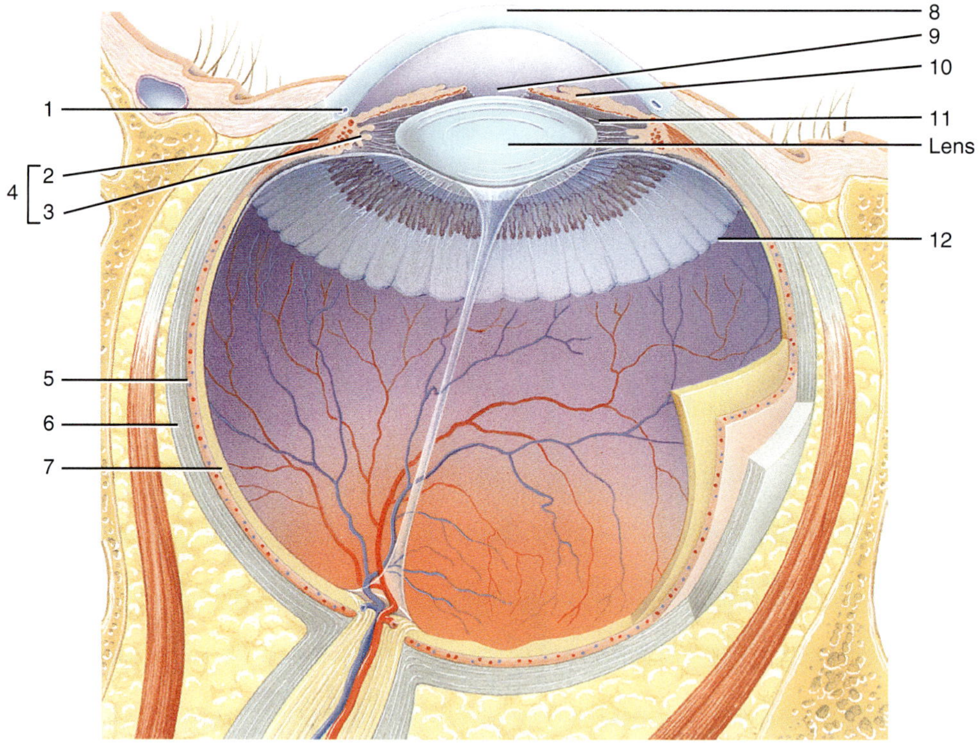

- choroid
- ciliary body (SIL-ee-air-ec)
- ciliary muscle
- ciliary process
- cornea (KOR-nee-ah)
- iris
- ora serrata (ser-RAH-tah)
- pupil
- retina
- sclera (SKLER-ah)
- scleral venous sinus
- suspensory ligament

1 ____________ 4 ____________ 7 ____________ 10 ____________

2 ____________ 5 ____________ 8 ____________ 11 ____________

3 ____________ 6 ____________ 9 ____________ 12 ____________

FIGURE 19B.3 Structure of the eyeball.

ACTIVITY 2 Structure of the Eyeball

1 Label the eyeball structures in Figure 19B.3.

2 Identify these structures on an eye model or chart.

3 Pronounce the terms as you point to them.

Interior of the Eyeball

Lens divides the interior of the eyeball into an anterior cavity and a vitreous chamber (posterior cavity).

Anterior cavity—space anterior to the lens
- **anterior chamber**—space between the cornea and the iris
- **posterior chamber**—space between the iris and the lens
- **aqueous humor** (*aqua* = water; *humor* = moist)—liquid in the anterior cavity produced by capillaries in the ciliary process
- **scleral venous** sinus (canal of Schlemm)—drains the aqueous humor into the blood

Vitreous chamber (posterior cavity)—larger space between the lens and the retina
- **vitreous body** (humor)—jelly-like substance that holds the retina flat against the choroid

CLINICAL NOTE: GLAUCOMA *is caused by an increase in pressure within the eye called intraocular pressure. Blockage of the scleral venous sinus prevents drainage of aqueous humor, increasing the amount in the anterior cavity that causes increased intraocular pressure.*

ACTIVITY 3 Anterior and Posterior Cavities of the Eye

1 Label the interior spaces and structures of the eyeball in Figure 19B.4.

2 Identify these spaces and structures on a model or chart.

3 Pronounce the terms as you point to them.

- anterior cavity
- anterior chamber
- lens
- posterior chamber
- scleral venous sinus
- vitreous chamber

1 ______________________

2 ______________________

3 ______________________

4 ______________________

5 ______________________

6 ______________________

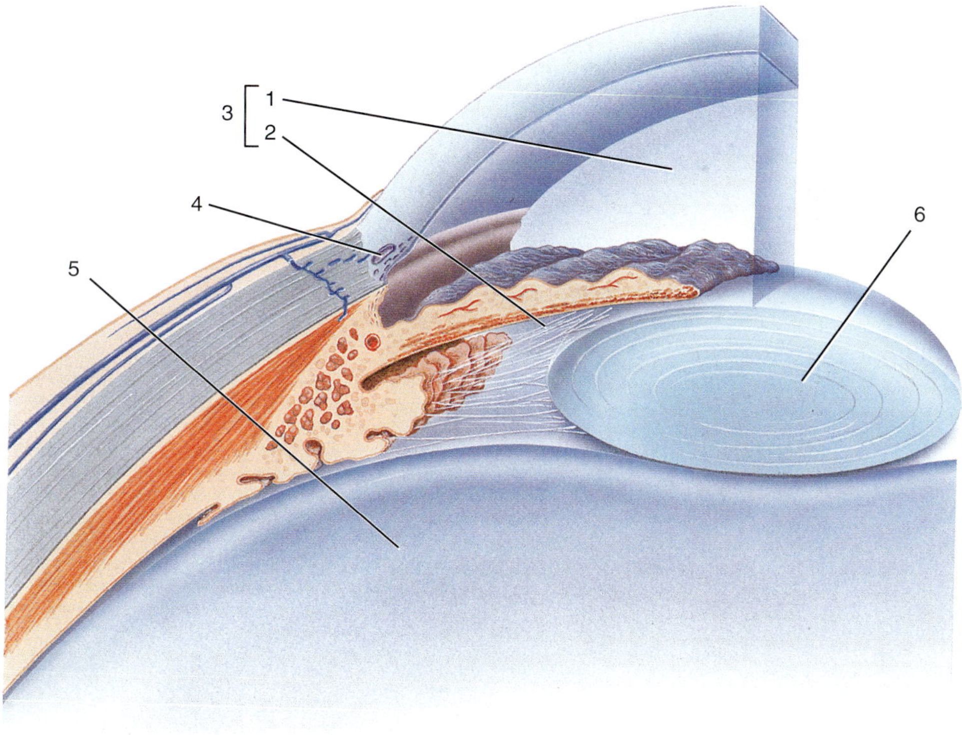

FIGURE 19B.4 Anterior and posterior cavities of the eyeball.

ACTIVITY 4 Dissection of Cow Eye

LAB SAFETY: *Use safety glasses and remember to properly dispose of any removed waste tissue as directed by your instructor. Always clean your dissection tools, tray, and lab surfaces as directed.*

1 Obtain a laboratory tray, blunt probe, scalpel, scissors, and disposable gloves.

2 Using gloves, obtain a cow eye and rinse it to remove excess preservative.

3 The posterior portion of the eye may be encased in adipose tissue. Carefully remove the adipose tissue protecting the optic nerve.

4 Identify the external eye structures: **cornea, sclera, optic nerve,** and **extrinsic eye muscles.** Refer to Figure 19B.5a. The preservative causes the cornea to change from being transparent and smooth to opaque and wrinkled.

5 Using the point of a scalpel, punch an opening ¼ inch posterior to the cornea through the very tough sclera. Be careful not to squeeze the eyeball too tightly or liquid may squirt out. Use the scissors to cut an incision all the way around the eyeball, separating it into two parts.

6 Carefully separate the anterior and posterior parts of the eyeball so the **vitreous body** remains in the posterior part of the eyeball and the **lens** in the anterior part.

7 Carefully remove the lens, noting the transparent **suspensory ligaments** that are attached to the lens.

8 Using Figure 19B.5b, identify the following structures in the anterior portion of the eyeball: **pupil, iris,** and **ciliary muscle.**

9 Carefully remove the vitreous body from the posterior portion of the eyeball. Refer to Figure 19B.5b to identify the structures in the posterior portion of the eyeball. The **retina,** a thin beige layer, will probably separate from the choroid. The only point of attachment of the retina to the wall of the eyeball is at the **optic disc.**

10 Pull the retina away from the **choroid,** the dark middle layer of the eyeball that contains the pigment melanin. The choroid of the cow's eye has an iridescent reflecting surface called the **tapetum lucidum** that is not found in humans. The tapetum lucidum reflects light within the eye and enables animals to see in low light conditions.

11 Separate the choroid from the **sclera.** Observe how the three coats or tunics—the **retina, choroid,** and **sclera**—form the wall of the eyeball.

12 Discard the eye as instructed by your instructor.

13 Clean your dissecting tray and equipment and return to the proper place.

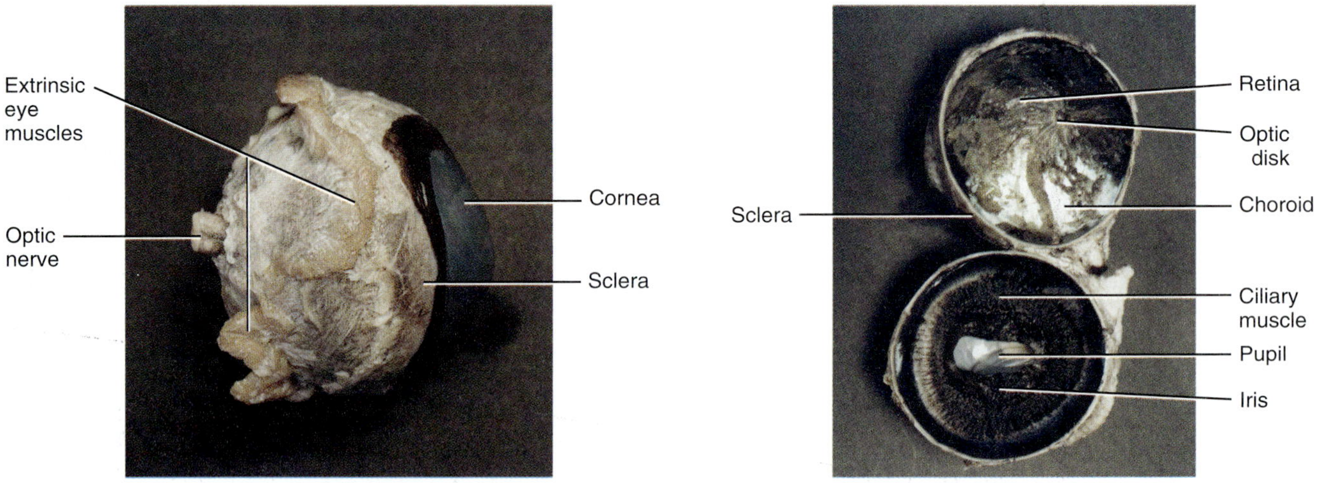

(a) External structures

(b) Anterior and posterior sections

FIGURE 19B.5 Cow eye dissection.

3. Anatomy of the Retina

The neural portion of the retina is an outgrowth of the brain and contains three layers of neurons: the photoreceptor layer (deepest cell layer), the bipolar cell layer (middle layer), and the ganglion cell layer (the superficial cell layer). The **photoreceptor cell layer** contains the rods and cones. **Rods** are used in night vision and respond to low levels of light, allowing us to perceive shades of gray, black, and white. Visual acuity with rods is low. **Cones** require brighter light for stimulation, but allow us to see color and provide high visual acuity. The rods and cones synapse with the bipolar neurons in the **bipolar cell layer,** which synapses on the ganglion cells in the **ganglion cell layer.** Axons from the ganglion cells extend through the optic disc and leave the eyeball as the optic nerve. The **optic disc** does not contain photoreceptors and forms the **blind spot** of the retina. It is also the site where the central retinal artery and vein enter and leave the retina, and the only place where the retina is secured to the other layers of the eyeball.

The **macula lutea** (*macula* = flat spot; *lutea* = yellow), the site of macular degeneration, is in the center of the neural portion of the retina. In the middle of the macula lutea is the **central fovea** (fovea centralis). This area of the retina has the highest density of cones of any area of the retina and is not covered by ganglion and bipolar cell layers. Therefore, this area has the highest visual acuity (sharpness of vision) of any area of the retina. When we look at an object, the light rays reflected from the object are focused onto the central fovea.

The retina can be viewed with an **ophthalmoscope.** The ophthalmoscope illuminates the interior of the eye, and the retina appears red from the many blood vessels. Blood vessels can be seen branching from the optic disc while the circular macula lutea appears dark because of the absence of blood vessels. The central fovea is in the middle of the macula lutea.

ACTIVITY 5 Anatomy of the Retina

1. Label the structures of the retina in Figure 19B.6a and Figure 19B.6b.
2. Label the structures of the retina as observed with an ophthalmoscope in Figure 19B.7.
3. Optional activity: View retina with ophthalmoscope. Instructions will be provided by your instructor.
4. Observe a longitudinal section of the eyeball in Figure 19B.8a, and label the photomicrograph in Figure 19B.8b.
5. Examine a slide showing a cross-section through an eyeball.
   - Using the low-power objective lens, find the posterior surface of the eyeball and identify the **sclera, choroid,** and **retina.** Place the retina in the center of the field of view and switch to the high-power objective lens.
   - Using the high-power objective lens, identify the **pigmented epithelium of the retina** and the **neural layer of the retina.** Within the neural layer of the retina, identify the **ganglion layer,** the **bipolar layer,** and the **photoreceptor layer.**

- central fovea
- central retinal artery
- central retinal vein
- optic disc
- optic nerve

1 ____________________

2 ____________________

3 ____________________

4 ____________________

5 ____________________

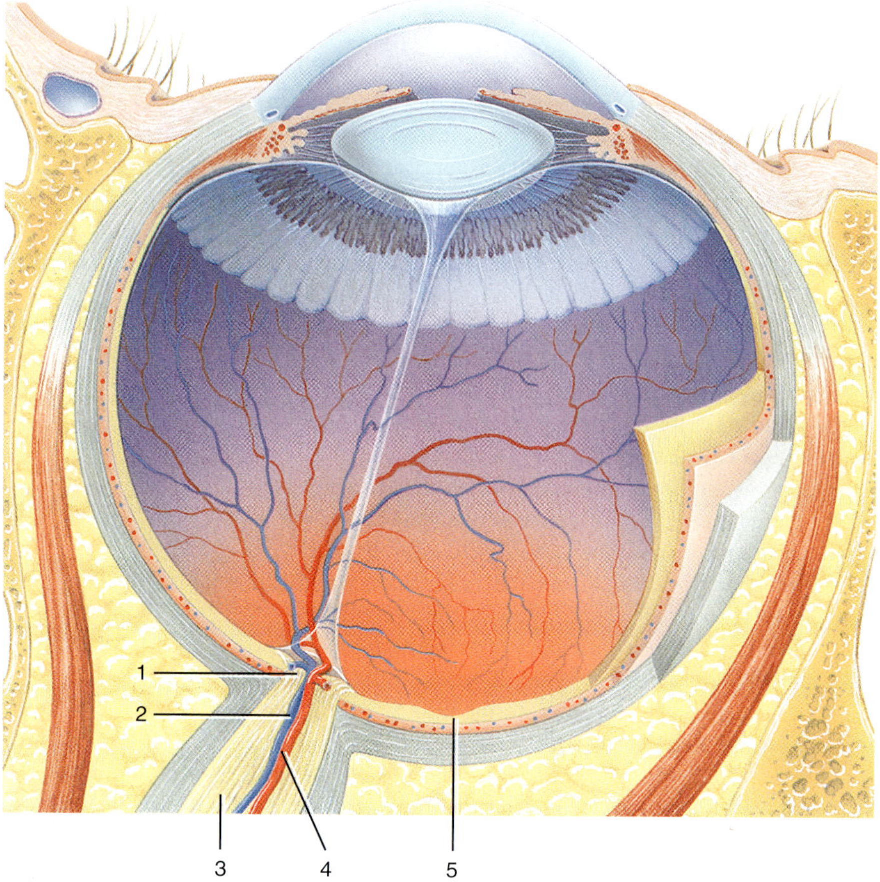

(a) Transverse section of eyeball

- bipolar cell layer
- ganglion cell layer
- neural portion of retina
- optic nerve fibers (axons)
- photoreceptor layer
- pigmented epithelium of retina

6 ____________________

7 ____________________

8 ____________________

9 ____________________

10 ____________________

11 ____________________

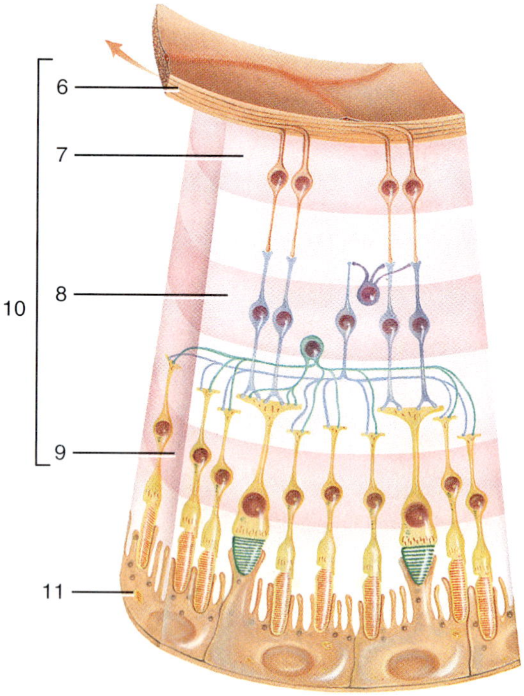

(b) Microscopic structure of retina

FIGURE 19B.6 Anatomy of the retina.

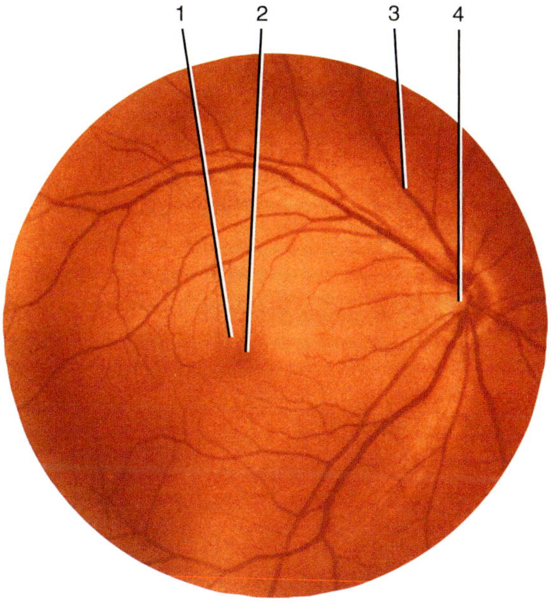

- blood vessel
- central fovea
- macula lutea
- optic disc

1 ______________________

2 ______________________

3 ______________________

4 ______________________

FIGURE 19B.7 **Normal retina viewed with an ophthalmoscope.**

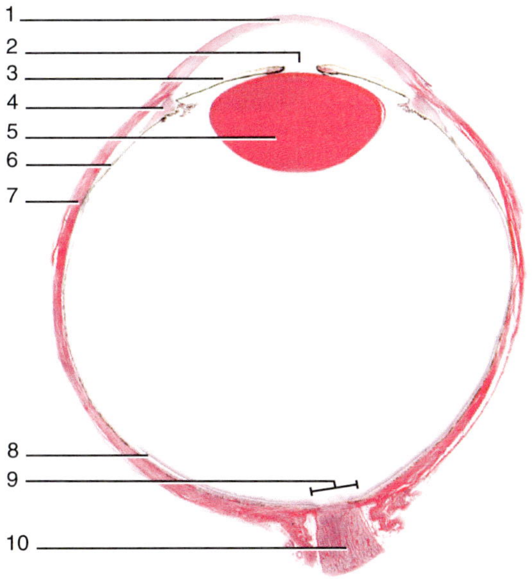

(a) Longitudinal section, 5x

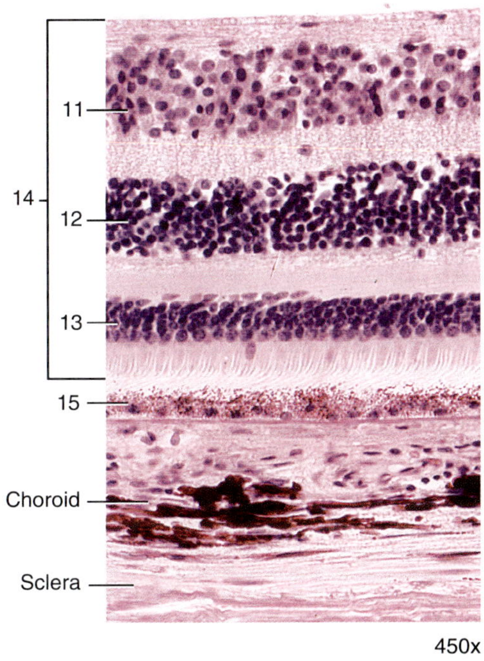

(b) Retina

(a) Section of eyeball
- choroid
- ciliary body
- cornea
- iris
- lens
- optic disc
- optic nerve
- pupil
- retina
- sclera

1 ______________________ 6 ______________________

2 ______________________ 7 ______________________

3 ______________________ 8 ______________________

4 ______________________ 9 ______________________

5 ______________________ 10 ______________________

(b) Section of posterior eyeball
- bipolar layer
- ganglion cell layer
- neural portion of retina
- photoreceptor layer
- pigmented epithelium of retina

11 ______________________

12 ______________________

13 ______________________

14 ______________________

15 ______________________

FIGURE 19B.8 **Photomicrograph of the eyeball.**

4. Visual Tests

Visual acuity tests measure the ability of the lens to focus light reflected from an object on the central fovea of the retina. The lens can **accommodate** or change shape to bend light rays to focus them on the central fovea. At 20 feet, light rays from an object are nearly parallel and do not have to bend as much to focus on the central fovea. At this distance, the lens is flattened and the refractive power (ability to bend light rays) of the lens is lowest. To observe objects closer than 20 feet, the lens must change shape or accommodate to focus the light rays on the central fovea. The lens bulges to increase the refractive power. Individuals that have normal distance vision and near vision are **emmetropic,** individuals that have normal distance vision but blurry near vision are **hyperopic** (farsighted), and individuals who have blurry distance vision but normal near vision are **myopic** (nearsighted).

As we age, the ability of the lens to accommodate diminishes and the ability to focus on very close objects decreases, a condition called **presbyopia** (*presby-* = old). The **near point of vision** is the closest distance that a person can focus on an object. The average near point of vision is 10 cm for a young adult, 20 cm for an adult in their 40's, and 80 cm for someone in their 60's.

Astigmatism is caused by irregularities in the curvature of the cornea or lens. This causes parts of an image to be blurry.

ACTIVITY 6 Visual Tests

1 **Distance visual acuity** is measured using a **Snellen eye chart** (provided by your instructor). *If you wear eyeglasses or contacts, remove them to determine visual acuity without correction or wear them to determine visual acuity with correction.*
- Have subject stand 20 feet from the Snellen eye chart that is placed in a well lighted area, and cover left eye with hand.
- Have subject read the smallest line of letters s/he can without squinting. If the subject can correctly read half or more of the letters, then ask the subject to read the letters on the next smaller line.
- Record the number of the line with the smallest-sized letters read with half or greater accuracy in Table 19B.2.
- Cover the right eye and repeat the procedure.
- A value of 20/20 indicates that the subject has normal vision. A value of 20/40 indicates that the subject sees at 20 feet what a person who has normal vision sees at 40 feet. This is not as good as normal vision. A value of 20/15 indicates that the subject sees at 20 feet what a person with normal vision sees at 15 feet. This is better than normal vision.

2 **Near visual acuity** is measured using a **Snellen acuity card** (Fig. 19B.9).
- Have subject hold the Snellen acuity card 14 inches from his/her face. The card should be illuminated with the light source either behind or above the subject. Instruct the subject to cover his/her left eye with his/her hand.
- Repeat the steps used to measure distance visual acuity test. Start with the second bulleted step.

3 Measure your **near point of vision** and compare it with the average for your age.
- Have the subject hold the Snellen visual acuity card (Figure 19B.9) 14 inches from his/her face.
- Have the subject cover his/her left eye and read letters from a line above his/her near visual acuity.

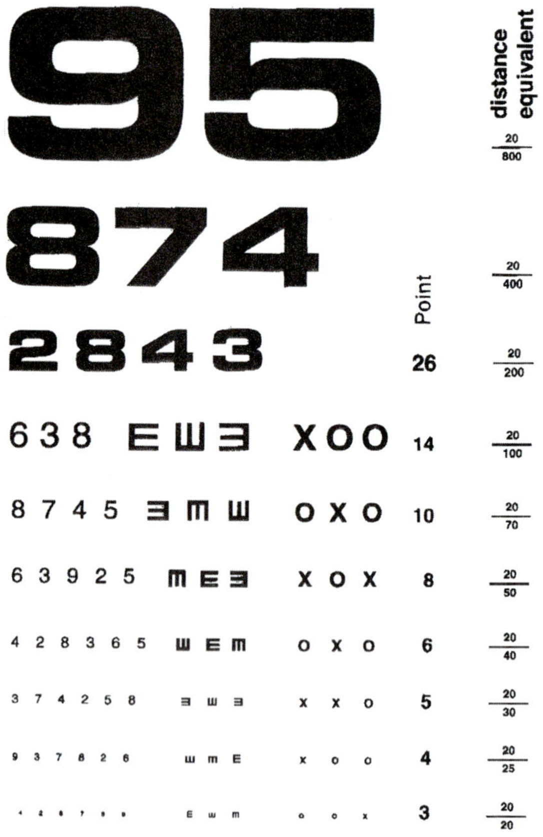

FIGURE 19B.9 Snellen acuity card.

- Instruct the subject to slowly move the chart closer to his/her face until the letters are blurry.
- Measure the distance from the card to the subject's eye in centimeters.
- Record the value into Table 19B.2.

4 Determine whether you have **astigmatism.**
- Remove corrective lenses.
- Cover the right eye and look at the center of the astigmatism chart in Figure 19B.10.
- If all the radiating lines are equally sharp and dark, you do not have astigmatism. However, if some lines are lighter or less distinct than others, you have astigmatism.
- Cover the left eye and repeat the procedure.

5 Answer the discussion questions with your lab group.

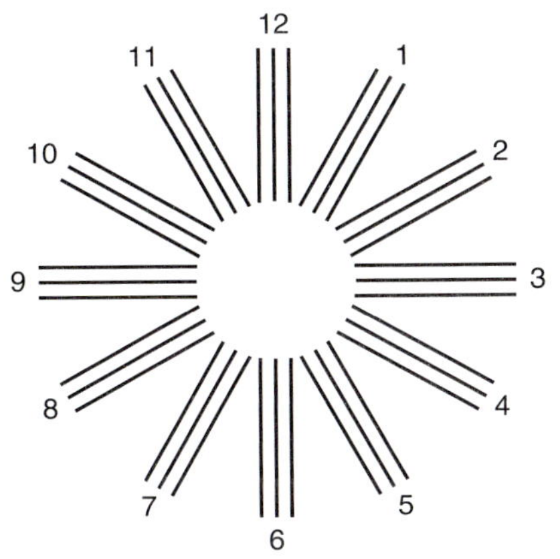

FIGURE 19B.10 Astigmatism chart.

CLINICAL NOTE: *To obtain an accurate acuity test, professionals also count the number of letters a patient missed on the line recorded as the best vision. For example, if the best vision was 20/40, and the patient missed 2 letters on that line, it would be recorded as $20/40^{(-2)}$. If a patient read 2 letters on the 20/15 line, it would be recorded as $20/15^{(+2)}$.*

DISCUSSION QUESTIONS: VISUAL TESTS

1 Why must the subject stand 20 feet from the Snellen eye chart to test distance vision?

2 Why must the subject hold the Snellen acuity card close to his/her eyes to test near vision?

TABLE 19B.2 Visual Test Results

TEST	RESULTS
Visual acuity tests (corrected or uncorrected)	Distance vision Left eye Right eye
	Near vision Left eye Right eye
Near point of vision (corrected or uncorrected)	
Astigmatism	Left eye Right eye

B. The Ear, Hearing, and Equilibrium

MATERIALS

- ear models or charts
- skull, tuning forks, cotton balls
- compound microscope, lens paper, and prepared slides of the cochlea, macula, and crista ampullaris
- swivel chair or stool

1. Anatomy of the Ear

The ear is divided into three regions: the external (outer) ear, the middle ear, and the internal (inner) ear.

External ear—outer ear

- **auricle**—external feature of the ear composed of a **helix** (rim) and a **lobule**
- **external auditory canal**—conducts sound waves from the auricle to the tympanic membrane
- **tympanic membrane** (*tympan-* = drum)—eardrum; separates outer and middle ear

Middle ear—air-filled cavity located in temporal bone; extends from the tympanic membrane to the oval window

- **auditory ossicles**—small bones within the cavity that are connected by synovial joints
  - **malleus**—outer most bone; connects to the tympanic membrane and incus
  - **incus**—middle bone; connects to malleus and stapes
  - **stapes**—innermost bone; connects to the incus and oval window
- **oval window**—membrane-covered opening separating the middle and inner ear
- **round window**—membrane-covered opening between middle ear and cochlea
- **auditory tube** (pharyngotympanic or Eustachian tube)—connects middle ear to the nasopharynx (part of throat near the nasal cavity); equalizes air pressure of middle ear with atmospheric air

ACTIVITY 7 Anatomy of the External and Middle Ear

1 Label the structures of the external and middle ear in Figure 19B.11.

2 Identify the structures on a model or chart.

3 Pronounce the terms as you point to them.

4 Identify the area of the temporal bone that houses the middle and internal ear on the skull.

- auditory tube
- auricle
- external auditory canal
- external ear
- helix (HEE-liks)
- incus (INK-us)
- internal ear
- lobule
- malleus (MAL-ee-us)
- middle ear
- stapes attached to oval window (STAY-peez)
- tympanic membrane (tim-PAN-ik)

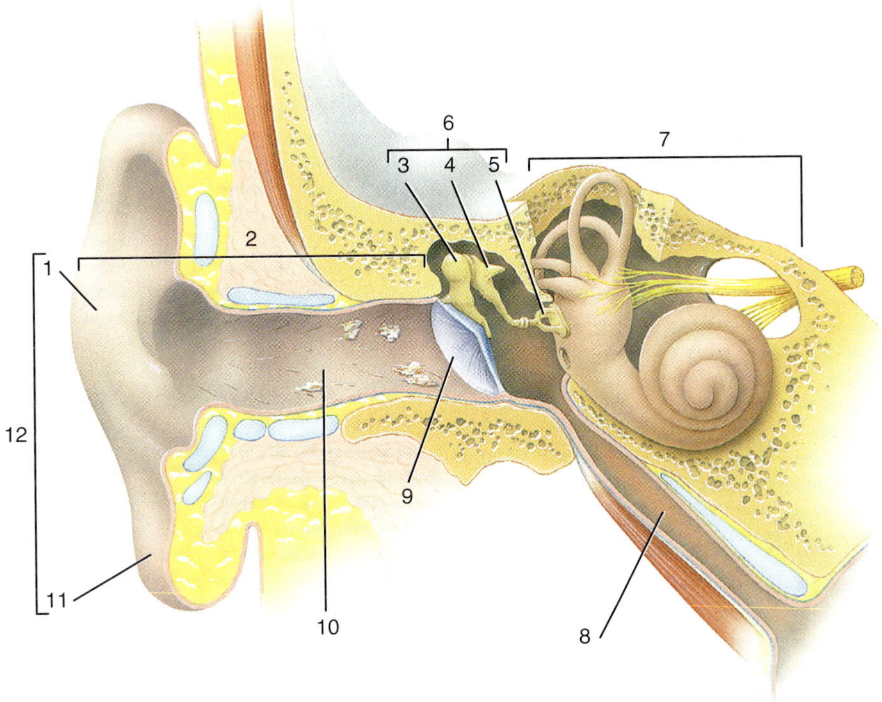

1 ____________________ 5 ____________________ 9 ____________________

2 ____________________ 6 ____________________ 10 ____________________

3 ____________________ 7 ____________________ 11 ____________________

4 ____________________ 8 ____________________ 12 ____________________

FIGURE 19B.11 **Anatomy of the external and middle ear.**

Internal ear—It is housed within the temporal bone. It consists of cavities within the bone called the **bony labyrinth** that encloses a series of connected membranous sacs, the **membranous labyrinth.** The bony labyrinth contains a fluid called **perilymph** that surrounds the membranous labyrinth. **Endolymph** is the fluid within the membranous labyrinth. The bony labyrinth has three main regions: the vestibule, the semicircular canals, and the cochlea.

- **Vestibule**—middle section of bony labyrinth that contains two sacs of membranous labyrinth
  utricle (*utricle* = little bag)—posterior section of membranous labyrinth within vestibule, houses equilibrium receptors.
  saccule—(*saccule* = little sac) anterior section of membranous labyrinth within vestibule that is continuous with utricle; houses equilibrium receptors.
- **Anterior, lateral, and posterior semicircular canals**—three bony canals posterior to vestibule that project posteriorly, laterally, and superiorly from the vestibule; each canal is at right angles to the other two
  ampulla—widened end of each semicircular canal
  semicircular ducts—section of membranous labyrinth within semicircular canals; connects with utricle and contains equilibrium receptors
- **Cochlea**—spiral section of bony labyrinth anterior to the vestibule
  cochlear duct—section of membranous labyrinth within the cochlea; connected to the saccule and houses the receptors for hearing

The **vestibulocochlear nerve** (cranial nerve VIII) has two branches: The **vestibular branch** that carries nerve impulses generated by equilibrium receptors and the **cochlear branch** that carries nerve impulses generated by the hearing receptors.

ACTIVITY 8 Anatomy of the Internal (Inner) Ear

1 Label the structures of the internal ear in Figure 19B.12.
2 Identify the structures on a model or chart.
3 Pronounce the terms as you point to them.

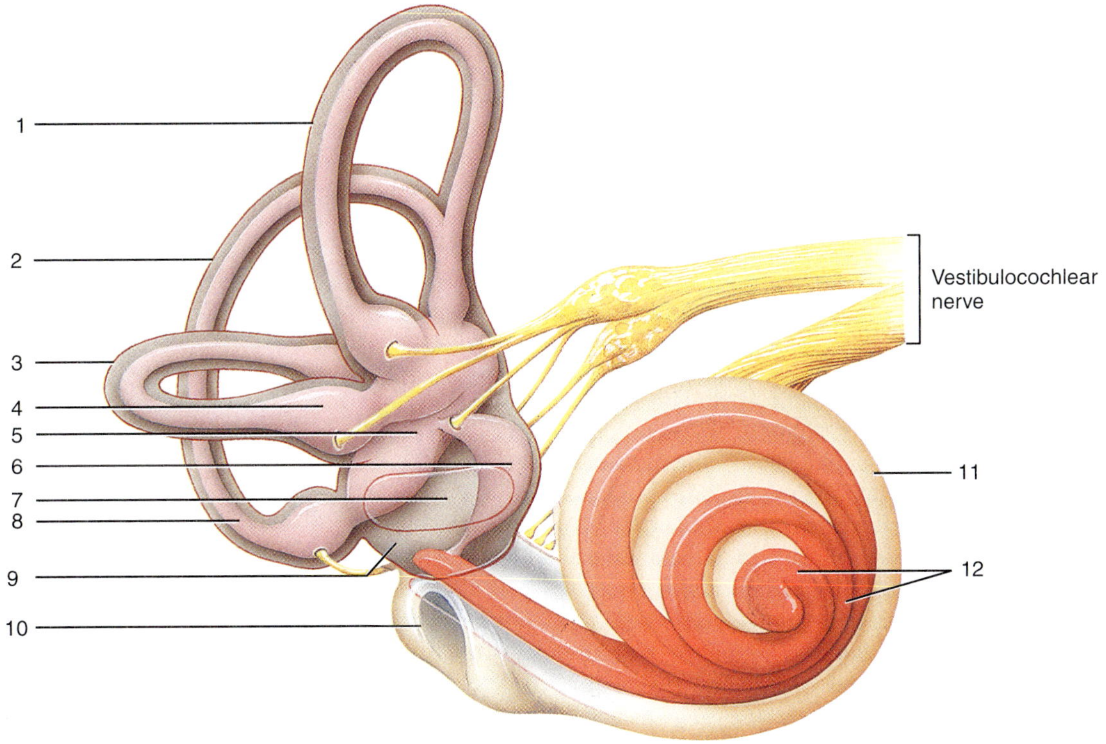

- ampulla
- anterior semicircular canal
- cochlea (COKE-lee-uh)
- cochlear duct
- lateral semicircular canal
- membranous semicircular duct
- oval window
- posterior semicircular canal
- round window
- saccule (SAK-yool)
- utricle (YOU-trih-cul)
- vestibule

1 ____________________ 7 ____________________

2 ____________________ 8 ____________________

3 ____________________ 9 ____________________

4 ____________________ 10 ____________________

5 ____________________ 11 ____________________

6 ____________________ 12 ____________________

FIGURE 19B.12 **Anatomy of the internal ear.**

2. Microscopic Anatomy of the Cochlea and the Spiral Organ of Corti

The cochlea is a spiral cavity that resembles the space within a snail shell. The cochlea makes three turns around a bony core. A section through the cochlea shows three channels: the scala vestibule, the cochlear duct (scala media), and the scala tympani. The **scala vestibuli** is part of the cochlea and is superior to the cochlear duct. It is separated from the cochlear duct by the **vestibular membrane.** The **scala tympani** is also part of the cochlea and is posterior to the cochlear duct. It is separated from the cochlear duct by the **basilar membrane.** The scala vestibuli and scala tympani are continuous with one another and are filled with perilymph. The **cochlear duct,** part of the membranous labyrinth, houses the spiral organ of Corti and is filled with endolymph.

The **spiral organ of Corti** sits on the basilar membrane. It contains hair cells (receptors for hearing) and supporting cells. The hair cells have a **hair bundle** composed of stereocilia at their apical end. Superior to and in contact with the sterocilia is the **tectorial membrane** (*tector* = covering). The basal end of the hair cells synapse with sensory and motor neurons from the cochlear branch of the vestibulocochlear nerve.

Movement of the basilar membrane, caused by perilymph movement, forces the hair bundle into the tectoral membrane and bends the stereocilia. This results in a generation of nerve impulses in the sensory neurons.

ACTIVITY 9 Microscopic Anatomy of the Cochlea and Spiral Organ of Corti

1 Label the structures of the cochlea and spiral organ of Corti in Figure 19B.13.

2 Identify the structures on a model or chart.

3 Pronounce the terms as you point to them.

4 Examine a slide showing a cross section through the cochlea.
- Using the low-power objective, identify the **basilar membrane, cochlear duct, spiral organ of Corti, scala tympani, scala vestibuli,** and **vestibular membrane.**
- Using the high-power objective, identify the **basilar membrane, hair bundle, hair cells,** and **tectoral membrane.**

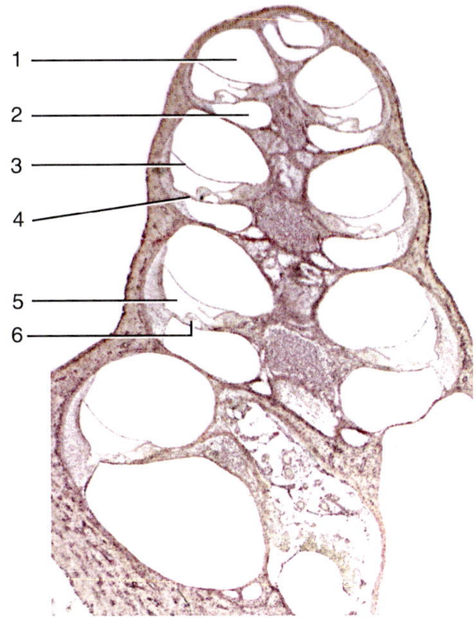

20x

(a) Cross-section through cochlea

- basilar membrane (BAY-sih-lur)
- cochlear duct
- spiral organ of Corti
- scala tympani (SCAY-lah)
- scala vestibuli
- vestibular membrane

1 ____________________

2 ____________________

3 ____________________

4 ____________________

5 ____________________

6 ____________________

- basilar membrane
- cochlear duct
- hair cells
- tectoral membrane
- vestibular membrane

7 ____________________

8 ____________________

9 ____________________

10 ____________________

11 ____________________

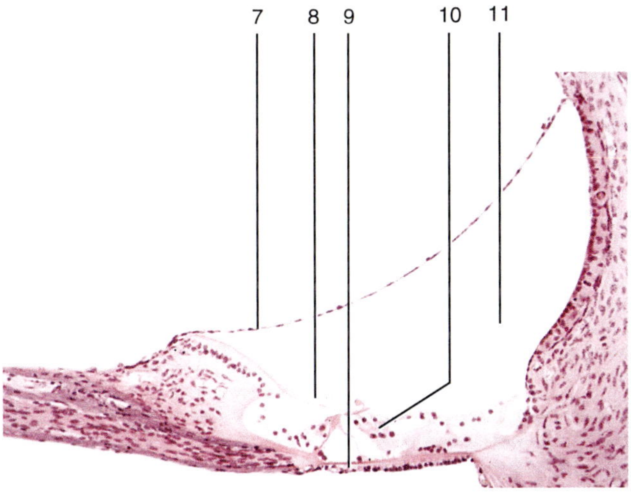

110x

(b) Cross-section through spiral organ of Corti

FIGURE 19B.13 Photomicrographs of the cochlea and spiral organ of Corti.

3. Microscopic Anatomy of the Equilibrium Receptors of the Internal Ear

There are two types of equilibrium receptors, the maculae located in the utricle and saccule and the crista located in the membranous semicircular ducts within the ampullae. The **maculae** provide information on head position (static equilibrium), as well as linear acceleration and deceleration, a type of dynamic equilibrium. The maculae consist of **hair cells** with **hair bundles** and **supporting cells.** The hair bundles are in contact with a gelatinous membrane, the **otolithic membrane.** (*oto* = stone), which contains calcium carbonate crystals, **otoliths.** Movement of the head causes movement of the otoliths and otolithic membrane, which bends the hair bundles. The direction of movement will determine if the hair cells release more or less neurotransmitter to the associated sensory neurons.

The **crista** (ampullaris) detects rotational acceleration and deceleration, a type of dynamic equilibrium. Each crista consists of **hair cells** and **supporting cells.** The hair bundles of the hair cells are covered by a gelatinous structure called the **cupula.** When the head moves, movement of endolymph pushes the cupula causing the hair cells to bend. Bending of the hair bundles results in generation of nerve impulses in the vestibular branch of the vestibulocochlear nerve.

ACTIVITY 10 Microscopic Anatomy of the Macula and Crista

1. Label the structures of the macula and crista in Figure 19B.14.
2. Identify the structures on a model or chart.
3. Pronounce the terms as you point to them.
4. Examine the demonstration slide showing a cross section through the crista with the high-power objective. Identify the **cupula** and **hair cells.**

- hair bundle
- hair cell
- otoliths (OH-toe-liths)
- otolitic membane
- vestibular branches of vestibulocochlear nerve

1 ______________________

2 ______________________

3 ______________________

4 ______________________

5 ______________________

- cupula (KYOU-pyul-uh)
- hair bundle
- hair cell

6 ______________________

7 ______________________

8 ______________________

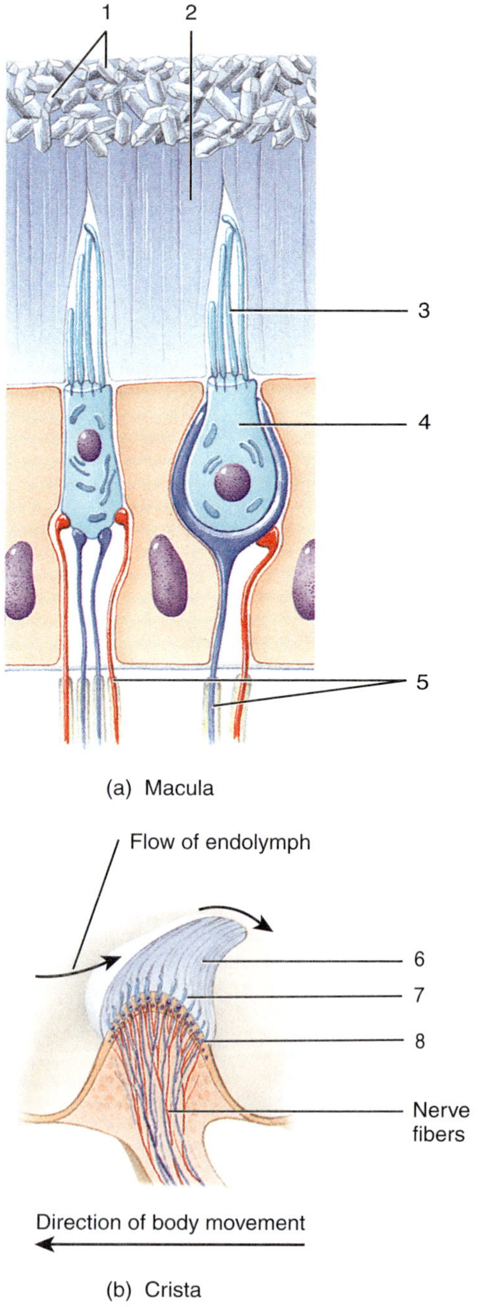

FIGURE 19B.14 Microscopic anatomy of the macula and crista.

4. Auditory and Equilibrium Tests

Hearing loss can be either conduction deafness or sensorineural deafness. **Conduction deafness** can be caused by decreased ability to conduct energy of sound waves through the external and middle ear to hearing receptors in the inner ear. Ear wax buildup, damage to tympanic membrane, or fusion of auditory ossicles may cause conduction deafness. **Sensorineural deafness** can be caused by damage to hair cells in the spiral organ, damage to the cochlear branch of the vestibulocochlear nerve, or damage of the neural pathways to the auditory cortex.

Inflammation of or injury to equilibrium receptors results in an inability to maintain body position, vertigo, and/or dizziness. Vertigo is the sensation of circular motion either of oneself or external objects, while dizziness is often used to describe faintness, unsteadiness or lightheadiness. Severe vertigo may be accompanied by **nystagmus**-rapid, involuntary movement of eyeballs.

ACTIVITY 11 Auditory and Equilibrium Tests

Unilateral conduction deafness can be mimicked by placing a cotton ball in one external auditory canal.

1 Test for unilateral (one-side only) deafness using the **Weber test.**
- Have the subject sit with head erect and facing forward.
- Strike a tuning fork (middle C preferably) and place it medially on the subject's forehead (bone conduction).
- Ask the subject if the sound is equally loud in both ears or louder in one ear. Circle the result in Table 19B.3.
- If the sound is equally loud in both ears, the subject either has normal hearing or equal hearing loss in both ears. If the subject hears the sound louder in one ear, then the subject may have either conduction deafness in that ear or sensorineural deafness in the opposite ear.
- To determine if the subject has conduction deafness or sensorineural deafness, conduct the Rinne test.

2 Test for conduction or sensorineural deafness using the **Rinne test.**
- Have the subject sit with head erect and facing forward.
- Strike a tuning fork and place it on the subject's right mastoid process to test hearing by **bone conduction.**
- Ask the subject to tell you when s/he can no longer hear the sound, then place the still-vibrating tuning fork close to his/her right ear to test hearing by air conduction. If the subject can hear the tuning fork again when it is placed next to his/her ear, the subject does not have conduction deafness in that ear. If the subject cannot hear the tuning fork again, then the subject may have conduction deafness in that ear.
- Circle the results in Table 19B.3 if normal.
- To verify conduction deafness, test the same ear again. This time you are testing hearing by **air conduction** first.
- Strike the tuning fork again and place the tuning fork close to the subject's ear.
- Ask the subject to tell you when s/he can no longer hear the sound, then place the tuning fork on the subject's mastoid process (bone conduction). If the subject hears the sound again, s/he has conduction deafness in that ear. Record whether the subject has

TABLE 19B.3 Results of Weber, Rinne, and Barnay Tests

TEST	RESULTS (CIRCLE YOUR RESULTS)		
Weber test	Equal loudness in both ears = normal hearing or equal hearing loss or Sound is louder in right ear = conduction deafness in right ear or sensorineural deafness in left ear or Sound is louder in left ear = conduction deafness in left ear or sensorineural deafness in right ear		
Rinne test	Right ear: conduction deafness or no conduction deafness Left ear: conduction deafness or no conduction deafness		Name semicircular canal stimulated
Barnay test	Head slightly forward: Eyes move	____________	____________
	Head toward shoulder: Eyes move	____________	____________
	Head on chin: Eyes move	____________	____________

normal hearing in that ear or conduction hearing loss by circling the results in Table 19B.3.
- Repeat this procedure for the left ear.

3 Conduct balance test to evaluate **static equilibrium** receptors.
- Have the subject stand in front of a wall or blackboard with their arms at his/her sides. The subject cannot lean against the wall or support him/herself in any manner.
- Tell the subject to stand perfectly still. If subject is in front of a blackboard or whiteboard, mark the outline of his/her shoulders to help determine when s/he sways.
- Tell the subject to close his/her eyes and observe movement in the shoulders. Notice that, although the subject may sway slightly, posture is always corrected. Signals from the maculae are helping the subject to maintain posture. If the maculae are not functioning, the subject will not be able to maintain posture and will exhibit large swaying movements or will fall.

4 Conduct **Barany's test** to evaluate function of semicircular canals and **dynamic equilibrium** receptors.
- Choose a subject for this demonstration who does not readily experience dizziness or become nauseated when rotated. If the subject experiences nausea during the demonstration, immediately stop rotation.
- Choose two people who are prepared to support the subject after inducing vertigo and dizziness.
- Provide the subject with a chair or stool that can be rotated. Have the subject sit on the chair and hold onto the arms or seat for safety. Decide how the subject will position his/her legs during rotation to ensure safety and prevent interference. Position 3–4 students around the chair to prevent the subject from falling off the chair.
- Tell the subject to slightly tilt his/her head forward, focus on a distant object, and keep both eyes open during the rotation.
- Carefully turn the chair or stool clockwise (to the right). Complete 10 turns, one turn per 2 seconds and stop suddenly. **Be prepared to support the subject until vertigo and/or dizziness has passed.** The subject will still experience rotation, indicating that the semicircular canals are functioning. Endolymph continues to move within the membranous semicircular ducts for a short time after rotation has stopped.
- Observe which way the subject's eyeballs are moving immediately after stopping rotation. Record direction in Table 19B.3.

  Lateral movement of the eyes indicates stimulation of the crista ampullaris in the lateral semicircular canals.

  Vertical movement of the eyes indicates stimulation of the crista ampullaris in the anterior semicircular canals.

  Rotational movement of the eyes indicates stimulation of the crista ampullaris in the posterior semicircular canals.
- Repeat the demonstration with the subject's head tilted toward one shoulder, and then again with the subject's chin resting on his/her chest.

C. The Nose and Olfaction

MATERIALS

- skull, stopwatch, cotton balls
- clove oil, peppermint oil, or cinnamon oil

The nose contains the receptors for the sense of smell or olfaction (*olfact-* = smell). Olfactory receptors are found within the olfactory epithelium, a specialized area of the epithelium lining the nasal cavity. The **olfactory epithelium** covers the inferior surface of the cribiform plate, the superior nasal concha, and the upper part of the middle nasal concha.

The olfactory epithelium contains olfactory receptor cells, supporting cells, basal stem cells, and ducts of olfactory glands. The **olfactory receptor cells** are bipolar neurons whose dendritic end is imbedded in the mucus layer covering the surface of the olfactory epithelium and whose axons form the **olfactory nerves.** The olfactory receptors are located on **olfactory hairs** that project from the dendrites of the olfactory receptor cells.

Olfactory nerves pass through olfactory foramina in the **cribiform plate** and synapse on neurons in the **olfactory bulb.** Nerve impulses then travel along the **olfactory tract** to the lateral olfactory area of the cerebral cortex.

Olfactory receptors adapt to odors very quickly. This explains why when we are trying to determine the source of an odor, we often lose the smell before we find it. If we leave the area and return, we can smell the odor again.

ACTIVITY 12 Structure of the Olfactory Epithelium and Olfactory Adaptation

1 Label the structures of the olfactory epithelium in Figure 19B.15.

2 Identify the following areas on a skull: location of **olfactory epithelium** and the **olfactory foramina** in the cribiform plate.

3 Observe olfactory adaptation. Instructions on next page.

4 Answer discussion questions about olfactory adaptation with your lab partners.

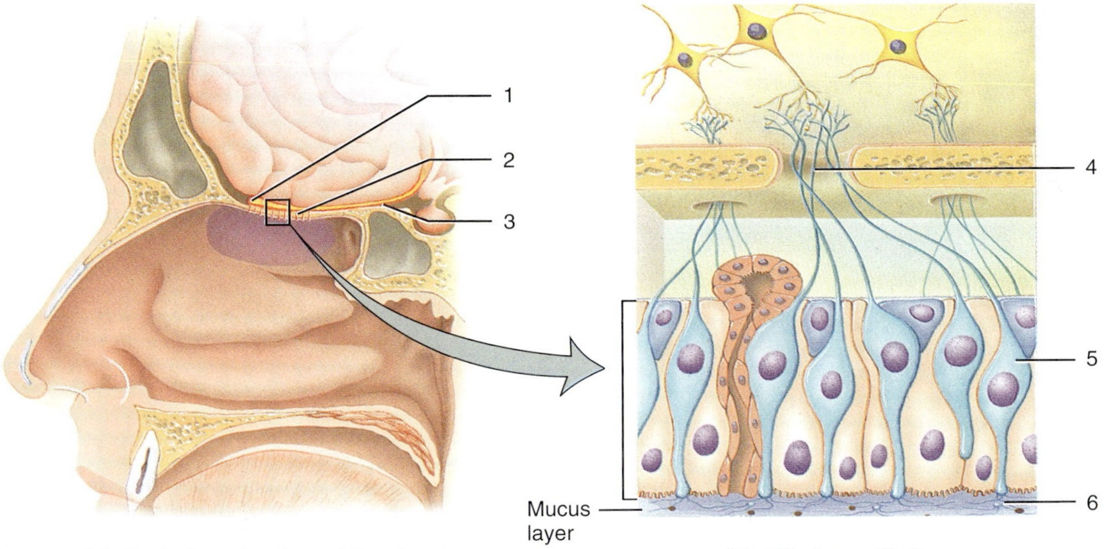

(a) Sagittal section through head showing olfactory structures

(b) Olfactory epithelium

- cribriform plate (CRIB-rin-form)
- olfactory bulb (OHL-fak-tore-ee)
- olfactory tract

- olfactory hairs
- olfactory nerves
- olfactory receptor cell

1 ______________________

2 ______________________

3 ______________________

4 ______________________

5 ______________________

6 ______________________

FIGURE 19B.15 Olfactory structures.

Olfactory Adaptation

1. Choose a subject, a timer, an experimentor (holds vial under subject's nose), and a recorder.
2. Have the subject plug one nostril with cotton and close both eyes.
3. Hold a container of cloves just under the open nostril (time 0) and ask the subject to inhale through the open nostril and exhale through the mouth.
4. Ask the subject to tell you when the odor has disappeared, note the time, and record in Table 19B.4. Instruct the subject to immediately pull out the cotton in the other nostril and inhale (vial still under nose).
5. Ask the subject if s/he can smell cloves. Record the result in Table 19B.4.
6. Repeat the experiment with another distinct smell, such as peppermint or cinnamon. Avoid irritating odors.

? DISCUSSION QUESTIONS: OLFACTORY ADAPTATION

1 Is the time of adaptation the same for all odors?

2 After the nostril was unplugged, explain why the subject was able to smell the odor again.

D. The Taste Buds and Gustation

MATERIALS

- compound microscope, lens paper, prepared slides of taste buds
- mirror, ½-inch cubes of apple, banana, cheese, and carrot

Taste buds, which are found on the tongue, soft palate, pharynx (throat), and larynx, are microscopic, onion-shaped structures that contain gustatory cells, gustatory hairs, and supporting cells. Each **gustatory** (*gust-* = taste) **cell** has one **gustatory hair** that projects through an opening, the **taste pore,** on the apical end of the taste bud. **Gustatory receptors** are located on the gustatory hairs. The basal end of gustatory cells synapse onto the dendritic end of sensory neurons. Axons from the sensory neurons contribute fibers to the facial nerve (cranial nerve VII), glossopharyngeal nerve (IX), or vagus nerve (X), depending on the location of the taste bud.

Taste buds on the tongue are located in **papillae,** elevated structures that give the tongue its rough appearance. There are three types of papillae: vallate (circumvallate), fungiform, and filiform. **Vallate** (circumvallate) **papillae** are the largest papillae and form an inverted V at the posterior of the tongue. **Fungiform papillae** are mushroom-shaped and are scattered over the surface of the tongue. **Filiform papillae** are slender pointed projections that cover the surface of the tongue and give the tongue a rough texture. Taste buds are found in all vallate papillae and most fungiform papillae, but rarely in filiform papillae.

TABLE 19B.4 Results of Olfactory Adaptation Experiment

ODOR	TIME TO ADAPTATION (SEC)	CAN SUBJECT SMELL ODOR AFTER NOSTRIL UNPLUGGED?
Cloves		
Peppermint		
Cinnamon		

There are four primary taste sensations: sweet, bitter, salty, and sour, and a possible fifth, MSG (monosodium glutamate). Gustatory receptors most sensitive to sweet and salty sensations are found on the tip of the tongue, while bitter sensations are in the back and sour sensations on the sides of the tongue. Other taste sensations are a mixture of these four. Smell, temperature, and texture (tactile sensation) contribute to our sense of taste. A person with a cold often has a loss of taste due to a loss of smell. Cold french fries are not as tasty as hot ones, and mushy apples are not as good as crisp ones.

ACTIVITY 13 Gustatory Structures and Sensations

1 Label the gustatory structures in Figure 19B.16a and Figure 19B.16b, and Figure 19B.16c.

2 Examine a microscope slide of a vallate papillae.

- Using the low-power objective, identify the taste bud in the wall of the papillae.
- Using the high-power objective, identify the **taste pore, gustatory hairs,** and **gustatory receptor cells** forming the wall of the taste bud.

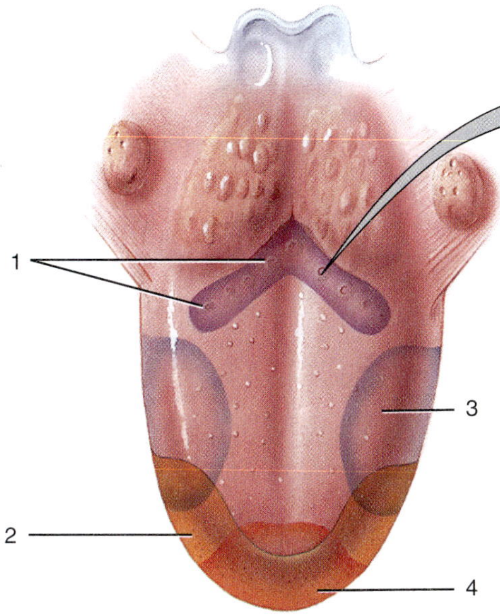

(a) Taste areas

- bitter
- salty
- sour
- sweet

1 ______________________

2 ______________________

3 ______________________

4 ______________________

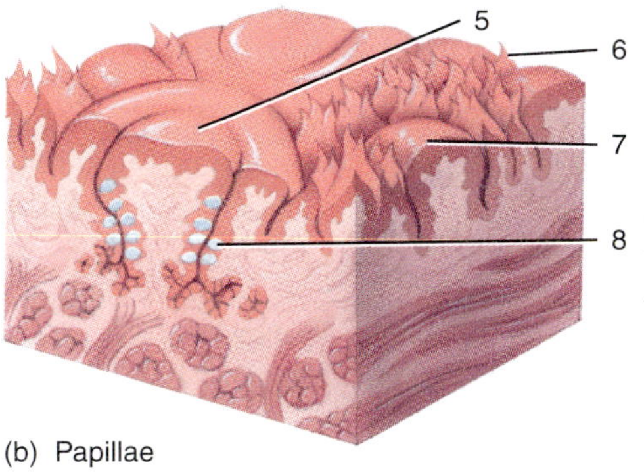

(b) Papillae

- vallate papillae
- filiform papillae
- fungiform papillae
- taste bud

5 ______________________

6 ______________________

7 ______________________

8 ______________________

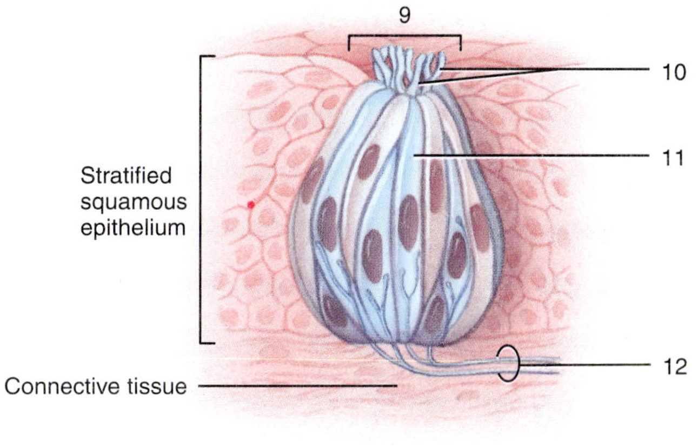

(c) Taste bud

- sensory axons
- gustatory hairs
- gustatory receptor cell
- taste pore

9 ______________________

10 ______________________

11 ______________________

12 ______________________

FIGURE 19B.16 **Gustatory structures.**

3 Use a mirror to identify fungiform and filiform papillae on your tongue. Try to see vallate papillae on the back of the tongue.

4 Examine the contribution of texture and smell to the sense of taste. Since many labs do not allow eating or drinking, this activity may be done in another area or at home.
- Choose a subject, an experimenter (who will give the food cubes to the subject), and a recorder. The subject will first try to identify food by texture only (rolling food on surface of tongue), then by taste (chewing food increases the amount of chemicals dissolved in saliva and capable of interacting with taste receptors), and finally with the addition of smell.
- Place ½-inch cubes of carrot, banana, apple, raw potato, and cheese on a plate.
- Have the subject pinch both nostrils, close both eyes, and open his/her mouth. Randomly choose one of the cubes and place it in the subject's mouth.
- Instruct the subject to roll the food around the surface of the tongue and attempt to identify the food. If identification is correct, check the texture only column next to the food in Table 19B.5.
- Instruct the subject to chew the food and attempt to identify the food. If identification is correct, check texture and taste column in Table 19B.5.
- Instruct the subject to open both nostrils and attempt to identify the food. If identification is correct, check the texture, taste, and smell column in Table 19B.5.
- Repeat procedure with the other food cubes.

TABLE 19B.5 Results of Experiment: Contribution of Texture and Smell to Taste

FOOD	TEXTURE ONLY	TEXTURE AND TASTE	TEXTURE, TASTE, AND SMELL
Carrot			
Banana			
Apple			
Raw potato			
Cheese			

Subject ______________________ Date ______________ Section ______________

EXERCISE 19B

REVIEWING YOUR KNOWLEDGE

A. Accessory Eye Structures

Choose structure that corresponds to each statement.

a. bulbar conjunctiva
b. lacrimal canals
c. lacrimal gland
d. lacrimal sac
e. nasolacrimal duct
f. palpebral conjunctiva

____ **1.** Drains tears into nasal cavity

____ **2.** Produces tears

____ **3.** Membrane that covers the inner surface of eyelid

____ **4.** Tears from surface of eye drain into here

B. Extrinsic Eye Muscles

Choose muscle that applies to each statement.

a. inferior oblique
b. inferior rectus
c. lateral rectus
d. medial rectus
e. superior oblique
f. superior rectus

____ **1.** Moves eyeball superiorly

____ **2.** Moves eyeball laterally

____ **3.** Moves eyeball inferiorly

____ **4.** Moves eyeball medially

____ **5.** Moves eyeball laterally and inferiorly

____ **6.** Moves eyeball laterally and superiorly

C. Eye Structures

Choose structure that applies to each statement. More than one structure may apply to a statement and a structure may be used more than once.

a. anterior cavity
b. anterior chamber
c. choroid
d. ciliary body
e. ciliary muscle
f. ciliary process
g. cornea
h. iris
i. lens
j. ora serrata
k. posterior chamber
l. pupil
m. retina
n. sclera
o. scleral venous sinus
p. suspensory ligaments
q. vitreous chamber

____ **1.** Produces aqueous humor

____ **2.** Structures that are part of vascular tunic

____ **3.** Contains photoreceptors

____ **4.** Controls the size of the pupil

____ **5.** Drains aqueous humor from the anterior chamber

____ **6.** Structures that are part of the fibrous tunic

____ **7.** Most anterior part of the eyeball

____ **8.** Anterior boundary of retina

____ **9.** Attaches lens to ciliary body

____ **10.** Changes shape to focus light on retina

____ **11.** Location of aqueous humor

____ **12.** White, tough, outer layer of eyeball

Answer the following questions:

13. Why does the retina pull easily away from the back of the eyeball?

14. Name the instrument used to view the retina during a physical exam.

15. Name the two layers of the retina.

D. Anatomy of the Retina

Choose the structure that corresponds to each statement.

a. bipolar cell layer
b. central fovea
c. cones
d. ganglion cell layer
e. macula lutea
f. optic disc
g. photoreceptor layer
h. rods

____ **1.** Has the highest density of cones in the retina

____ **2.** Axons form optic nerve

____ **3.** Does not contain photoreceptors; blind spot

____ **4.** Photoreceptor that allows us to see color

____ **5.** Contains rods and cones

____ **6.** Light rays strike this layer of the retina first

E. Visual Acuity Tests

1. Define accommodation.

2. A 10-year-old patient's distance visual acuity was tested and determined to be 20/80. Explain what that means.

3. A 60-year-old man has to hold his newspaper at arm's length to read it. What condition does he have?

4. A person with ________________ has blurry near vision but normal distance vision.

5. A person with ________________ does not see everything within a visual field clearly; some parts are blurry.

6. A person with ________________ has normal near vision but blurry distance vision.

F. External and Middle Ear Structures

Choose structure that applies to each statement. More than one structure may apply to a statement, and a structure may be used more than once.

auditory tube	incus	stapes
auricle	lobule	round window
external auditory canal	malleus	tympanic membrane
external ear	middle ear	
helix	oval window	

______________ **1.** Auditory ossicle attached to tympanic membrane

______________ **2.** Equalizes air pressure in middle ear with external air pressure

______________ **3.** External ear structures

______________ **4.** Ear drum

______________ **5.** External feature of ear that contains the helix and lobule

______________ **6.** Stapes is attached to this membrane-covered opening

______________ **7.** Middle auditory ossicle

______________ **8.** Small bones of middle ear that are connected by synovial joints

G. Internal Ear Structures

Choose structure that applies to each statement. More than one structure may apply to a statement, and a structure may be used more than once.

ampulla	oval window	semicircular canals
cochlea	perilymph	semicircular ducts
cochlear duct	round window	utricle
endolymph	saccule	vestibule

______________ **1.** Interconnected components of membranous labyrinth

______________ **2.** Fluid found within all bony labyrinth structures

______________ **3.** Sections of the membranous labyrinth found within vestibule

______________ **4.** Section of the membranous labyrinth that contains hearing receptors

______________ **5.** Sections of the membranous labyrinth that contain equilibrium receptors

______________ **6.** Interconnected components of bony labyrinth

H. Microscopic Anatomy of the Cochlea, Spiral Organ of Corti, Macula, and Crista

Choose a structure that applies to each statement. More than one structure may apply to a statement, and a structure may be used more than once.

basilar membrane
cochlear duct
crista
cupula
hair bundle
hair cells
macula
otolithic membrane
scala tympani
scala vestibuli
spiral organ of Corti
supporting cells
tectorial membrane
vestibular membrane

________________ **1.** Receptor for hearing

________________ **2.** Receptor(s) that contain(s) hair bundles, hair cells, and supporting cells

________________ **3.** Components of macula

________________ **4.** Membrane separating the superior chamber of cochlea from cochlear duct

________________ **5.** Structure(s) that bends stereocilia of hair cells

________________ **6.** Spiral organ of Corti sits on this membrane

________________ **7.** Equilibrium receptors

________________ **8.** Endolymph found in this structure

________________ **9.** Perilymph found in these structures

________________ **10.** Equilibrium receptor found within ampullae of semicircular canals

I. Auditory and Equilibrium Tests

1. What causes nystagmus?

2. What causes conduction deafness?

3. What causes sensorineural deafness?

4. If a vibrating tuning fork is placed on the mastoid process, who would "hear" the sound, someone with normal hearing, someone with conduction deafness, or someone with sensorineural deafness? Circle all that apply.

5. Inability to maintain posture while standing would indicate a problem with which equilibrium receptor?

J. Olfaction

Choose a structure that applies to each statement.

cribiform plate
superior portion of nasal cavity
olfactory hair
olfactory nerve
olfactory receptor cells

____________________ **1.** Bipolar neurons

____________________ **2.** Part of olfactory receptor cell that contains the olfactory receptors

____________________ **3.** Formed of bipolar neuron axons

____________________ **4.** Olfactory nerves pass through this structure before synapsing onto olfactory bulb

____________________ **5.** Identify the location of the olfactory epithelium.

K. Taste

Choose a structure that applies to each statement. More than one structure may apply to a statement, and a structure may be used more than once.

filiform papillae
fungiform papillae
pharynx
soft palate
gustatory cell
gustatory hair
supporting cell
taste buds
taste pore
vallate papillae

____________________ **1.** Contain taste buds

____________________ **2.** Part of gustatory cell that contains gustatory receptor

____________________ **3.** Opening in taste bud through which gustatory hair projects

____________________ **4.** Components of taste bud

____________________ **5.** Mushroom-shaped projections on tongue

____________________ **6.** Projections that form inverted V on back of tongue

7. Identify where on the tongue the receptors most sensitive to each of the four taste sensations are located.

8. What other sensations contribute to the sensation of taste?

Name ______________________ Date ______________ Subject ________________

EXERCISE **19B**

USING YOUR KNOWLEDGE

The Eye and Vision

1. Strabismus, a misalignment of the eyeball caused by an imbalance in the extrinsic eye muscles, is also called lazy eye or wandering eye. Identify the extrinsic eye muscle that would cause lateral strabismus of the right eye.

2. Where in the nasal cavity does the nasolacrimal duct empty?

3–4. Name all the accessory eyeball structures, fluids, and retinal layers that light passes through before it hits the photoreceptors.

5. Explain why the retina can detach from the eyeball with just a blow to the back of the head.

6. Is the retinal area in Figure 19B.17 the macula lutea, fovea centralis, or optic disc? Explain your choice.

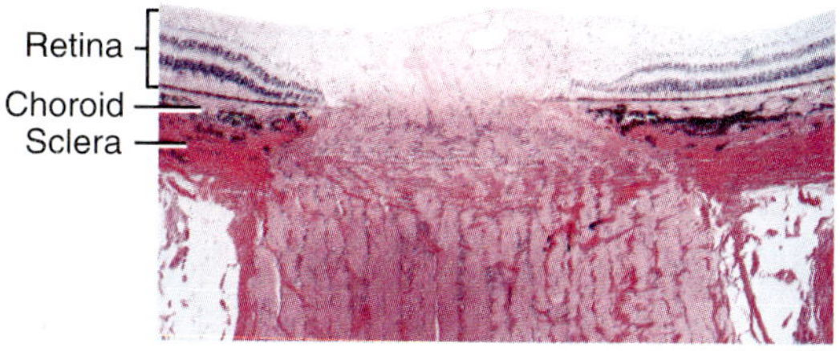

FIGURE 19B.17 Retinal area.

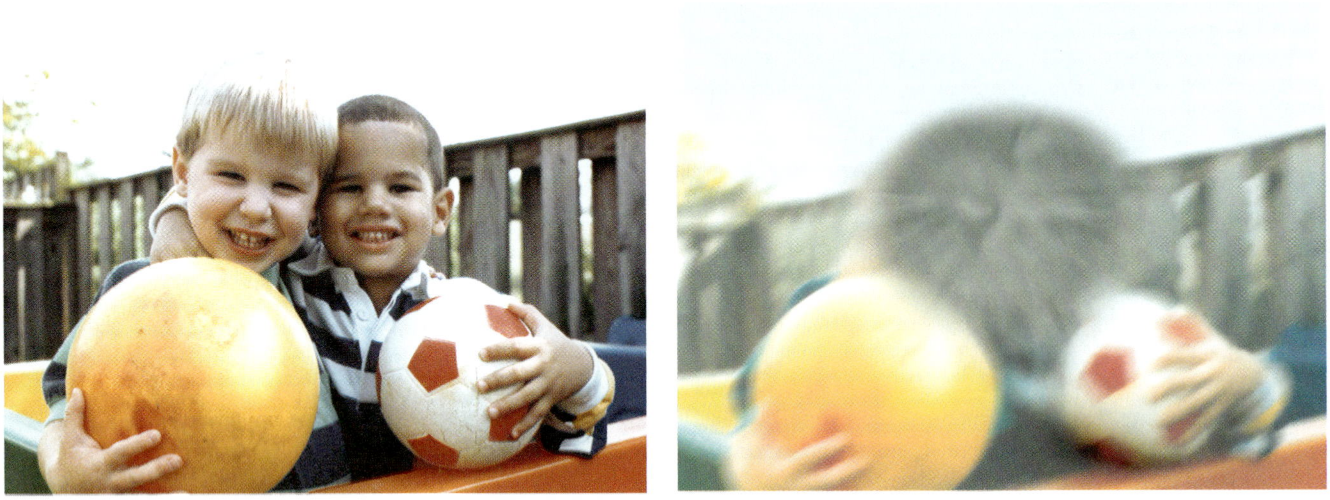

(a) Normal (b) Abnormal

FIGURE 19B.18 **Visual fields.**

7. Explain why a pituitary tumor may affect vision.

8. A 10-year-old male has 20/20 distance vision, and 20/60 near vision. What refraction abnormality does he have?

9. Using your text book or another source, research how and why glaucoma and macular degeneration affect vision. Compare Figure 19B.18a and Figure 19B.18b and identify whether the visual field in Figure 19B.18b is representative of a person with macular degeneration or glaucoma.

10. Explain why the condition represented in Figure 19B.18b causes loss of vision in the center of the field of vision and blurriness in the periphery.

11. What structure keeps a contact lens on the cornea and prevents it from becoming lodged on the posterior surface of the eyeball?

The Ear, Hearing, and Balance

12–13. Sound waves enter the external auditory canal and cause vibrations in structures and fluids of the ear. Identify in order the structures and fluids that vibrate in the pathway from the external auditory canal to the spiral organ of Corti.

14. Diving to the bottom of a deep pool will sometimes cause discomfort in the middle ear. Explain the cause of this discomfort.

15. What do the receptor cells for hearing, static equilibrium, and dynamic equilibrium have in common?

16. Would the receptors for equilibrium work in space (0 gravity)?

17. Describe a series of movements that would stimulate all semicircular duct receptors and if repeated may cause vertigo. (Hint: Think of a carnival ride that causes vertigo.)

Olfaction and Gustation

18. Why do we sniff when we wish to smell something better?

19. When you lick ice cream off an ice cream cone, which papillae are involved in scraping the ice cream off the cone?

20. Licking cold ice cream off an ice cream cone stimulates a variety of sensory receptors associated with the tongue. Name all the sensory receptors involved.

ANSWER KEY

Exercise 1

Figure 1.1

1. skull
2. face
3. armpit
4. forearm
5. wrist
6. thigh
7. ankle
8. chest
9. arm
10. abdomen
11. groin
12. pelvis
13. foot
14. shoulder
15. back
16. hand
17. buttock
18. leg
19. head
20. neck

Figure 1.2

1. cranial
2. facial
3. cervical
4. acromial
5. axillary
6. brachial
7. antecubital
8. antebrachial
9. carpal
10. digital
11. palmar
12. femoral
13. patellar
14. crural
15. tarsal
16. digital
17. pedal
18. pubic
19. manual
20. inguinal
21. coxal
22. umbilical
23. pectoral
24. sternal
25. mental
26. oral
27. nasal
28. buccal
29. otic
30. orbital
31. frontal
32. occipital
33. scapular
34. vertebral
35. olecranal
36. gluteal
37. popliteal
38. sural
39. fibular (peroneal)
40. plantar
41. calcaneal
42. lumbar

Directional Terms: Complete the sentence.

1. anterior
2. superior
3. medial
4. distal
5. ipsilateral
6. superficial

Figure 1.3

1. superior
2. posterior
3. anterior
4. proximal

5. distal
6. inferior

Figure 1.4

1. frontal or coronal section
2. sagittal section
3. transverse section

Exercise 2

Figure 2.1

1. digestive
2. nervous
3. endocrine
4. lymphatic and immune
5. integumentary
6. muscular
7. cardiovascular
8. respiratory
9. reproductive
10. skeletal
11. urinary

Activity 2: Organ Systems and Organs

1. a, 2. b, 3. c, 4. c, 5. d, 6. b, 7. b, 8. a, 9. c, 10. b

Figure 2.2

1. dorsal cavity
2. cranial cavity
3. vertebral canal
4. ventral cavity
5. thoracic cavity
6. diaphragm
7. abdominopelvic cavity
8. abdominal cavity
9. pelvic cavity
10. thoracic cavity
11. mediastinum
12. pleural cavity
13. pericardial cavity
14. diaphragm
15. abdominopelvic cavity
16. abdominal cavity
17. brim of pelvis
18. pelvic cavity

Table 2.2

Cranial cavity: brain
Vertebral canal: spinal cord
Thoracic cavity: trachea, bronchi, lungs; heart, aorta, venae cavae; esophagus
Pleural cavities: lungs
Pericardial cavity: heart
Abdominal cavity: stomach, pancreas, liver, gall bladder, small intestine, large intestine, appendix, kidneys, ureters, spleen, adrenal glands
Pelvic cavity female: urinary bladder, urethra, ovaries, uterus, vagina
Pelvic cavity male: urinary bladder, male reproductive duct system

Figure 2.3

1. parietal pericardium
2. pericardial cavity
3. visceral pericardium
4. visceral pleura
5. pleural cavity
6. parietal pleura
7. visceral pericardium
8. pericardial cavity
9. parietal pericardium
10. visceral pleura
11. pleural cavity
12. parietal pleura

Figure 2.4

1. parietal peritoneum
2. peritoneal cavity
3. visceral peritoneum
4. visceral peritoneum
5. peritoneal cavity
6. parietal peritoneum

Figure 2.5

1. RLQ
2. all 4 quadrants
3. mainly RUQ
4. LLQ and RLQ
5. LUQ
6. all 4 quadrants
7. LUQ
8. mainly LUQ

Exercise 3

Activity 1 Discussion Questions: Cell Specialization

1. 1st b; 2nd d, 3rd a, 4th c
2. a. spindle shaped; nucleus
   b. irregular shape with processes that extend from cell body; nucleus
   c. oval with a flagellum; nucleus and flagellum
   d. round; none
   e. round; nucleus
3. a. is tapered to nestle with other like cells to contract together
   b. has processes to obtain and send nerve impulses
   c. has flagellum and is tapered for movement
   d. biconcave to bend to go through capillaries
   e. has nucleus to synthesize enzymes to fight bacteria and viruses
4. size and shape

Activity 2 Discussion Questions: Cheek smear

1. to see cell structure
2. nucleus
3. normally bacteria are seen
4. no
5. no

Activity 3 Discussion Questions: Diffusion

1. potassium permanganate
2. it has smaller molecules

Figure 3.5

1. hypotonic
2. hypertonic

Activity 4 Discussion Questions: Dialysis Bag

1. Water moved into dialysis bag.
2. Distilled water is more hypotonic to the hypertonic dialysis bag solution. The water moved into the dialysis bag.
3. To track the movement of sucrose solution
4. Net water movement will stop when the two solutions become isotonic.
5. Yes
6. Distilled water from the beaker moved into the dialysis bag faster because of its low MW.

Activity 5: Osmosis in Living Cell

1. isotonic; hypertonic; hypotonic
2. not change shape; swell; crenate
3. hypotonic

Figure 3.6 Osmosis in RBCs

a. normal shape, isotonic solution
b. swollen, hypotonic solution
c. crenated, hypertonic solution

Activity 5 Discussion Questions: Osmosis in RBCs

1. no
2. yes
3. Water would enter the RBCs, but slower than if the cells are in distilled water.
4. hypertonic and hypotonic solutions

Activity 6: Discussion Questions: Filtration

1. plasma membrane of a cell
2. hydrostatic pressure
3. yes; filtration was faster at the beginning.

Activity 7: Discussion Question: Phagocytosis

1. Irregular with cytoplasmic processes that change as it moves

Figure 3.8

a. interphase
b. prophase
c. metaphase
d. anaphase
e. telophase

Exercise 4

Discussion Questions: Epithelial Tissue

1. No, cells in apical layer are thin and flat and cells in basal layer are cuboidal
2. Connective tissue has much more extracellular space than epithelial cells. Extracellular space cannot be observed in epithelial cells using the light microscope.

Figure 4.2

1. epithelial tissue
2. connective tissue
3. nucleus of connective tissue cell
4. nucleus of epithelial cell

Figure 4.4

1. fibers
2. ground substance
3. nuclei of connective tissue cells

Discussion Questions: Connective Tissue

1. Loose arrangement of fibers
2. No, the tissue contains a greater volume of extracellular matrix than cell volume.

Figure 4.6

1. entire width of muscle cell
2. nucleus of striated muscle cell
3. striation

Discussion Questions: Muscle Tissue

1. There is less extracellular space between muscle cells than between connective tissue cells.
2. Skeletal muscle cells are wider and longer than connective tissue cells.
3. Consider magnification

Figure 4.8

1. process of multipolar neuron
2. nucleus of multipolar neuron
3. cell body of multipolar neuron
4. neuroglia

Discussion Questions: Nervous Tissue

1. Neuroglial cells are smaller than multipolar neurons.
2. Processes from neurons.

Figure 4.11

1. nucleus of simple squamous epithelial cell
2. cell membrane of simple squamous epithelial cell
3. cytoplasm of simple squamous epithelial cell

Figure 4.12

1. nucleus of connective tissue cell
2. connective tissue
3. simple squamous epithelium
4. nucleus of simple squamous epithelial cell

Figure 4.14

1. simple cuboidal epithelium
2. apical surface of simple cuboidal epithelial cell
3. lumen of kidney tubule

4. nucleus of simple cuboidal epithelial cell
   Answer to question: The tubules are not straight, but contain many curves. Parts of a tubule may be perpendicular to plane of section (appear circular in section), parallel to plane of section (long oval in section), or oblique to plane of section (short oval).

Figure 4.16

1. microvilli on apical surface of simple columnar epithelial cell
2. nucleus of simple columnar epithelial cell
3. simple columnar epithelium
4. connective tissue

Figure 4.18

1. nucleus of squamous epithelial cell
2. stratified squamous epithelium
3. nucleus of epithelial cell in basal layer of epithelium
4. connective tissue

Figure 4.20

1. nucleus of transitional epithelial cell in apical layer
2. nucleus of transitional epithelial cell in basal layer
3. transitional epithelium
4. connective tissue

Figure 4.22

1. goblet cell
2. nucleus of ciliated columnar epithelial cell
3. cilia on apical surface of columnar epithelial cell
4. pseudostratified ciliated columnar epithelium
5. connective tissue

Figure 4.24

1. collagen fiber
2. elastic fiber
3. connective tissue cells (fibroblasts or lymphocytes)
4. mast cells

Figure 4.25

1. connective tissue cell
2. fiber

Figure 4.27

1. reticular fiber
2. reticulocyte

Figure 4.29

1. nucleus of adipocyte
2. lipid storage area

Figure 4.31

1. fibroblast
2. collagen fiber bundle

Figure 4.33

1. fibroblast
2. collagen fiber bundles running in different directions
3. parallel collagen fiber bundles

Figure 4.35

1. fibroblast
2. elastic fiber

Figure 4.37

1. extracellular matrix
2. lacuna
3. nucleus of chondrocyte

Figure 4.39

1. lamella
2. canaliculi
3. lacuna
4. central canal

Figure 4.41

1. red blood cell
2. nucleus of white blood cell
3. platelet

Exercise 5

Figure 5.1

1. dermal papillae
2. epidermis
3. papillary layer of dermis
4. reticular layer of dermis
5. hypodermis

Figure 5.2

1. stratum corneum
2. stratum lucidum
3. stratum granulosum
4. stratum spinosum
5. stratum basale

Figure 5.3

1. hair shaft
2. hair root
3. sebaceous gland
4. arrector pili muscle
5. hair follicle
6. hair bulb
7. eccrine sweat gland
8. papilla of hair
9. apocrine sweat gland

Figure 5.4

1. sebaceous gland
2. hair follicle

3. hair root
4. hair bulb
5. papillae of hair

Discussion Questions: Eccrine Gland Density

1. Right palm and forehead had the highest density; right anterior forearm the lowest.
2. Areas with greatest density of eccrine sweat glands will have the most sweat during exercise or nervousness.

Figure 5.5

1. free edge
2. nail body
3. lunula
4. eponychium
5. nail matrix
6. nail root
7. eponychium
8. lunula
9. nail body
10. free edge
11. hyponychium

Exercise 6

Figure 6.1

a. short
b. flat
c. irregular
d. sesamoid
e. long

Figure 6.2

1. proximal epiphysis
2. diaphysis
3. distal epiphysis
4. articular cartilage
5. epiphyseal line
6. compact bone
7. medullary cavity
8. yellow marrow
9. periosteum
10. nutrient artery
11. endosteum
12. spongy bone

Activity 3 Discussion Questions: Fresh Long Bone

1. shiny
2. Articular cartilage keeps bones from rubbing and reduces friction at joints.
3. dull

Figure 6.3

1. osteocyte
2. lacuna
3. periosteum
4. central canal
5. perforating canal
6. canaliculi
7. concentric lamellae
8. osteon
9. blood vessels
10. trabeculae
11. spongy bone
12. compact bone
13. concentric lamella
14. lacunae
15. central canal
16. canaliculi

Figure 6.4

1. trabeculae
2. osteocyte in lacuna
3. interstitial lamellae

Activity 5 Discussion Questions: Chemical Composition of Bone

1. not flexible at all
2. increased hardness
3. collagen/organic matter
4. osteoporosis
5. increased flexiblity
6. not hard; very soft
7. calcium phosphate/minerals/salts
8. rickets

Figure 6.5

1. chondrocyte
2. lacuna
3. extracellular matrix
4. lacuna
5. chondrocyte
6. elastic fiber
7. lacuna
8. chondrocyte
9. collagen fiber

Figure 6.6

1. elastic cartilage
2. fibrocartilage
3. fibrocartilage
4. fibrocartilage
5. hyaline cartilage
6. hyaline cartilage
7. hyaline cartilage
8. elastic cartilage
9. hyaline cartilage

Exercise 7

Figure 7.2

1. parietal bone
2. coronal suture

3. squamous suture
4. temporal bone
5. lambdoid suture
6. occipital bone
7. frontal bone
8. sphenoid bone
9. ethmoid bone
10. lacrimal bone
11. nasal bone
12. zygomatic bone
13. maxilla
14. mandible

Figure 7.3

1. frontal bone
2. coronal suture
3. parietal bone
4. sagittal suture
5. lambdoid suture
6. occipital bone

Figure 7.4

1. maxilla
2. vomer
3. sphenoid bone
4. occipital bone
5. zygomatic bone
6. palatine bone
7. temporal bone

Figure 7.5

1. parietal bone
2. occipital bone
3. frontal bone
4. ethmoid bone
5. sphenoid bone
6. temporal bone
7. lambdoid suture

Figure 7.6

1. parietal bone
2. sphenoid bone
3. ethmoid bone
4. lacrimal bone
5. inferior nasal concha
6. vomer
7. frontal bone
8. squamous suture
9. temporal bone
10. nasal bone
11. zygomatic bone
12. maxilla
13. mandible

Figure 7.7

1. frontal bone
2. sphenoid bone
3. zygomatic bone
4. ethmoid bone
5. lacrimal bone
6. maxilla

Figure 7.8

1. supraorbital foramen
2. orbit of eye
3. inferior orbital fissure
4. perpendicular plate of ethmoid
5. mental foramen of mandible
6. supraorbital margin
7. superior orbital fissure
8. middle nasal concha

Figure 7.9

1. external auditory meatus
2. mastoid process
3. zygomatic process of temporal bone
4. condylar process (mandibular condyle)
5. ramus of mandible
6. body of mandible

Figure 7.10

1. palatine process of maxilla
2. palatine bone
3. hard palate
4. foramen ovale
5. jugular foramen
6. occipital condyle
7. hypoglossal foramen
8. mandibular fossa
9. foramen lacerum
10. carotid foramen (canal)
11. stylomastoid foramen
12. mastoid process
13. foramen magnum

Figure 7.11

1. crista galli
2. olfactory foramina
3. cribriform plate
4. sella turcica
5. foramen ovale
6. internal auditory (acoustic) meatus
7. foramen magnum
8. lesser wing of sphenoid
9. optic foramen
10. greater wing of sphenoid
11. foramen rotundum
12. foramen lacerum
13. jugular foramen

Figure 7.12

1. frontal sinus
2. ethmoidal sinus
3. sphenoidal sinus
4. maxillary sinus

Figure 7.13

1. perpendicular plate of ethmoid
2. septal cartilage
3. vomer

Figure 7.14

1. anterior fontanel
2. posterior fontanel
3. posterior fontanel (occipital)
4. posterolateral fontanel (mastoid)
5. anterior fontanel (frontal)
6. anterolateral fontanel (sphenoid)

Figure 7.15

1. cervical curve
2. thoracic curve
3. lumbar curve
4. sacral curve
5. cervical vertebrae
6. thoracic vertebrae
7. lumbar vertebrae
8. sacrum
9. coccyx

Figure 7.17

1. superior articular facet
2. transverse foramen
3. transverse process
4. lamina
5. dens (odontoid process)
6. spinous process
7. body
8. transverse process
9. bifurcated spinous process
10. pedicle

Figure 7.18

1. transverse process
2. facet for articular part of tubercle
3. superior articular facet
4. superior demifacet
5. facet for articular part of tubercle
6. slanted spinous process
7. superior demifacet
8. inferior demifacet

Figure 7.19

1. pedicle
2. superior articular process
3. transverse process
4. vertebral foramen
5. body
6. hatchet-shaped spinous process
7. inferior articular facet

Figure 7.20

1. intervertebral foramen
2. nucleus pulposus
3. annulus fibrosus
4. intervertebral disc
5. herniation
6. nucleus pulposus
7. annulus fibrosus

Figure 7.21

1. sacral ala
2. sacral base
3. sacral promontory
4. sacral foramen
5. coccyx
6. sacral canal
7. superior articular facet
8. auricular surface (for sacroiliac joint)

Figure 7.22

a. scoliosis
b. kyphosis
c. lordosis

Figure 7.23

1. suprasternal notch (jugular)
2. manubrium
3. body of sternum
4. xiphoid process
5. sternum
6. costal cartilage
7. sternal angle
8. true ribs
9. floating ribs
10. false ribs

Figure 7.24

1. facet for articular part of tubercle
2. tubercle (nonarticular)
3. articular part of tubercle
4. head of rib
5. demifacet of vertebra
6. tubercle (nonarticular)
7. intervertebral foramen
8. inferior demifacet of vertebra
9. head of rib
10. superior demifacet of vertebra
11. body of rib

Exercise 8

Figure 8.1

1. acromial end (extremity)
2. sternal end (extremity)
3. acromion
4. coracoid process
5. glenoid cavity
6. axillary border
7. subscapular fossa
8. vertebral border

9. supraspinous fossa
10. infraspinous fossa
11. acromion
12. spine of scapula
13. glenoid cavity

Figure 8.2

1. greater tubercle
2. intertubercular groove
3. lesser tubercle
4. lateral epicondyle
5. capitulum
6. head
7. anatomical neck
8. deltoid tuberosity
9. coronoid fossa
10. medial epicondyle
11. trochlea
12. olecranon fossa
13. medial epicondyle
14. lateral epicondyle

Figure 8.3

1. head of radius
2. styloid process of radius
3. olecranon (process)
4. trochlear notch (semilunar)
5. coronoid process
6. styloid process of ulna
7. ulna
8. radius

Figure 8.4

1. carpals
2. metacarpals
3. 5th proximal phalanx
4. 5th middle phalanx
5. 5th distal phalanx

Figure 8.5

1. ilium
2. greater sciatic notch
3. ischium
4. ischial spine
5. lesser sciatic notch
6. obturator foramen
7. ischial tuberosity
8. iliac crest
9. anterior superior iliac spine
10. acetabulum
11. pubis

Figure 8.6

1. iliac crest
2. ilium
3. ischial spine
4. pelvic brim
5. pubic symphysis
6. false pelvis
7. true pelvis
8. pubis
9. ischial spine
10. false pelvis
11. sacroiliac joint
12. sacrum
13. coccyx
14. true pelvis
15. pubis

Figure 8.7

1. head of femur
2. greater trochanter
3. neck
4. lesser trochanter
5. medial epicondyle
6. medial condyle
7. linea aspera
8. lateral epicondyle
9. lateral condyle

Figure 8.8

1. lateral condyle
2. head of fibula
3. fibula
4. lateral malleolus
5. medial condyle
6. tibial tuberosity
7. tibia
8. medial malleolus

Figure 8.9

1. calcaneus
2. talus
3. 2nd proximal phalanx
4. 2nd middle phalanx
5. 2nd distal phalanx
6. tarsals
7. metatarsals
8. phalanges
9. calcaneus
10. tibia
11. lateral malleolus of fibula
12. talus
13. tarsals
14. metatarsals
15. phalanges

Exercise 9

Figure 9.1

1. synovial
2. synovial
3. cartilaginous
4. synovial

5. fibrous
6. fibrous
7. cartilaginous
8. cartilaginous
9. synovial
10. synovial
11. fibrous
12. fibrous

Figure 9.2

1. synarthrosis
2. amphiarthrosis
3. diarthrosis
4. amphiarthrosis
5. diarthrosis
6. diarthrosis
7. diarthrosis
8. diarthrosis
9. amphiarthrosis
10. synarthrosis

Figure 9.3

1. articular bone
2. synovial fluid
3. synovial cavity
4. articular cartilage
5. fibrous capsule
6. synovial membrane
7. articular capsule

Figure 9.4

1. articular cartilage of femur
2. fibular collateral ligament
3. lateral meniscus
4. posterior cruciate ligament
5. anterior cruciate ligament
6. medial meniscus
7. tibial collateral ligament
8. patellar ligament
9. fibrous capsule
10. articular cartilage
11. synovial cavity with synovial fluid
12. bursae
13. infrapatellar fat pad
14. patellar ligament

Figure 9.5

1. flexion
2. extension
3. hyperextension
4. hyperextension
5. extension
6. flexion
7. flexion
8. extension
9. flexion
10. extension
11. hyperextension
12. hyperextension
13. extension
14. flexion
15. flexion
16. extension

Figure 9.6

1. abduction
2. adduction
3. circumduction
4. abduction
5. adduction
6. circumduction
7. adduction
8. abduction
9. abduction
10. adduction

Figure 9.7

1. rotation
2. lateral rotation
3. medial rotation

Figure 9.8

1. elevation
2. depression
3. protraction
4. retraction
5. pronation
6. supination

Figure 9.9

1. inversion
2. eversion
3. dorsiflexion
4. plantar flexion

Exercise 10

Figure 10.1

1. epimysium
2. perimysium
3. fascicle
4. endomysium
5. muscle fiber

Figure 10.2

1. endomysium
2. skeletal muscle fiber
3. fascicle
4. perimysium
5. width of skeletal muscle fiber
6. nuclei
7. striations

Figure 10.3

1. nucleus
2. intercalated disc
3. width of cardiac muscle cell
4. branch of cardiac muscle cell

Figure 10.4

1. width of cardiac muscle cell
2. nucleus
3. branches of cardiac muscle cell
4. intercalated disc

Figure 10.5

1. nucleus
2. width of smooth muscle cell

Figure 10.6

1. smooth muscle layer
2. connective tissue
3. epithelial layer
4. nucleus of smooth muscle fiber in cross-section
5. nucleus of smooth muscle fiber in longitudinal section

Figure 10.7

1. triad
2. sarcolemma
3. myofibril
4. t-tubule
5. terminal cisternae
6. sarcoplasmic reticulum
7. sarcomere
8. thin filament
9. thick filament
10. actin
11. tropomyosin
12. troponin
13. myosin cross-bridges
14. myosin tails

Figure 10.8

1. myofibril
2. t-tubule
3. sarcoplasmic reticulum
4. sarcolemma
5. sarcomere

Figure 10.9

1. dense bodies
2. nucleus
3. intermediate filaments

Exercise 11

Figure 11.2

1. Z disc
2. M line
3. H zone
4. I band
5. A band

Discussion Questions: Sarcomere Structure

1. No. Filament length does not change, but there is greater overlap of thin and thick filaments when the muscle fiber contracts (shortens).
2. No. By definition, the A band is the length of the thick filaments and since filament length does not change, A band length does not change.
3. Yes. The I band contains the portion of the thin filaments that does not overlap with thick filaments. When a muscle fiber contracts, thin filaments are pulled over the thick filaments, so there is more overlap of thin and thick filaments and a shorter I band.
4. Yes. The H zone is the portion of the thick filaments that does not overlap with thin filaments. As thin filaments are pulled over thick filaments, this zone becomes smaller and eventually disappears when muscle is fully contracted.
5. Fully relaxed because the H zone is still present.

Figure 11.3

1. axon terminal
2. synaptic end bulb
3. synaptic vesicle with neurotransmitter
4. synaptic cleft
5. motor end plate
6. receptors

Figure 11.4

1. skeletal muscle fibers
2. axon terminal with synaptic end bulbs
3. motor neuron axon

Discussion Questions: Observation of Unfused Tetanus, Recruitment, and Fatigue

1. Incomplete tetanus and asynchronous contractions allow you to maintain a contraction over time.
2. Motor unit recruitment. More motor units recruited, more cross-bridges attached and more force generated.
3. More motor units contracting at a given time, as motor units fatigue, less motor units to take over. Therefore it takes less time to fatigue all motor units.

Activity 4: Recording Muscle Contraction

1. Force = 1.5 g; latent period = 30 msec; contraction period = 50 msec; relaxation period = 80 msec (160 msec if count time to baseline)

Exercise 12

Skeletal Muscle Names

1. orbicularis—direction of fibers (circular); oculi—location (eye)
2. biceps—number of origins (two); brachii—location (arm)
3. rectus—orientation of muscle (muscle parallel to body midline); femoris—location (thigh)
4. gluteus—location (buttocks); maximus—muscle size (largest)
5. deltoid—shape (triangular)
6. sternocleidomastoid—origin and insertion (sterno- and cleido- indicate origin on sternum and clavicle; mastoid indicates insertion on mastoid process).

Figure 12.1

1. frontalis
2. orbicularis oculi
3. zygomaticus major
4. zygomaticus minor
5. orbicularis oris
6. masseter
7. buccinator
8. orbicularis oris
9. frontalis
10. occipitalis
11. orbicularis oculi
12. masseter
13. zygomaticus minor
14. zygomaticus major
15. buccinator
16. temporalis
17. lateral pterygoids
18. medial pterygoids
19. orbicularis oris
20. buccinator

Figure 12.2

1. trapezius
2. sternocleidomastoid
3. levator scapulae
4. platysma
5. digastric, anterior belly
6. stylohyoid
7. digastric, posterior belly
8. omohyoid
9. sternocleidomastoid
10. sternohyoid
11. mylohyoid
12. scalenes
13. levator scapulae

Figure 12.3

1. pectoralis major
2. serratus anterior
3. external obliques
4. pectoralis minor
5. internal intercostals
6. external intercostals
7. internal obliques
8. transverse abdominis
9. rectus abdominis

Figure 12.4

1. deltoid
2. trapezius
3. teres minor
4. teres major
5. infraspinatus
6. latissimus dorsi
7. rhomboid minor
8. supraspinatus
9. teres minor
10. infraspinatus
11. teres major
12. rhomboid major

Figure 12.5

1. biceps brachii
2. brachialis
3. triceps brachii, lateral head
4. triceps brachii, long head
5. triceps brachii, medial head

Figure 12.6

1. pronator teres
2. flexor carpi radialis
3. brachioradialis
4. palmaris longus
5. flexor carpi ulnaris
6. supinator
7. flexor digitorum profundus
8. flexor pollicis longus
9. extensor carpi radialis longus
10. flexor carpi ulnaris
11. extensor carpi radialis brevis
12. extensor carpi ulnaris
13. extensor digiti minimi
14. extensor digitorum
15. supinator
16. extensor pollicis longus

Figure 12.7

1. sartorius
2. rectus femoris
3. tensor fasciae latae
4. vastus intermedius
5. vastus medialis
6. vastus lateralis
7. iliacus
8. psoas major
9. pectineus
10. gracilis
11. adductor longus
12. adductor magnus

13. adductor brevis
14. adductor magnus
15. gracilis
16. gluteus maximus
17. gluteus medius
18. semitendinosus
19. semimembranosus
20. biceps femoris
21. gluteus minimus
22. piriformis

Figure 12.8

1. extensor digitorum longus
2. tibialis anterior
3. fibularis (peroneus) longus
4. gastrocnemius
5. soleus
6. flexor digitorum longus
7. tibialis anterior
8. extensor digitorum longus
9. fibularis longus
10. soleus
11. gastrocnemius
12. gastrocnemius
13. soleus
14. flexor hallucis longus
15. flexor digitorum longus

Skeletal Muscle Actions

Muscles of Facial Expression and Mastication

1. orbicularis oris
2. orbicularis oculi
3. occipitalis
4. zygomaticus major
5. frontalis
6. zygomaticus minor
7. platysma
8. lateral pterygoid
9. buccinator
10. temporalis
11. masseter
12. medial pterygoid

Muscles that Move the Head, Vertebral Column, and Abdominal Wall

1. trapezius
2. splenius capitus
3. scalenes
4. sternocleidomastoid
5. rectus abdominis
6. external oblique
7. internal oblique
8. transverse abdominis
9. erector spinae

Muscles that Act on the Thoracic Cage

1. internal intercostals
2. pectoralis minor
3. scalenes
4. external intercostals
5. diaphragm

Muscles that Move the Scapula

1. pectoralis minor
2. serratus anterior
3. levator scapulae
4. rhomboid major
5. rhomboid minor
6. trapezius

Muscles that Move the Arm

1. teres major
2. pectoralis major
3. latissimus dorsi
4. deltoid

Muscles that Move the Forearm

1. triceps brachii
2. brachialis
3. biceps brachii
4. brachioradialis
5. pronator
6. supinator

Muscles that Move the Forearm, Wrist, and Hand

1. flexor carpi radialis
2. flexor carpi ulnaris
3. palmaris longus
4. flexor digitorum superficialis
5. extensor carpi radialis longus
6. extensor carpi radialis brevis
7. extensor carpi ulnaris
8. extensor digitorum
9. abductor pollicis
10. extensor pollicis

Muscles that Move the Thigh

1. pectineus
2. adductor brevis
3. adductor longus
4. adductor magnus
5. gracilis
6. psoas major
7. iliacus
8. tensor fasciae latae
9. gluteus maximus
10. gluteus medius
11. gluteus minimus

Muscles that Move the Leg

1. rectus femoris
2. vastus lateralis
3. vastus medialis
4. vastus intermedius
5. biceps femoris

6. semitendinosus
7. semimembranosus
8. sartorius

Muscles that Move the Ankle and Foot

1. flexor digitorum longus
2. gastrocnemius
3. soleus
4. fibularis (peroneus) longus
5. extensor digitorum longus
6. tibialis anterior
7. flexor hallucis longus

Exercise 13

Table 13.1

1. Schwann cells—pns
2. ependymal cells—cns
3. microglia—cns
4. astrocytes—cns
5. satellite cells—pns
6. oligodendrocytes—cns

Figure 13.1

1. microglia
2. astrocytes
3. ependymal cells
4. oligodendrocytes
5. satellite cells
6. Schwann cell

Figure 13.2

1. axon terminal
2. Schwann cell
3. node of Ranvier
4. axon collateral
5. axon
6. dendrites
7. cell body
8. axon hillock
9. trigger zone
10. myelin sheath of Schwann cell

Figure 13.3

1. processes
2. cell body
3. dendrites
4. axon
5. axon hillock
6. cell body
7. nucleus

Figure 13.4

1. unipolar
2. multipolar
3. bipolar
4. sensory neuron
5. interneuron
6. motor neuron

Figure 13.5

1. process
2. satellite cell
3. nucleus
4. neuron cell body
5. neuron cell body
6. nucleus
7. process

Figure 13.6

1. cytoplasm of Schwann cell
2. axons
3. node of Ranvier
4. cytoplasm of Schwann cells
5. axon
6. myelin sheath
7. gray matter
8. white matter

Figure 13.7

1. neurilemma
2. myelin sheath
3. node of Ranvier
4. axon

Exercise 14

Figure 14.1

1. cerebrum
2. cerebellum
3. diencephalon
4. brain stem

Figure 14.2

1. superior colliculus
2. inferior colliculus
3. corpora quadrigemina
4. cerebral peduncle
5. pons
6. medulla oblongata
7. brain stem
8. pons
9. medulla oblongata
10. midbrain

Figure 14.3

1. cerebellar hemispheres
2. vermis
3. folia
4. superior colliculus
5. inferior colliculus
6. cerebellar cortex (gray matter)

7. arbor vitae (white matter)
8. folia
9. cerebellar peduncle
10. pons
11. medulla oblongata
12. brain stem

Figure 14.4

1. pineal gland
2. thalamus
3. hypothalamus
4. diencephalon
5. mammillary body
6. pineal gland
7. thalamus
8. intermediate mass
9. hypothalamus
10. infundibulum

Figure 14.5

1. insula
2. cerebral cortex (gray matter)
3. white matter
4. corpus callosum
5. fornix
6. basal nuclei (gray matter)
7. projection fibers
8. association fibers
9. corpus callosum (commissural fibers)
10. fornix (association fibers)

Figure 14.6

1. frontal lobe
2. lateral cerebral sulcus
3. precentral gyrus
4. central sulcus
5. postcentral gyrus
6. temporal lobe
7. parietal lobe
8. transverse fissure
9. parieto-occipital sulcus
10. occipital lobe
11. frontal lobe
12. longitudinal fissure
13. precentral gyrus
14. central sulcus
15. postcentral gyrus
16. parietal lobe
17. gyrus
18. sulcus
19. gray matter
20. white matter
21. longitudinal fissure

Figure 14.7

1. primary visual cortex
2. primary somatosensory cortex
3. central sulcus
4. primary motor cortex
5. primary gustatory cortex
6. Broca's speech area
7. primary auditory cortex
8. Wernicke's area

Figure 14.8

1. meningeal layer of dura mater
2. superior sagittal sinus
3. periosteal layer of dura mater
4. arachnoid villus
5. parietal bone
6. arachnoid mater
7. subarachnoid space
8. pia mater
9. cerebral cortex
10. white matter
11. falx cerebri

Figure 14.9

1. lateral ventricles
2. interventricular foramen
3. third ventricle
4. cerebral aquaduct
5. fourth ventricle
6. central canal of spinal cord
7. superior sagittal sinus
8. arachnoid villus
9. subarachnoid space
10. lateral ventricle
11. choroid plexus
12. third ventricle
13. cerebral aquaduct
14. fourth ventricle
15. central canal

Exercise 15

Figure 15.1

1. pia mater
2. dura mater
3. epidural space
4. subarachnoid space
5. arachnoid mater web-like projection

Figure 15.2

1. cervical enlargement
2. lumbar enlargement
3. conus medullaris
4. cauda equina
5. filum terminale

Figure 15.3

1. spinal nerve
2. posterior (dorsal) root ganglion
3. posterior (dorsal) root
4. posterior median sulcus
5. central canal

6. anterior (ventral) root
7. anterior median fissure

Figure 15.4

1. axon of motor neuron
2. cell body of motor neuron
3. anterior white column
4. anterior gray horn
5. lateral white column
6. lateral gray horn
7. posterior gray horn
8. posterior white column
9. gray commissure
10. axon of sensory neuron
11. cell body of sensory neuron

Figure 15.5

1. posterior (dorsal) root
2. lateral white column
3. central canal
4. posterior median sulcus
5. posterior white column
6. posterior gray horn
7. posterior (dorsal) root ganglion
8. anterior (ventral) root
9. anterior gray horn
10. anterior white column
11. gray commissure
12. anterior median fissure

Exercise 16

Figure 16.1

1. abducens
2. facial
3. vestibulocochlear
4. glossopharyngeal
5. vagus
6. olfactory tract
7. optic
8. oculomotor
9. trochlear
10. trigeminal
11. hypoglossal
12. accessory

Figure 16.2

1. olfactory tract
2. trigeminal
3. optic
4. oculomotor
5. abducens

Discussion Questions: Cranial Nerves of Sheep Brain

1. Olfactory bulbs on the sheep brain are larger because sheep have a more acute sense of smell.
2. Olfactory tracts do not contain axons of sensory neurons. Olfactory nerves travel from olfactory receptor cells in superior nasal epithelium through olfactory foramina in cribriform plate of ethmoid and synapse on olfactory bulbs.

Exercise 17A

Figure 17A.1

1. spinal nerve
2. epineurium
3. perineurium
4. fascicle
5. endoneurium
6. axon

Figure 17A.2

1. perineurium
2. axon
3. myelin sheath
4. endoneurium

Figure 17A.3

1. spinal nerve
2. anterior (ventral) ramus
3. posterior (dorsal) ramus
4. rami communicantes
5. sympathetic ganglion
6. sympathetic ganglion
7. spinal nerve
8. intervertebral foraman
9. anterior (ventral) ramus
10. posterior (dorsal) ramus
11. rami communicantes

Figure 17A.4

1. sacral plexus
2. lumbar plexus
3. brachial plexus
4. cervical plexus
5. cervical nerves
6. thoracic nerves
7. lumbar nerves
8. sacral nerves
9. coccygeal nerve

Figure 17A.5

1. axillary nerve
2. musculocutaneous nerve
3. median nerve
4. ulnar nerve
5. radial nerve
6. phrenic nerve

Figure 17A.6

1. obturator
2. pudendal
3. femoral
4. sciatic
5. tibial
6. common fibular (peroneal)

Exercise 17B

Table 17B.1

somatic, spinal nerve reflex
autonomic, cranial nerve reflex
autonomic, cranial nerve reflex
somatic, spinal nerve reflex

Figure 17B.1

1. integrating center
2. sensory neuron axon
3. sensory neuron cell body
4. sensory receptor
5. effector
6. motor neuron axon
7. motor neuron cell body

Discussion Questions: Reflex Arc

1. polysynaptic
2. ipsilateral

Figure 17B.2

1. receptor
2. sensory neuron
3. integrating center for patellar reflex arc
4. motor neuron for patellar reflex arc
5. effector for patellar reflex arc
6. integrating center for reciprocal innervation
7. motor neuron for reciprocal innervation
8. effector for reciprocal innervation

Discussion Questions: Patellar Reflex

1. ipsilateral
2. inhibits
3. reinforces and intensifies the response

Discussion Questions: Biceps Reflex

1. musculocutaneous nerve
2. triceps brachii

Discussion Questions: Triceps Reflex

1. radial nerve
2. biceps brachii

Discussion Questions: Achilles Reflex

1. tibial nerve
2. tibialis anterior

Activity 6: Plantar Flexion

2. tibial nerve

Exercise 18

Figure 18.1

1. right sympathetic trunk ganglia
2. splanchnic nerves
3. left sympathetic trunk ganglia
4. prevertebral ganglia

Figure 18.2

1. sensory receptor
2. sensory neuron (afferent)
3. interneuron
4. preganglionic motor neuron
5. autonomic ganglion
6. postganglionic motor neuron
7. visceral effector

Discussion Questions: Pupillary Light Reflex

1. autonomic
2. optic nerve
3. oculomotor nerve
4. polysynaptic
5. both

Discussion Questions: Lie Detector Test and the ANS

1. The type of test done in class will give erroneous results because data collection is inaccurate.
2. Some people have learned to lie without feeling emotion or lie without showing ANS responses.

Exercise 19A

Figure 19A.1

1. type I cutaneous mechanoreceptor
2. corpuscle of touch
3. type II cutaneous mechanoreceptor
4. hair root plexus
5. laminated (Pacinian) corpuscle
6. muscle spindle
7. tendon organ

Figure 19A.2

1. third order neuron
2. second order neuron
3. first order neuron
4. third order neuron
5. second order neuron
6. first order neuron

Discussion Questions: Sensory Pathways

1. unipolar
2. posterior (dorsal) root ganglion
3. posterior (dorsal) horn of spinal cord

4. thalamus
5. medulla oblongata
6. spinal cord

Discussion Questions: Tactile Sensitivity

1. fingertip
2. back of leg
3. fingertip
4. back of leg
5. fingertip
6. back of leg

Discussion Questions: Adaptation of Sensory Receptors

1. less than 1 minute
2. Receives decreased number of signals
3. (a) some rapidly and some slowly (b) some rapidly and some slowly (c) not at all (d) not at all

Discussion Questions: Referred pain

1. elbow, forearm, hand
2. ulnar

Exercise 19B

Figure 19B.1

1. conjunctival fold
2. palpebral conjunctiva
3. bulbar conjunctiva
4. lacrimal gland
5. lacrimal canals
6. lacrimal sac
7. nasolacrimal duct

Table 19B.1

inferior oblique—moves eye superiorly and laterally
inferior rectus—moves eye inferiorly
lateral rectus—moves eye laterally
medial rectus—moves eye medially
superior oblique—moves eye inferiorly and laterally
superior rectus—moves eye superiorly

Figure 19B.2

1. superior oblique
2. superior rectus
3. lateral rectus
4. medial rectus
5. inferior oblique
6. inferior rectus

Figure 19B.3

1. scleral venous sinus
2. ciliary muscle
3. ciliary process
4. ciliary body
5. choroid
6. sclera
7. retina
8. cornea
9. pupil
10. iris
11. suspensory ligaments
12. ora serrata

Figure 19B.4

1. anterior chamber
2. posterior chamber
3. anterior cavity
4. scleral venous sinus
5. vitreous chamber
6. lens

Figure 19B.6

1. optic disc
2. central retinal vein
3. optic nerve
4. central retinal artery
5. central fovea
6. optic nerve fibers
7. ganglion cell layer
8. bipolar cell layer
9. photoreceptor layer
10. neural portion of retina
11. pigmented epithelium of retina

Figure 19B.7

1. macula lutea
2. central fovea
3. blood vessel
4. optic disc

Figure 19B.8

1. cornea
2. pupil
3. iris
4. ciliary body
5. lens
6. choroid
7. sclera
8. retina
9. optic disc
10. optic nerve
11. ganglion cell layer
12. bipolar cell layer
13. photoreceptor layer
14. neural portion of retina
15. pigmented epithelium of retina

Discussion Questions: Visual Tests

1. To accommodate the lens of the eye for distance vision.
2. To accommodate the lens of the eye for near vision.

Figure 19B.11

1. helix
2. external ear
3. malleus
4. incus
5. stapes attached to oval window
6. middle ear
7. internal ear
8. auditory tube
9. tympanic membrane
10. external auditory canal
11. lobule
12. auricle

Figure 19B.12

1. anterior semicircular canal
2. posterior semicircular canal
3. lateral semicircular canal
4. ampulla
5. utricle
6. saccule
7. oval window
8. membranous semicircular duct
9. vestibule
10. round window
11. cochlea
12. cochlear duct

Figure 19B.13

1. scala vestibuli
2. scala tympani
3. vestibular membrane
4. basilar membrane
5. cochlear duct
6. spiral organ of Corti
7. vestibular membrane
8. tectorial membrane
9. basilar membrane
10. hair cells
11. cochlear duct

Figure 19B.14

1. otoliths
2. otolithic membrane
3. hair bundle
4. hair cell
5. vestibular branches of vestibulocochlear nerve
6. cupula
7. hair bundle
8. hair cell

Figure 19B.15

1. olfactory bulb
2. cribiform plate
3. olfactory tract
4. olfactory nerves
5. olfactory receptor cell
6. olfactory hairs

Figure 19B.16

1. bitter
2. salty
3. sour
4. sweet
5. vallate papillae
6. filiform papillae
7. fungiform papillae
8. taste bud
9. taste pore
10. gustatory hairs
11. gustatory receptor cell
12. sensory axons

Discussion Questions: Olfactory Adaptation

1. Similar
2. The receptors on that side have not adapted.

Exercise 20

Figure 20.1

1. pineal gland
2. parathyroid glands
3. adrenal glands
4. pancreas
5. hypothalamus
6. pituitary gland
7. thyroid gland
8. thymus
9. ovaries
10. testes

Figure 20.2

1. hypothalamus
2. infundibulum
3. anterior pituitary
4. posterior pituitary
5. hypothalamus
6. infundibulum
7. anterior pituitary
8. posterior pituitary
9. posterior pituitary
10. anterior pituitary

Figure 20.3

1. right lobe of thyroid gland
2. thyroid cartilage of larynx
3. left lobe of thyroid gland
4. isthmus of thyroid gland
5. trachea
6. left parathyroid glands
7. thyroid gland
8. right parathyroid glands
9. trachea

Figure 20.4

1. thyroid gland
2. parathyroid gland
3. colloid-filled follicle
4. follicular cell
5. parafollicular cell

Discussion Question: Thyroid and Parathyroid Glands

1. Storage space for thyroglobulin is much greater due to the large follicles. Calcitonin and PTH are stored only within the small parafollicular cells and principal cells respectively.

Figure 20.5

1. right adrenal gland
2. left adrenal gland
3. kidney
4. capsule
5. adrenal cortex
6. adrenal medulla
7. capsule
8. zona glomerulosa
9. zona fasciculata
10. zona reticularis
11. adrenal medulla
12. adrenal cortex

Figure 20.6

1. tail of pancreas
2. body of pancreas
3. head of pancreas
4. exocrine or acinar cells
5. pancreatic islet

Exercise 21A

Figure 21A.2

1. base of heart
2. right lung
3. left lung
4. apex of heart
5. fibrous pericardium
6. diaphragm
7. fibrous pericardium
8. parietal layer of visceral pericardium
9. pericardial cavity
10. visceral layer of serous pericardium
11. endocardium
12. myocardium

Figure 21A.3

1. right atrium
2. coronary sulcus
3. right ventricle
4. auricle of left atrium
5. anterior interventricular sulcus
6. left ventricle
7. left auricle
8. coronary sulcus
9. left ventricle
10. adipose tissue
11. posterior interventricular sulcus
12. right auricle
13. right ventricle

Figure 21A.4

1. superior vena cava
2. right pulmonary artery
3. ascending aorta
4. pulmonary trunk
5. right pulmonary veins
6. inferior vena cava
7. aortic arch
8. ligamentum arteriosum
9. left pulmonary artery
10. descending aorta
11. left pulmonary veins
12. aortic arch
13. ligamentum arteriosum
14. left pulmonary artery
15. left pulmonary veins
16. coronary sinus
17. superior vena cava
18. ascending aorta
19. right pulmonary artery
20. right pulmonary veins
21. inferior vena cava

Figure 21.5

1. pulmonary (semilunar) valve
2. right atrium
3. coronary sinus opening
4. tricuspid valve
5. right ventricle
6. trabeculae carneae
7. left atrium
8. aortic (semilunar) valve
9. bicuspid valve (mitral)
10. chordae tendineae
11. interventricular septum
12. papillary muscle
13. left ventricle

Activity 6

Oxygen-Poor Blood Vessels

1. pulmonary arteries
2. pulmonary trunk
3. venae cavae

Oxygen-Rich Blood Vessels

4. aorta
5. pulmonary veins

Trace blood flow

1. right atrium
2. tricuspid valve
3. right ventricle
4. pulmonary (semilunar) valve
5. pulmonary trunk
6. right and left pulmonary arteries
7. pulmonary capillaries
8. pulmonary veins
9. left atrium
10. bicuspid valve
11. left ventricle
12. aortic (semilunar) valve
13. aorta
14. systemic arteries
15. systemic capillaries
16. systemic veins
17. venae cavae

Figure 21A.7

1. posterior interventricular branch
2. marginal branch
3. right coronary artery
4. left coronary artery
5. circumflex branch
6. anterior atrioventricular branch (LAD)
7. small cardiac vein
8. middle cardiac vein
9. coronary sinus
10. great cardiac vein

Activity 8: Dissection of a Sheep Heart

8. The three cusps are half moon shaped and have no chordae tendineae.
10. Two main cusps that are counted; yes; yes; lesser number; left ventricle is thicker to pump blood through the systemic circulation

Figure 21A.9

1. cardiac muscle fiber
2. intercalated discs
3. branching fiber
4. nucleus

Exercise 21B

Discussion Questions: Heart Sounds, Heart Rate, and Pulse Rate

1. Lubb occurs when ventricles contracting.
2. They should be the same.
3. The pause is shorter after exercise.
4. Differences in recovery time may be due to age, health, and physical condition.

Figure 21B.2

1. Purkinje fibers in right ventricle
2. right bundle branch
3. AV bundle (of His)
4. AV node
5. SA node
6. left bundle branch
7. Purkinje fibers in left ventricle

Figure 21B.4

1. P wave
2. P-Q interval
3. QRS complex
4. S-T segment
5. T wave
6. Q-T segment

Figure 21B.5

(a) bradycardia 50 squares = 2 sec/beat = 30 beats/min
(b) NSR 25 squares = 1 sec/beat = 60 beats/min
(c) tachycardia 13 squares = 0.52 sec/beat = 120 beats/min

Activity 5: Calculate Lengths of the ECG Segments

PQ interval = 4.5 squares = 0.18 sec
QRS complex = 3 squares = 0.12 sec
QT interval = 14 squares = 0.56 sec
Relaxation period = 11 squares = 0.44 sec
Heart rate = 53 bpm

Discussion Questions: Calculate Lengths of the ECG Segments

1. QT is abnormal; QRS is long but not over 0.12 sec
2. The relaxation period decreases when heart rate increases and increases when heart rate decreases.

Exercise 22

Figure 22.1

1. endothelium
2. basement membrane
3. internal elastic lamina
4. tunica interna
5. smooth muscle
6. external elastic lamina
7. tunica media
8. tunica externa

Figure 22.2

(b) is vasoconstricted

Figure 22.3

1. capillary
2. arteriole

Figure 22.4

1. intercellular cleft
2. vesicles involved in transcytosis
3. fenestration

Figure 22.5

1. endothelium
2. basement membrane
3. valve
4. smooth muscle
5. tunica externa
6. tunica interna
7. tunica media

Figure 22.6

1. lumen of artery
2. tunica interna
3. tunica media
4. tunica externa
5. tunica externa
6. tunica media
7. tunica interna
8. lumen of vein

Discussion Questions: Regulation of Blood Pressure

1. Supine position. Head is not higher than heart, it does not take as much pressure to drive blood to head. Pressure increases when standing to provide enough pressure to overcome gravity and deliver blood to brain.
2. BP and heart rate increase. BP changed by increasing cardiac output.

Exercise 23

Figure 23.1

1. right common carotid artery
2. right subclavian artery
3. brachiocephalic trunk
4. ascending aorta
5. right coronary artery
6. left common carotid
7. left subclavian artery
8. aortic arch
9. left coronary artery

Figure 23.2

1. basilar artery
2. internal carotid artery
3. vertebral artery
4. middle cerebral artery
5. anterior cerebral artery
6. posterior communicating artery
7. posterior cerebral artery
8. external carotid artery
9. common carotid artery
10. brachiocephalic trunk
11. anterior cerebral artery
12. middle cerebral artery
13. internal carotid artery
14. posterior communicating artery
15. posterior cerebral artery
16. basilar artery
17. vertebral artery
18. anterior communicating artery

Figure 23.3

1. subclavian artery
2. axillary artery
3. brachial artery
4. radial artery
5. ulnar artery

Figure 23.4

1. celiac trunk
2. suprarenal
3. gonadal
4. common iliac
5. thoracic aorta
6. superior mesenteric
7. renal
8. abdominal aorta
9. inferior mesenteric

Figure 23.5

1. left gastric artery
2. celiac trunk
3. common hepatic artery
4. splenic artery

Figure 23.6

1. common iliac
2. external iliac
3. internal iliac
4. femoral
5. popliteal
6. anterior tibial
7. posterior tibial
8. fibular (peroneal)
9. dorsal artery of the foot (dorsalis pedis)

Figure 23.7

1. superior vena cava
2. coronary sinus
3. inferior vena cava

Figure 23.8

1. vertebral vein
2. internal jugular vein
3. external jugular vein
4. subclavian vein
5. brachiocephalic vein

TABLE 24.4

BLOOD TYPE	TYPE A	TYPE B	AB TYPE	O TYPE
Antigen on RBCs	A	B	A, B	neither A or B
Antibody in plasma	anti-B	anti-A	none	anti-A; anti-B
Compatible donor	A; O	B; O	A; B; AB; O	O
Incompatible donor	B; AB	A; AB	none	A; B; AB

Figure 23.9

1. subclavian vein
2. axillary vein
3. brachial veins
4. basilic vein
5. cephalic vein
6. radial veins
7. median cubital vein
8. ulnar veins

Figure 23.10

1. right brachiocephalic vein
2. left brachiocephalic vein
3. superior vena cava
4. azygous
5. hepatic veins
6. right suprarenal
7. right renal
8. right gonadal
9. inferior vena cava
10. right common iliac
11. right internal iliac
12. right external iliac
13. accesory hemiazygous
14. hemiazygous
15. left suprarenal vein
16. left renal vein
17. left gonadal vein
18. left common iliac vein
19. left internal iliac vein
20. left external iliac vein

Figure 23.11

1. hepatic vein
2. hepatic portal vein
3. superior mesenteric vein
4. splenic vein
5. inferior mesenteric vein

Figure 23.12

1. external iliac vein
2. femoral vein
3. great saphenous vein
4. anterior tibial veins
5. small saphenous vein
6. posterior tibial veins
7. femoral vein
8. popliteal vein
9. great saphenous vein
10. posterior tibial veins
11. small saphenous veins
12. fibular (peroneal) veins

Figure 23.13

1. right pulmonary artery
2. right pulmonary vein
3. left pulmonary artery
4. pulmonary trunk
5. left pulmonary vein

Figure 23.14

1. foramen ovale
2. ductus venosus
3. umbilical vein
4. umbilical arteries
5. placenta
6. ductus arteriosus
7. ligamentum arteriosum
8. fossa ovalis
9. ligamentum venosum
10. ligamentum teres
11. medial umbilical ligaments

Exercise 24

Figure 24.1

1. plasma
2. RBCs
3. WBCs and platelets

Discussion Questions: Hematocrit

1. Tube (a)—45% = normal
   Tube (b)—22% = anemia

Discussion Questions: Hemoglobin Content of Blood

2. Lower
3. RBCs could have different amounts of hemoglobin

Discussion Questions: Coagulation Time

1. Longer than normal coagulation time
2. Coagulation time would be longer.

Exercise 25

Figure 25.1

1. palatine tonsil
2. submandibular node
3. cervical node
4. thymus
5. intestinal node
6. appendix
7. red bone marrow
8. axillary node
9. mammary node
10. thoracic node
11. spleen
12. aggregated lymphatic follicle (Peyer's patches)
13. iliac node
14. inguinal node
15. palatine tonsil
16. pharyngeal tonsil
17. lingual tonsil

Figure 25.2

1. tissue cell
2. interstitial fluid
3. blood capillary (with plasma)
4. lymphatic capillary (with lymph)
5. interstitial fluid
6. opening into lymphatic capillary
7. tissue cell
8. lymph in lymphatic capillary

Figure 25.3

1. right lymphatic duct
2. lymphatic vessel in arm
3. thoracic duct in thorax
4. cisterna chyli
5. lymphatic vessel in leg
6. thoracic duct draining into subclavian vein
7. area drained by right lymphatic duct
8. area drained by thoracic duct
9. right jugular trunk
10. right lymphatic duct
11. right subclavian duct
12. cisterna chyli
13. thoracic duct
14. thoracic (left lymphatic) duct in thorax

Figure 25.4

1. trabecular sinus
2. afferent vessels
3. valve
4. subcapsular sinus
5. cortex
6. medulla
7. medullary sinus
8. efferent vessels
9. hilus
10. capsule
11. trabeculae
12. cortex
13. medulla
14. capsule
15. germinal center in lymphatic nodule
16. reticulocytes
17. reticular fiber

Figure 25.5

1. splenic artery
2. splecnic vein
3. hilus
4. capsule
5. red pulp
6. trabeculae
7. white pulp

Figure 25.6

1. e
2. e
3. e
4. c
5. e
6. e
7. a, b, d
8. e
9. e
10. e
11. e
12. e

Exercise 26

Figure 26.1

1. pharynx
2. right primary bronchus
3. lungs
4. nose
5. nasal cavity
6. larynx
7. trachea

Figure 26.2

1. internal nares
2. superior nasal concha
3. middle nasal concha
4. inferior nasal concha
5. superior nasal meatus
6. middle nasal meatus
7. inferior nasal meatus
8. external nares
9. hard palate
10. middle meatus
11. nasal septum

12. inferior meatus
13. middle concha
14. inferior concha

Figure 26.3

1. nasopharynx
2. oropharynx
3. laryngopharynx
4. pharyngeal tonsil
5. orifice of the auditory tubes
6. uvula
7. palatine tonsil
8. lingual tonsil
9. internal nares
10. soft palate

Figure 26.4

1. epiglottis
2. thyroid cartilage
3. cricoid cartilage
4. epiglottis
5. thyroid cartilage
6. cricoid cartilage
7. arytenoid cartilage
8. cricoid cartilage
9. epiglottis
10. ventricular folds
11. vocal folds
12. thyroid cartilage
13. ventricular folds
14. vocal folds
15. glottis

Figure 26.5

1. trachea
2. right primary bronchus
3. carina
4. right secondary bronchus
5. diaphragm
6. larynx
7. tracheal cartilage
8. left primary bronchus
9. left tertiary bronchus
10. bronchiole
11. primary bronchus
12. secondary bronchus
13. tertiary bronchus
14. terminal bronchiole
15. respiratory bronchiole
16. alveolar sac

Figure 26.6

1. respiratory bronchiole
2. alveolar ducts
3. alveolar sac
4. alveoli

Figure 26.7

1. apex
2. superior lobe
3. middle lobe
4. inferior lobe
5. base
6. apex
7. superior lobe
8. cardiac notch
9. inferior lobe
10. base
11. superior lobe
12. hilus
13. middle lobe
14. inferior lobe
15. superior lobe
16. inferior lobe
17. hilus
18. cardiac notch

Figure 26.8

1. visceral pleura
2. parietal pleura
3. pleural cavity
4. diaphragm
5. right lung
6. left lung
7. visceral pleura
8. pleural cavity
9. parietal pleura
10. pericardium

Figure 26.9

1. lumen of esophagus
2. trachealis muscle
3. lumen of trachea
4. epithelial lining of trachea
5. tracheal cartilage
6. respiratory bronchiole
7. simple squamous epithelium
8. alveolar ducts
9. alveoli
10. alveolar sac

Questions: Microscopic Anatomy of Respiratory System

1. elastic connective tissue
2. hyaline cartilage

Figure 26.10

1. sternocleidomastoid
2. scalenes
3. pectoralis minor
4. rectus abdominis
5. external oblique
6. internal oblique
7. transverse abdominis

8. internal intercostals
9. external intercostals
10. diaphragm

Table 26.2

external intercostals—increase diameter
internal intercostals—decrease diameter
sternocleidomastoids—increase diameter
scalenes—increase diameter
pectoralis minors—increase diameter
diaphragm—increases length
abdominal muscles—decrease length

Figure 26.11

a. expiration
b inspiration

Figure 26.12

1. parietal pleura and thoracic wall
2. trachea
3. bronchus
4. lungs and visceral pleura
5. intrapleural cavity
6. diaphragm

Table 26.3

1. decreased
2. increased
3. deflated
4. out of balloons
5. increased
6. decreased
7. inflated
8. into balloons

Questions: Bell Jar Demonstration

1. serous fluid; larger than pleural cavity
2. (a) subatmospheric (If rubber membrane is not sealed to bell jar, then pressure inside bell jar might be atmospheric.) (b) subatmospheric
3. (a) It would increase and become atmospheric. (b) Lung size decreases. (c) Pneumothorax.
4. two separate pleural cavities
5. The trachea and bronchi provide a patent, semirigid airway. The bronchial tree has many branches.
6. The thorax increases in size with inspiration and decreases with expiration.

Figure 26.13

FVC = 3.1 L
FEV_1 = 1.9 L
FEV_1/FVC ratio = 0.61

Questions: Bicarbonate and Hydrogen Ion Formation

1. hydrogen ion concentration
2. increase
3. increase
4. (a) Decrease. (b) Exhaled air has a greater carbon dioxide concentration than atmospheric air. More carbon dioxide dissolves, in water, causing more carbonic acid to be formed. The carbonic acid dissociates into bicarbonate and hydrogen ions, causing the pH to decrease.
5. Increased blood carbon dioxide levels will decrease pH. The increased hydrogen ion concentration of blood will stimulate chemoreceptors, causing an increased breathing rate.

Exercise 27A

Figure 27A.1

1. salivary glands
2. pharynx
3. esophagus
4. liver
5. gallbladder
6. large intestine
7. mouth
8. teeth
9. tongue
10. stomach
11. pancreas
12. small intestine
13. anus

Figure 27A.2

1. mucosa
2. submucosa
3. serosa
4. muscularis

Figure 27A.3

1. retroperitoneal organs
2. lesser omentum
3. mesentery
4. greater omentum
5. mesocolon
6. parietal peritoneum
7. visceral peritoneum
8. peritoneal cavity
9. falciform ligament
10. greater omentum
11. lesser omentum
12. greater omentum (reflected)
13. mesocolon
14. mesentery

Figure 27A.4

1. hard palate
2. soft palate
3. uvula
4. cheek
5. vestibule
6. superior lip
7. fauces

8. palatine tonsil
9. tongue
10. gingiva (gums)
11. inferior labial frenulum
12. inferior lip

Figure 27A.5

1. nasopharynx
2. soft palate
3. uvula
4. fauces
5. oropharynx
6. laryngopharynx
7. esophagus
8. hard palate
9. oral cavity
10. tongue

Figure 27A.6

1. lower esophageal sphincter
2. cardia
3. body
4. lesser curvature
5. pyloric sphincter
6. esophagus
7. fundus
8. longitudinal muscle layer
9. circular muscle layer
10. oblique muscle layer
11. greater curvature
12. rugae
13. pylorus

Figure 27A.7

1. duodenum
2. ascending colon
3. jejunum
4. ileum
5. stomach
6. transverse colon
7. descending colon
8. rectum
9. right colic flexure
10. ascending colon
11. ileum
12. ileocecal sphincter
13. cecum
14. appendix
15. rectum
16. transverse colon
17. left colic flexure
18. descending colon
19. teniae coli
20. epiploic appendages
21. haustra
22. sigmoid colon
23. anal canal
24. anus
25. rectum
26. anal canal
27. internal anal sphincter
28. external anal sphincter
29. anal column
30. anus

Figure 27A.8

1. parotid gland
2. parotid duct
3. opening of parotid duct
4. opening of sublinguinal duct
5. sublinguinal gland
6. submandibular duct
7. submandibular gland
8. crown
9. neck
10. root
11. enamel
12. dentin
13. gingiva
14. blood supply
15. pulp cavity with pulp
16. cementum
17. root canal
18. peridontal ligament
19. nerve
20. apical foramen
21. molars
22. premolar
23. cuspids
24. inscisors
25. tongue
26. lingual frenulum

Figure 27A.9

1. right hepatic duct
2. cystic duct
3. gall bladder
4. duodenum
5. hepatopancreatic ampulla
6. falciform ligament
7. left lobe of liver
8. left hepatic duct
9. common hepatic duct
10. common bile duct
11. accessory pancreatic duct
12. tail of pancreas
13. body of pancreas
14. pancreatic duct
15. head of pancreas
16. jejunum
17. hepatopancreatic ampulla
18. duodenal papilla
19. common bile duct
20. pancreatic duct
21. quadrate lobe
22. left lobe of liver
23. caudate lobe

24. right lobe
25. gall bladder

Figure 27A.10

1. circular layer of smooth muscle fibers
2. longitudinal layer of smooth muscle fibers
3. stratified squamous epithelium
4. lamina propria
5. mucosa
6. submucosa
7. muscularis
8. serosa
9. gastric pits
10. simple columnar epithelium
11. lamina propria
12. gastric glands
13. simple columnar epithelium
14. goblet cell
15. villus
16. lamina propria
17. intestinal glands
18. duodenal glands
19. acini
20. pancreatic islet
21. heptocytes
22. sinusoids
23. central vein

Figure 27A.11

1. bile canaliculus
2. hepatic vein
3. central vein
4. sinusoids
5. portal triad
6. bile duct
7. hepatocytes
8. branch of hepatic portal vein
9. branches of hepatic artery

Exercise 27B

Discussion Questions: Digestion of Starch

1. Less sugar produced by whole cracker. Whole cracker had smaller surface area for amylase to act on.
2. 7.4
3. Tubes with amylase at pH 7.4
4. No, not all starch was converted to sugar
5. Yes, the tubes without amylase and the tubes with amylase and HCl
6. More sugar would appear in tubes with amylase at pH 7.4.
7. The tubes with amylase and HCl

Discussion Questions: Bile Emulsification

1. Tube 2
2. No, it doesn't break down fat. It suspends it in the watery medium so it can be broken down by water soluable lipase.
3. Increases surface area of fats

Exercise 28

Figure 28.1

1. peritoneum
2. right kidney
3. renal capsule
4. adipose capsule
5. renal fascia
6. left kidney
7. renal hilus

Figure 28.2

1. renal medulla
2. renal cortex
3. renal column
4. renal capsule
5. renal pyramid
6. renal papilla
7. minor calyx
8. major calyx
9. renal artery
10. renal vein
11. renal hilus
12. renal pelvis in renal sinus

Discussion Questions: Location and Gross Anatomy of the Kidney

1. ribs 11 and 12
2. right kidney; liver forces the right kidney lower.

Figure 28.3

1. internal urethral sphincter
2. ureters
3. detrusor muscle of urinary bladder
4. ureteral openings
5. trigone
6. internal urethral orifice
7. urethra
8. external urethral sphincter
9. external urethral orifice

Figure 28.4

1. rectum
2. anus
3. ureter
4. urinary bladder
5. ureteral opening
6. internal urethral orifice
7. prostatic urethra
8. membranous urethra
9. spongy urethra
10. external urethral opening
11. urogenital diaphragm
12. rectum
13. anus
14. uterus
15. urinary bladder

16. internal urethral orifice
17. urethra
18. urogenital diaphragm
19. external urethral orifice
20. vagina

Discussion Questions: Ureters, Urinary Bladder, and Urethra

1. No, it is covered by visceral peritoneum.

Figure 28.5

1. glomerular capsule
2. proximal convoluted tubule
3. ascending limb of loop of Henle
4. descending limb of loop of Henle
5. distal convoluted tubule
6. collecting duct
7. papillary duct
8. glomerulus
9. glomerular capsule
10. renal corpuscle
11. peritubular capillaries
12. efferent arteriole
13. afferent arteriole

Figure 28.6

1. afferent arteriole
2. efferent arteriole
3. vasa recta
4. peritubular capillaries
5. interlobular artery
6. interlobar artery
7. arcuate artery
8. segmental artery
9. renal artery
10. renal vein
11. interlobar vein
12. arcuate vein
13. interlobular vein

Discussion Questions: Blood Flow through the Kidney

1. segmental and interlobar arteries and interlobar veins
2. interlobar arteries and veins
3. arcuate arteries and veins
4. interlobular arteries and veins, afferent and efferent arterioles, glomerulus, peritubular capillaries

Figure 28.8

1. proximal and distal convoluted tubules
2. renal corpuscle
3. loops of Henle and collecting ducts
4. glomerulus
5. parietal layer of glomerular capsule
6. capsular space

Discussion Questions: Histology of the Kidney

1. Filtration
2. PCT needs extra area of brush border for reabsorption

Figure 28.9

1. lamina propria
2. transitional epithelium
3. lumen
4. mucosa
5. muscularis
6. adventitia

Discussion Question: Histology of Ureters, Urinary Bladder, and Urethra

1. Stratified squamous epithelium offers more protection from external environment.

Exercise 29A

Figure 29A.1

1. cremaster muscle
2. dartos muscle
3. scrotum
4. tunica albuginea of testis

Figure 29A.2

1. efferent duct
2. seminiferous tubules
3. straight tubules
4. rete testis
5. tunica albuginea
6. lobule
7. septum

Figure 29A.3

1. ductus (vas) deferens
2. epididymis
3. spermatic cord
4. blood vessels and nerves

Figure 29A.4

1. ampulla of vas deferens
2. ejaculatory duct
3. prostate gland
4. membranous urethra
5. epididymis
6. testis
7. scrotum
8. ductus (vas) deferens
9. prostatic urethra
10. spongy (penile) urethra
11. penis
12. external urethral orifice

Figure 29A.5

1. seminal vesicle
2. prostate gland
3. prostatic urethra
4. membranous urethra
5. ductus (vas) deferens
6. ampulla of ductus deferens
7. ejaculatory duct
8. bulbourethral gland
9. spongy (penile) urethra

Figure 29A.6

1. seminal vesicle
2. prostate gland
3. bulbourethral gland

Figure 29A.7

1. prostate gland
2. prostatic urethra
3. membranous urethra
4. corpus spongiosum penis
5. corpora cavernosa penis
6. spongy (penile) urethra
7. glans penis
8. bulbourethral gland
9. prepuce
10. external urethral orifice
11. corpora cavernosa penis
12. corpus spongiosum penis
13. spongy (penile) urethra

Figure 29A.8

1. spermatogonium
2. spermatozoa (n)
3. spermatid (n)
4. secondary spermatocyte (n)
5. primary spermatocyte (2n)
6. spermatozoa
7. late spermatid
8. early spermatid
9. secondary spermatocyte
10. Sertoli cells
11. primary spermatocyte
12. spermatogonium
13. basement membrane
14. Leydig cells

Discussion Question

1. 4

Figure 29A.9

1. lumen
2. tails of sperm
3. basement membrane
4. Leydig cells
5. interstitial space

Figure 29A.10

1. acrosome
2. nucleus
3. mitochondria
4. head
5. midpiece
6. tail (flagellum)

Exercise 29B

Figure 29B.1

1. uterine tube
2. infundibulum
3. ampulla
4. isthmus
5. fimbriae
6. suspensory ligament
7. ovary
8. ovarian ligament

Figure 29B.2

1. uterine cavity
2. myometrium of uterus
3. vaginal canal
4. ovary
5. round ligament
6. cervix
7. urinary bladder

Figure 29B.3

1. uterine cavity
2. endometrium
3. myometrium
4. perimetrium
5. round ligament
6. internal os
7. cervical canal
8. cervix
9. rugae of vagina
10. fundus of uterus
11. broad ligament
12. body of uterus
13. external os
14. vagina

Figure 29B.4

1. anus
2. vaginal orifice
3. pubic symphysis
4. mons pubis
5. clitoris
6. external urethral orifice
7. labium minus
8. labium majus

Figure 29B.5

1. labia majora
2. labia minora
3. hymen
4. anus
5. mons pubis
6. prepuce
7. clitoris
8. external urethral orifice
9. vaginal orifice

Figure 29B.6

1. lobule with alveoli
2. mammary duct
3. lactiferous sinus
4. lactiferous duct
5. adipose tissue
6. areola
7. nipple

Figure 29B.7

1. secondary oocyte
2. sperm cell
3. ovum
4. zygote
5. oogonium
6. primary oocyte
7. 1st polar body
8. 2nd polar body
9. meiosis I
10. meiosis II

Figure 29B.8

1. primordial follicles
2. primary follicles
3. secondary follicle
4. secondary oocyte
5. Graafian (mature) follicle
6. ovulated secondary oocyte
7. corpus luteum
8. corpus albicans
9. primordial follicles
10. ovarian cortex
11. primary oocyte
12. granulosa cells
13. follicular fluid in antrum
14. granulosa cells
15. primary oocyte

Figure 29B.9

1. endometrium
2. endometrial gland
3. stratum functionalis
4. stratum basalis
5. myometrium

PHOTO CREDITS

Preface: P.2: Courtesy Olympus America, Inc.

Exercise 1: 1.6a,b: Mark Nielsen. 1.8a: Simon Fraser, Royal Victoria Infirmary, Newcastle Upon Tyne/Photo Researchers. 1.8b: Alfred Pasieka/Photo Researchers. 1.8c: Mark Nielsen.

Exercise 2: 2.6a: © Benedet/Phototake. 2.6b,d: CNRI/Phototake. 2.6c: Geoff Tompkinson/Photo Researchers.

Exercise 3: 3.2a: Courtesy Michael Ross, University of Florida. 3.2b: Carolina Biological/Visuals Unlimited. 3.2c: M. Abbey/Photo Researchers. 3.2d: Michael Abbey/Visuals Unlimited. 3.3: Bruce Iverson/Photo Researchers. 3.6a,b,c: David Phillips/Photo Researchers. 3.8a–e: Courtesy Michael Ross, University of Florida.

Exercise 4: 4.2, 4.4, 4.6, 4.8, 4.11, 4.12, 4.14, 4.16, 4.18, 4.20, 4.22, 4.24, 4.25, 4.27, 4.29, 4.31, 4.33, 4.35, 4.37, 4.39, 4.41: Courtesy Michael Ross, University of Florida. 4.42: 1, Biophoto Associates/Photo Researchers. 4.42: 2, 3, and 4, Ed Reschke. 4.43: 1, 2, 3, 9, 11, 13, 14, and 15, Biophoto Associates/Photo Researchers. 4.43: 4, 5, 8, 10, 12, Ed Reschke. 4.43: 6, Courtesy Michael Ross, University of Florida. 4.43: 7, Courtesy Andrew J. Kuntzman.

Exercise 5: 5.1, 5.2 and 5.4: Courtesy Michael Ross, University of Florida.

Exercise 6: 6.3b: Ed Reschke. 6.5a,b,c: Biophoto Associates/Photo Researchers. 6.7: Don W. Fawcett/Visuals Unlimited. 6.8: L. Bassett/Visuals Unlimited. Figure 6.9a: Mehau Kulyk/Photo Researchers. 6.9b: Scott Camazine and Sue Trainor/Photo Researchers. 6.10a,b: P. Motta/Photo Researchers.

Exercise 7: 7.2, 7.3, 7.4, 7.5, 7.6, 7.7, 7.8, 7.9, 7.10, 7.11, 7.15, 7.17, 7.18, 7.19, 7.21, 7.23 and 7.24: Mark Nielsen. 7.29a: Dept. of Clinical Radiology, Salisbury District Hospital/Photo Researchers. 7.29b: AFIP/Science Source/Photo Researchers. 7.30a,b: Courtesy Chaim J. Margolin.

Exercise 8: 8.1, 8.2, 8.3, 8.4, 8.5, 8.6, 8.7, 8.8 and 8.9: Mark Nielsen. 8.12a: Larry Mulvehill/Photo Researchers. 8.12b: © SIU/Visuals Unlimited. 8.12c: Mehau Kulyk/Photo Researchers. 8.13a: Jim Erickson/Corbis Stock Market. 8.13b: Dick Luria/Photo Researchers.

Exercise 9: 9.5, 9.6, 9.7, 9.8 and 9.9: John Wilson White. 9.10a,b,c: Mark Nielsen.

Exercise 10: 10.2, 10.4, 10.6 and 10.10a,b: Courtesy Michael Ross, University of Florida. 10.10c: Ed Reshke.

Exercise 11: 11.2: Courtesy Denah Appelt and Clara Franzini-Armstrong. 11.4b: Courtesy Michael Ross, University of Florida.

Exercise 12: 12.10a,b,c: © John Wiley and Sons.

Exercise 13: 13.3a: Courtesy Michael Ross, University of Florida. 13.3b: Jan Leesma/Custom Medical Stock Photo, Inc. 13.5a,b: Courtesy Michael Ross, University of Florida. 13.6 (left); © Glauberman/Photo Researchers. 13.6 (right): John D. Cunningham/Visuals Unlimited. 13.7: Courtesy Michael Ross, University of Florida.

Exercise 14: 14.1, 14.2, 14.4 and 14.5a: Mark Nielsen. 14.5b: N. Gluhbegovic and T. H. Williams, *The Human Brain: A Photographic Guide,* Harper and Row, Publishers, Inc. Hagerstown, MD, 1980. 14.6a: Fred Hossler/Visuals Unlimited. 14.10, 14.11, 14.12, 14.13, 14.18, 14.19 and 14.20: Mark Nielsen. 14.17: From Stephen A. Kieffer and E. Robert Heitzman, *An Atlas of Cross-Sectional Anatomy,* Harper and Row, Publishers, Inc.

Exercise 15: 15.5: © CABISCO/Visuals Unlimited. 15.6 and 15.8: Mark Nielsen.

Exercise 16: 16.1: © Ralph Hutchings. 16.2: Mark Nielsen.

Exercise 17: 17.2: Courtesy Michael Ross, University of Florida.

Exercise 19: 19B.5a,b: Courtesy William Radke, University of Central Oklahoma. 19B.7: Scott Camazine/Photo Researchers. 19B.8, 19B.13 and 19B.17: Courtesy Michael Ross, University of Florida. 19B.18a,b: Science VU-NEINIH/Visuals Unlimited.

Exercise 20: 20.2, 20.4, 20.5 and 20.6: Courtesy Michael Ross, University of Florida. 20.7: From *The Color Atlas of Anatomy,* 3e., by J. W. Rohen and C. Yokochi. Reprinted by permission of Lippincott Williams and Wilkins.

Exercise 21: 21A.8a,b: Mark Nielsen. 21A.8c: Courtesy William Radke, University of Central Oklahoma. 21A.9: Ed Reshke.

Exercise 22: 22.2a,b: From Phelps, P. C., and J. H. Luft. *Am. J. Anat.* 125:399, 1969. 22.3: T. Kuwabara-D. Fawcett/Visuals Unlimited. 22.4a: Don Fawcett/Visuals Unlimited. 22.4b: Biophoto Associates/Photo Researchers. 22.6: Carolina Biological/Visuals Unlimited.

Exercise 23: 23.18: CNRI/Photo Researchers.

Exercise 24: 24.2: From Lennart Nilsson, *Our Body Victorious,* Boehringer Ingelheim International GmbH. Reproduced with permission. 24.3a: Courtesy Michael Ross, University of Florida. 24.3b: Courtesy Michael Ross, University of Florida. 24.3c: 1, 2, 3, Courtesy Michael Ross, University of Florida. 24.3c: 4, John D. Cunningham/Visuals Unlimited. 24.3d: 1, 2, 3, Courtesy Michael Ross, University of Florida. 24.3d: 4, John D. Cunningham/Visuals Unlimited. 24.3e: 1, 2, Courtesy Michael Ross, University of Florida. 24.3e: 3, John D. Cunningham/Visuals Unlimited. 24.6: JC REVY/ISM/Phototake. 24.7: James Hayden/Phototake.

Exercise 25: 25.3d: Courtesy Michael Ross, University of Florida. 25.4b: Leroy, Biocosmos/Photo Researchers. 25.4c: Courtesy Michael Ross, University of Florida. 25.5b: Biophoto Associates/Photo Researchers. 25.6b: Arnold Brody/Photo Researchers.

Exercise 26: 26.9a: John Cunningham/Visuals Unlimited. 26.9b: Biophoto Associates/Photo Researchers. 26.11a,b: ©SIU/Visuals Unlimited. 26.14: CNRI/Science Photo Library/Photo Researchers. 26.15: CNRI/Phototake. 26.16a: Ed Reschke/Peter Arnold, Inc. 26.16b: Martin Rotker/Phototake. 26.16c: Ida Wyman/Phototake.

Exercise 27: 27A.10a,d and e: Courtesy Michael Ross, University of Florida. 27A.10b: Ed Reschke. 27A.10c: Willis/Biological Photo Service. 27A.12a: Alfred Pasieka/Photo Researchers. 27A.12b: CNRI/Science Photo Library/Photo Researchers.

Exercise 28: 28.7: Courtesy Dr. William Benyak. 28.8 and 28.9: Courtesy Michael Ross, University of Florida. 28.10: Clinical Radiology Dept., Salisbury District Hospital/Photo Researchers.

Exercise 29: 29A.9: Ed Reschke. 29B.8b,c: Biophoto Associates/Photo Researchers.

Exercise 29B: 29B.9: Andrew J. Kuntzman.